Also Available From the American Ac

By Dr Kenneth Ginsbu

Building Resilience in Children and Teens: Gi

Raising Kids to Thrive: Balancing Love With Expectation,
Protection With Trust

Reaching Teens: Strength-Based, Trauma-Sensitive, Resilience-Building
Communication Strategies Rooted in Positive Youth Development

Additional Books for Parents of Preteens and Teens

Achieving a Healthy Weight for Your Child: An Action Plan for Families

ADHD: What Every Parent Needs to Know

Autism Spectrum Disorder: What Every Parent Needs to Know

Building Happier Kids: Stress-busting Tools for Parents

Caring for Your School-Age Child: Ages 5–12

Family Fit Plan: A 30-Day Wellness Transformation

High-Five Discipline: Positive Parenting for Happy, Healthy,
Well-Behaved Kids

Parenting Through Puberty: Mood Swings, Acne, and Growing Pains

Quirky Kids: Understanding and Supporting Your Child With
Developmental Differences

Raising an Organized Child: 5 Steps to Boost Independence,
Ease Frustration, and Promote Confidence

You-ology: A Puberty Guide for EVERY Body

**For additional parenting resources,
visit the HealthyChildren bookstore at
https://shop.aap.org/for-parents.**

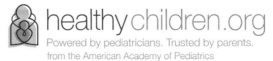

healthychildren.org
Powered by pediatricians. Trusted by parents.
from the American Academy of Pediatrics

Congrats—

You're Having a

Teen!

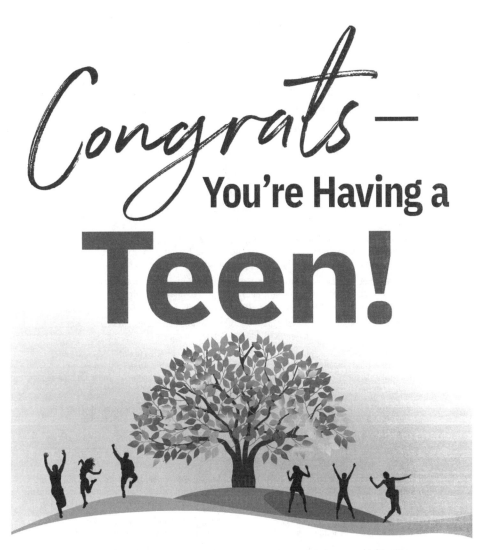

Strengthen Your Family
and Raise a Good Person

Kenneth R. Ginsburg, MD, MS Ed, FAAP

American Academy of Pediatrics

DEDICATED TO THE HEALTH OF ALL CHILDREN®

AMERICAN ACADEMY OF PEDIATRICS PUBLISHING STAFF

Mary Lou White, *Chief Product and Services Officer/SVP, Membership, Marketing, and Publishing*

Mark Grimes, *Vice President, Publishing*

Kathryn Sparks, *Senior Editor, Consumer Publishing*

Jason Crase, *Senior Manager, Production and Editorial Services*

Shannan Martin, *Production Manager, Consumer Publications*

Sara Hoerdeman, *Marketing Manager, Consumer Products*

Published by the American Academy of Pediatrics
345 Park Blvd
Itasca, IL 60143
Telephone: 630/626-6000
Facsimile: 847/434-8000
www.aap.org

The American Academy of Pediatrics is an organization of 67,000 primary care pediatricians, pediatric medical subspecialists, and pediatric surgical specialists dedicated to the health, safety, and well-being of all infants, children, adolescents, and young adults.

The information contained in this publication should not be used as a substitute for the medical care and advice of your pediatrician. There may be variations in treatment that your pediatrician may recommend based on individual facts and circumstances.

Statements and opinions expressed are those of the authors and not necessarily those of the American Academy of Pediatrics.

Any websites, brand names, products, or manufacturers are mentioned for informational and identification purposes only and do not imply an endorsement by the American Academy of Pediatrics (AAP). The AAP is not responsible for the content of external resources. Information was current at the time of publication.

The persons whose photographs are depicted in this publication are professional models. They have no relation to the issues discussed. Any characters they are portraying are fictional.

The publishers have made every effort to trace the copyright holders for borrowed materials. If they have inadvertently overlooked any, they will be pleased to make the necessary arrangements at the first opportunity.

This publication has been developed by the American Academy of Pediatrics. The contributors are expert authorities in the field of pediatrics. No commercial involvement of any kind has been solicited or accepted in development of the content of this publication. Disclosures: The author reports no conflicts of interest.

Every effort is made to keep *Congrats—You're Having a Teen! Strengthen Your Family and Raise a Good Person* consistent with the most recent advice and information available from the American Academy of Pediatrics.

Special discounts are available for bulk purchases of this publication. Email Special Sales at nationalaccounts@aap.org for more information.

Printed in the United States of America

9-474/0922   1 2 3 4 5 6 7 8 9 10

CB0130
ISBN: 978-1-61002-598-0
eBook: 978-1-61002-601-7
EPUB: 978-1-61002-599-7

Cover design by Daniel Rembert
Publication design by Peg Mulcahy

Library of Congress Control Number: 2021913067

What People Are Saying About
Congrats—You're Having a Teen!

How we talk about teenagers matters—and no one understands this better than Dr Kenneth Ginsburg. In *Congrats—You're Having a Teen!* Dr Ginsburg provides adults with a helpful and hopeful road map for enjoying and staying close to adolescents while guiding them through the fascinating, dynamic, and truly wonderful teenage years.

> Lisa Damour, PhD, author of *Untangled: Guiding Teenage Girls Through the Seven Transitions Into Adulthood* and *Under Pressure: Confronting the Epidemic of Stress and Anxiety in Girls*

Parenting books seem to replicate. How does one choose among points of view that are often at odds with one another? I've been a clinical psychologist for 40 years and know, with certainty, that there is one voice I can always depend on. Ken Ginsburg is my go-to expert on all things related to teens and parenting. Not only is he funny, wise, compassionate, and experienced, but he insists on viewing the developmental trajectory of both parents and teens through the lens of opportunity and growth—a very welcome antidote to the misplaced pessimism of so much thinking about teens. In a challenging, busy world where time and energy can feel scarce, *Congrats—You're Having a Teen!* is your one must-read book.

> Madeline Levine, PhD, author of *The Price of Privilege: How Parental Pressure and Material Advantage Are Creating a Generation of Disconnected and Unhappy Kids; Teach Your Children Well: Why Values and Coping Skills Matter More Than Grades, Trophies, or "Fat Envelopes";* and *Ready or Not: Preparing Our Kids to Thrive in an Uncertain and Rapidly Changing World*

Congrats—You're Having a Teen! is a treasure. If you want to "catch" the thoughts that prevent you from being the parent you want to be and replace them with productive thoughts—if you want the latest research on adolescence—if you want sound strategies to help your adolescent really thrive—and if you want to thrive as the parent of a teen—this is REALLY the book for you. Dr Ken Ginsburg is a national treasure!

> Ellen Galinsky, author of *Mind in the Making: The Seven Essential Skills Every Child Needs* and *The Breakthrough Years: Five Things Every Adolescent Wants Us to Know—and Why the Latest Research Says We Should Listen* and president, Families and Work Institute

Congrats—You're Having a Teen! is an essential, empowering guide that gives parents all the practical tools they need to leverage their teens' strengths and turn out thoughtful, ethical people. As a school counselor and therapist, I appreciate Dr Ginsburg's consistent, reassuring message that parenting is not about perfection and the teen years can be a time of joy, awe, gratitude, and opportunity. I am obsessed with this book and will be recommending it to every parent I know!

> Phyllis Fagell, licensed therapist, school counselor, and author of
> *Middle School Matters: The 10 Key Skills Kids Need to Thrive in Middle School and Beyond—and How Parents Can Help*

Dr Ginsburg is a beacon of light on the shores of the teen parenting adventure. His approach is paradigm shifting—teens are full of growth and potential and want to be connected to their parents. With a strength-based and compassionate lens, Dr Ginsburg uses his professional and personal experience—and wisdom—to guide parents, caretakers, educators, and professionals in understanding the complexities of teen development while providing tools to support healthy growth. This book keeps us focused on what matters most—love, connection, relationship, and seeing your teens for the unique people they are now while keeping our eye on the adult we want them to become. A must-read.

> Dan Peters, PhD, licensed psychologist, podcast host of *Parent Footprint with Dr. Dan*, author of *Make Your Worrier a Warrior: A Guide to Conquering Your Child's Fears,* and executive director, Summit Center

This book will change how you think about your teens—and how you think about yourself as a parent.

> KJ Dell'Antonia, *New York Times* best-selling author of *The Chicken Sisters* and *How to Be a Happier Parent: Raising a Family, Having a Life, and Loving (Almost) Every Minute*

As a pediatrician and mom, *Congrats—You're Having a Teen!* is the guidebook I will take on the journey of adolescence with my 13-year-old son and will gladly share the opportunity with families I serve. It is a transformative approach to parenting teens that beautifully focuses mindset toward opportunity, promotes parent-teen connection, and builds skills supportive of teen development into meaningful adulthood. I trust families will benefit greatly from the love and wisdom of adolescents imparted by Dr Ginsburg. His 7 truths about teens will guide my thoughts of adolescence forever.

> Candice W. Jones, MD, FAAP, author of *High Five Discipline: Positive Parenting for Happy, Healthy, Well-Behaved Kids*

Warning: this book might make you rethink some of your beliefs about teenagers. Along with busting myths, it offers practical guidance for being a better parent.

> Adam Grant, No. 1 *New York Times* best-selling author of *Think Again: The Power of Knowing What You Don't Know* and host of the TED podcast WorkLife

Ken Ginsburg and I are in total agreement: parenting adolescents is the most exciting and fascinating phase of parenthood, but if you don't yet agree, *Congrats—You're Having a Teen!* will convince you.

> Jessica Lahey, *New York Times* best-selling author of *The Gift of Failure: How the Best Parents Learn to Let Go So Their Children Can Succeed* and *The Addiction Inoculation: Raising Healthy Kids in a Culture of Dependence*

This work is dedicated to the life and legacy of Roderick Dupris of Bridger, South Dakota (1973–2021). I met Roderick when he was 9 years old and, even then, the depth of his sensitivity and caring nature was palpable. His life journey was not always smooth, but he remained grounded in the knowledge that he wanted to bring good to the world. In his last few years, he served the young people in his community and tribe as a youth development worker. He used the strength of his Lakota culture and the power of human connection to ensure that each young person felt authentically and deeply valued. He guided each of them to stay rooted in their strong cultural values and to be elevated by the knowledge that they mattered to their families, the community, and each other.

Equity, Diversity, and Inclusion Statement

The American Academy of Pediatrics is committed to principles of equity, diversity, and inclusion in its publishing program. Editorial boards, author selections, and author transitions (publication succession plans) are designed to include diverse voices that reflect society as a whole. Editor and author teams are encouraged to actively seek out diverse authors and reviewers at all stages of the editorial process. Publishing staff are committed to promoting equity, diversity, and inclusion in all aspects of publication writing, review, and production.

Contents

Acknowledgments

I am genuinely grateful and humbled that the American Academy of Pediatrics believes that I am worthy of transmitting knowledge and skills that will strengthen families. First, I must thank Mark Grimes and Carolyn Kolbaba for reaching out to me many years ago because they trusted that my work would benefit children, teens, and families. In recent years, I feel so fortunate that Kathryn Sparks has been my editorial partner. She has shepherded every step of *Congrats—You're Having a Teen!* with such care and skill. I am certain that the reason she has done such a masterful job with this book is because she passionately believes in the critical role parents play in raising good people.

I also must celebrate the core team at the Center for Parent and Teen Communication (CPTC) (Elyse Salek, MS Ed; Jill Baker, DrPH; Jacques Louis, MS; Eden Pontz; Andrew Pool, PhD; and Taylor Tropea) for their deep understanding of communication strategies that strengthen families. Their constant presence as supportive colleagues has enabled me to invest the energy in writing this book. Elyse Salek has been my close partner for more than a decade, and her presence has enabled me to accomplish so much more than I ever could have on my own. Dr Pool worked closely along-side me to ensure that the information included in this book is supported by research conducted by leading thinkers in positive youth development and character development. Our center is able to work to strengthen and deepen family connections because of the trust given to us to do so by the John Templeton Foundation; the Hive at Spring Point; Kathy Fields, MD, and Garry Rayant, DDS; the Funders for Adolescent Science Translation; and the Koret Foundation.

I am so appreciative of the experts who contributed to portions of this work or reviewed my words to ensure that I offered the most meaningful guidance I could. Joanna Lee Williams, PhD, also affiliated with CPTC, partnered with me on Chapter 7 ("The Largest Questions Life Offers: Identity Development"). Maria Veronica Svetaz, MD, MPH, and Tamera Coyne-Beasley, MD, MPH, crafted Chapter 30 ("Helping Our Teens Rise Above the Noise and Find Their Own Rhythm"). Roberto Montenegro, MD, PhD, also contributed to Chapter 30 by deepening our discussion on helping teens address microaggressions. Marvin Berkowitz, PhD, reviewed Chapter 31 ("A Bridge to the Future: A Generation Prepared to Do Good and Be Good") to ensure that I captured his essential wisdom on parenting children to have character strengths. Angela Duckworth, PhD, allowed me to incorporate her cutting-edge thinking into this chapter as well. William Damon, PhD, ensured that Chapter 32 ("Nurture Meaning and Purpose") fairly represented his decades of work on this critical subject. Some of the greatest experts who contributed to this work are young people them-selves. In my practice as well as in daily interactions with adolescents (a shout-out to the advisory board of CPTC and my teen neighbors!), I check in to make sure that I, as an advocate for young people, am fairly representing their views. I am particularly appreciative to Ayanna Dunlop who shared her wisdom with me on her generation's journey.

I could not possibly name all the leaders in youth development and adolescent health and well-being that have inspired me to take action and informed me how we might best make a difference in young lives. First, I offer my respect and gratitude to the leaders of the positive youth development and resilience movements who have inspired me. Rick Little and his team at the International Youth Foundation first elucidated the importance of the primary ingredients needed for healthy youth development—confidence, competence, character, connection, and contribution. Although I have modi-fied these a bit to include coping and control, they originated and solidified the core ideas. I have been honored to know Richard Lerner, PhD, of Tufts University, who was part of that team and is one of the great developmental psychologists of our time. Dr Lerner has spent decades demonstrating that positive youth development efforts indeed work and that caring is another core trait we must actively nurture through our own demonstrations of car-ing. I was originally moved to action by the words of Karen Pittman of the Forum for Youth Investment. She called for our nation to understand that "problem free is not fully prepared." Next, I have grown to understand how to foster authentic success from my colleagues at Challenge Success. The work of Denise Pope, PhD, and Madeline Levine, PhD, has been foundational in forming my perspective of what we must do to raise our children truly prepared to lead us into the future. I also must credit Nat Kendall-Taylor, PhD, and his team at FrameWorks Institute for reinforcing my drive and building my skills to tell the truths about adolescent development. It is these truths that will ensure that adults will know how much they matter in the lives of youth and will prevent young people from being undermined by harmful myths and false narratives about adolescence.

I have been blessed to work in regional, national, and international settings to promote resilience. I must highlight, however, the opportunity I have had to work with The Hive at Spring Point, an inspirational group of strength-based youth development organizations in Philadelphia, PA. I am learning from colleagues in each of these organizations how best to engage youth and families in strategies that will help them to THRIVE. We hope to take all that we are learning to help the people, programs, and systems that touch the lives of young people throughout the nation understand the power of respectful, loving adult relationships in the lives of youth. Joanna Berwind and The Hive at Spring Point are my partners along this journey. None of it would be possible without Joanna's vision for The Hive—to amplify voice, choice, and opportunity for all young people.

I am appreciative of the work that the John Templeton Foundation has done to explore how we can best equip youth to build character strengths. My understanding of how to prepare youth to be their best selves has been deeply enriched by the research they have supported and the network of colleagues they have created.

I thank my professional mentors, Gail B. Slap, MD, and Donald Schwarz, MD, FAAP, who have had the experience to guide me, the knowledge to enlighten me, and the passion and love of youth to transmit to me. Above all, they repeatedly demonstrated that they cared not just about my academic career but also about me. I thank the best teacher I ever had, Judith Lowenthal, PhD, who inspired me (when I was an adolescent) to grasp the potential in every young person. I am indebted to my colleagues at the Craig-Dalsimer Division of Adolescent Medicine at Children's Hospital of Philadelphia for teaching me so much about compassionate care and being uniformly supportive of these efforts. Our division is led by Carol Ford, MD, who cares deeply about work that supports youth and families.

My first mentors and first teachers, of course, were my parents, Arnold and Marilyn Ginsburg. I learned much of what I have come to see as good parenting in their home. I was also blessed to learn about the strength of family from my grandmother, Belle Moore, who demonstrated unconditional love better than anyone I have known, except for her daughter Marilyn. They were 2 of a kind. I hope that I have passed along in some small measure what I learned from them to my own daughters.

When it comes to parenting, I have lived with my mentor, my wife Celia Pretter. I look at my own young adult children, Ilana and Talia, and marvel at the depth of their compassion and their core goodness. In them, I see the investment of Celia's energy and commitment. From them, I continue to learn every day.

Above all, I thank the young people and their families who have let me into their lives. I have been privileged to witness the strength and resilience of our military-affiliated families through my work with the Military Child Education Coalition. I am consistently awed by the love I have seen in families who have entrusted me to serve their children at Children's Hospital of Philadelphia. I am moved by the resilience of many of my patients, but, in particular, the youth of Covenant House Pennsylvania, who serve as a constant reminder of the tenacity, strength, and essential goodness of the human spirit.

I Hear Congratulations Are in Order!
You're Having a Teen!

Congratulations! Welcome to this exciting time! The teen years will give you so much to celebrate. Raising 2 daughters of my own, I found adolescence to unfold a world of wonder and discovery. I genuinely believe that approaching these years as an opportunity to nurture their growth led to the strong and loving relationships that have endured into their young adulthood...and I hope for many years to come.

Congratulations?

The word "congratulations" is not usually associated with parenting teenagers. When you saw this title, didn't you assume this would be another book about adolescence steeped in sarcasm? Did you expect yet another "survival guide" to the teen years? Reflect on that for a moment. Your expectations of adolescents may have already been negatively flavored, and that can harm your relationship with your growing teen.

Far too many parents approach these years with dread, which is not surprising considering the uninvited "wisdom" offered from bystanders. A typical experience is at the grocery store or on the sidelines of a sporting event. A preteen nestles their head against a loving parent, and that moment is disrupted by a well-meaning stranger who says, "Get those hugs in while you can! That child is going to turn into a monster you won't recognize...and may not even like!" The problem is compounded when parents read books framed in the language of survival. This distorted view of adolescence as a time of storm and stress, trouble and turmoil fills parents with foreboding.

In turn, your child is sensitive to your unspoken signals that you fear their growth. Too many adolescents learn their stage of life is worthy of an eye roll and, worse yet, that they are disappointing their parents just by growing—a process they couldn't stop if they wanted to.

This book is part of a movement to create a better world for teens—one family at a time. It is unabashedly pro-teenager and unashamedly pro-parent. I hope to position you to be the essential guide your teen needs to make the most of this age of astounding opportunity and unrivaled growth.

We will celebrate adolescence but not be naive about the challenges the teen years *sometimes* bring to caregivers and young people alike. This book is a toolkit that will empower you with the skills to bring out the best in your teen and to strengthen your relationship. It will also prepare you with the strategies you'll need to bring your child back to being their best self if they do go astray. It is solidly committed to the notion that the best way to address a problem is to use mutually respectful communication to build on an existing strength. As a toolkit, this book is not meant to be a quick or light read. Rather, it is a rich resource that you will study and return to as different needs arise in your teen and as they reach different developmental stages.

Truth Telling and Myth Busting

My hope is that this book will fill you with excitement about adolescence and empower you with the skills to prepare your child to thrive as an adult. Let's start with some truth telling about teens.

- **Truth No. 1:** Adults are the most important people in the lives of young people, and teens like adults. In fact, adolescents care more about what their parents think than they care about anybody else's opinion (supported in Chapter 3).

- **Truth No. 2:** Adolescence is a time of astoundingly rapid brain development, and we can shape our children's future far into adulthood by nurturing that development (supported in Chapter 8).

- **Truth No. 3:** Adolescents are super learners, and they will learn more during this period of their life than at any other time that follows (supported in Chapters 8, 11, and 33).

- **Truth No. 4**: Young people care deeply about safety and want to avoid danger but need guidance as they learn about risk. Because adolescents are super learners, they are also driven to explore limits and to engage in experimentation. This makes sense because new knowledge is gained by expanding limits and peeking beyond the edges of what is already known (supported in Chapters 23 and 26–29).

- **Truth No. 5:** Teens can be as rational and thoughtful as adults. To take advantage of this capability, we need to talk to them calmly, in a manner that acknowledges their intelligence and recognizes that they are the experts in their own lives. Although they need the wisdom you've earned over the years, they hold unrivaled expertise on the lives and circumstances they navigate (supported in Chapters 8, 16, 18, and 27).

- **Truth No. 6:** Adolescents are driven by idealism and committed to repairing the world (supported in Chapter 31).

- **Truth No. 7:** The most important truth by far is that you, the parent, matter. In fact, you matter as much now to your teen's healthy development as when your child was a toddler (supported in Chapters 3, 14, and virtually the entire book!).

We need to state the truths explicitly because the teen years are surrounded by myths. You need to bring the undermining myths to consciousness to defend yourself against believing them and prevent your child from incorporating them into how they see themself. As you read each myth, reflect on this question: "Is this myth something I have been told or I have assumed to be true?" I suspect that, in many cases, the answer will be "yes," and that your view of teens may have been tainted as a result. Your work begins! I hope this book allows you to discard these false notions entirely and that you'll use the truths about teens to enable you to build the relationship both you and your teen deserve.

- **Myth No. 1:** Adolescents don't care what adults think and dislike their parents (refuted in Chapter 3).

- **Myth No. 2:** By adolescence, a young person's development is pretty much on autopilot (refuted in Chapters 6–11).

- **Myth No. 3:** Adolescents are lazy and don't care much about what they learn. They'd rather just hang out with friends and have fun (refuted in Chapters 11 and 22).

- **Myth No. 4:** Adolescents think they are invincible and are wired for risk (refuted in Chapter 28).

- **Myth No. 5:** Adolescents are driven by emotion, and it is hard to talk sense into them (refuted in Chapters 8, 10, and 18).

- **Myth No. 6:** Adolescents are self-centered and selfish (refuted in Chapters 31, 32, and 34).

- **Myth No. 7:** Teens prefer to figure things out on their own. Because they are inherently rebellious, they are uninterested in what their parents think, say, or do (refuted in Chapters 3 and 13).

Can these myths really do harm? Yes! If you believe these myths, you may believe that what you do doesn't matter. After all, if your child doesn't like you or care what you think, why engage? If you believe that your child is naturally inclined toward risk, why not just protect them with restrictions instead of guiding them to think for themself and making wise, healthy decisions? You could reasonably believe the best thing you can do for your child is protect them from themself, rather than invest in their developing wisdom. If you believe that teens can't be reasoned with, why would you even bother trying to guide them to think things through?

These myths hurt the way adults view and interact with adolescents, but, just as critically, they undermine the way adolescents view themselves. Christy Buchanan, PhD, of Wake Forest University, has demonstrated that parents' negative expectations of adolescence predict worse parent-child relationships and more risk-taking and difficult behavior over time. In other words, our attitudes create a self-fulfilling prophecy by shaping the way we interact with our teens and the way they end up behaving!

This book tells the truth about young people. It will help you see all that is good and right in your teen. That is the first essential step toward your adolescent holding themself to high standards. You *will* know how much you matter after reading this book!

In This Book You'll Learn...

- A comprehensive approach to parenting adolescents with a focus on effective communication.

- How to be a stabilizing force in your child's life during a time of rapid developmental changes. Understanding adolescent development will position you to communicate much more effectively with your teen.

- Strength-based communication strategies that focus on what is right about a person both to build on their existing strengths and to steer them away from concerning behaviors.

- Communication strategies that will strengthen your family now and in the future.

- How to stand by your children during challenging times and get them the support and resources they deserve to course correct.

- How much you and other adults matter in adolescents' lives. Adults joining together as guides for our youth is the key to our shaping a positive shared future!

Let's Start the Journey

This book takes you on a journey just as you will accompany your child on their trek into adulthood. Each section of this book offers you moments of reflection as well as opportunities to build your skills as their guide. Your teen needs you now as much as they ever did. Earlier in their life, they relied on you for their survival...now they rely on you to shape them into an adult who will lead us into the future.

Recognizing

Perhaps the most protective force in your child's life is you recognizing all that is good and right within them. There is more to recognize, however, than just your child's growing strengths. This is also a time to reinvest in yourself and to recognize how much you continue to matter to your family and those around you.

Honoring

Adolescence is a time of opportunity shaped by astounding growth in which young people's brains, bodies, emotions, and thinking capacities rapidly develop. When you understand and even honor these changes, your relationship will strengthen and you'll earn your role as an irreplaceable guide in your teen's journey toward adulthood.

Shaping

How you manage the good and the challenging moments in these adolescent years can shape your relationship now and throughout your child's life, far into their adult years. Healthy lifelong relationships are shaped by honest, open, respectful, and supportive communication and by an undeniable and unwavering presence that remains steady through the ups and downs of life.

Guiding

The best way to protect your child is to prepare them to deal with life's uncertainties while having the ability to savor life's joys. It is about building their resilience. Sometimes you'll get out of the way. Sometimes you'll watch closely. Sometimes you'll set and monitor rules. Sometimes you'll need to enforce a course correction. But always do it with your child knowing that you guide them because you care.

Bridging

Allow yourself to see and celebrate your teen's idealism. When you trust that your child might have the solutions, you are building our bridge to the

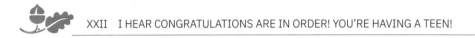

future. Honor their sense of wonder, and you'll support their passion for lifelong learning.

Restoring

Your child may pull away from you and make some unwise choices or even serious mistakes. You can work to restore your relationship and bring your child back to reconnect with their better and wiser self by leveraging the knowledge of all that is good and right about your child. Your child needs *you* to be their North Star.

More to Love

Your child's development will be breathtaking in adolescence. You'll get a glimpse of the adult your child is to become and be mesmerized by the changes they'll go through as they transition from being a child into someone prepared to independently navigate the world. However, no one makes this transition on their own; you'll be their guide along their journey. In fact, your unwavering, loving presence will give them the security and deep-seated sense of worth that will enable them to thrive through the best and the most challenging of times.

If you approach this phase with a sense of awe and gratitude, you'll find that, as your child grows in size and deepens their ability to consider life's complexities, there will be more of them to love.

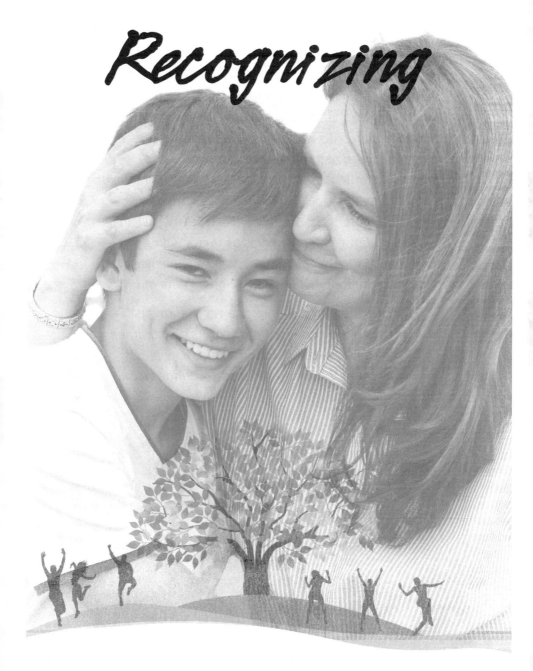

PART 1

Recognizing

―――⊗⊗⊗―――

Perhaps the most protective force in your child's life is your recognizing all that is good and right within them. Above all, it instills within your adolescent the deeply rooted knowledge that they are worthy of being loved. But it also enables you to guide them through challenges and bring them back when they have strayed away from their better self. Your knowledge of your tween or teen's essential goodness serves as their guiding force— their North Star—as their journey seeks to answer that most fundamental of life's questions: "Who am I?"

There is more to recognize, however, than just your child's growing strengths. This is also a time to reinvest in yourself and recognize how much you continue to matter to those around you.

―――⊗⊗⊗―――

CHAPTER 1

Recognizing Adolescence as a Time of Astounding Opportunity

hat words come to your mind when you think of teens?

The words that play out in our heads when we think of adolescents form a script that directly affects our attitude about them and our actions toward them. That is why it is so important that when you hear "teen" or "adolescent," the word "opportunity" is among the *first* words that come to your mind. It is even better if you emphasize the point by adding a word such as "astounding" or "wondrous" in front of the word "opportunity."

Every time the word "opportunity" pops up when you are thinking about your teen, you'll be reminded that because your child is full of **potential** they are deserving of your investment of time and commitment to learning. Hopefully, you'll seek advice from an indispensable expert: your teen. Your adolescent may lack the wisdom that comes from age, but they are already the expert on *their* life. Your teen is the person best able to offer you the guidance about what they need from you. But they'll only do so if you ask.

The Scripts in Our Head Don't Stay There

Given common undermining stereotypes about teens, "opportunity" may not *yet* be the way you frame adolescence. Other words such as "stubborn," "irrational," or even "risky" may come to mind first. It's critical to understand that the silent scripts that play in our minds affect the way our teens learn to see themselves. In other words, your attitudes affect the esteem your child is building, even if you think your thoughts and feelings are hidden from view.

This is because adolescents have a remarkable sensitivity to what others are feeling even when words remain unspoken and actions are controlled. If your child senses that your attitude about them changes as they become a teen, it could affect the expectations they set for themself. Their own internal script may read, "After all, if teens are supposed to be (fill in the blank), then shouldn't I be that way too?" This makes your positive perceptions particularly important because you remain a buffer against negative messages they may receive from others about teens. I dream of a world in which all adults see teens the way they deserve to be seen, but we are not there yet. You want your child to draw their sense of security and esteem from you, not from others who hold stereotyped and incorrect perceptions.

I Wish I Had Said...

When my girls were 12 years old, a colleague teasingly (but with enough sarcasm to sting) said to me, "Dr Ken, the world is watching; let's see how you do with your own teenagers." He said this because my love of teenagers was well known. Still, I was caught without a response better than a forced smile. Looking back, I wish I had said, "I'm looking forward to the opportunity." Now that it's nearly 14 years later, I want to reach out and tell him I made the most of that opportunity and had the joy of watching my little girls develop into wonderful young women.

Shifting Our Mindsets

Let's consider why we should move away from other initial thoughts that may come to mind when you hear the word "teen."

Might you focus first on the "changes" associated with this time? Adolescence *is* filled with a myriad of changes, so the word accurately describes what's happening during these years. However, I don't want "changes" to be the main way you frame these years because I want you to know how much your involvement matters. Changes can be things you passively observe while hoping for the best. I want you to approach these years ready for action. Also, while some of us savor changes, most of us are uneasy with the uncertainty associated with changes. I don't want your child's adolescence to be associated with anxiety, or even fear. But the fact that changes are coming is real—I hope to help you better understand the developmental changes of adolescence and to feel prepared to support your adolescent as they experience these changes. Some people associate the words "danger" or "rebellion" with these years. There are countless ways these undermining thoughts harm your teen. Above all, we know that young people tend to rise or lower themselves to our expectations. We must not allow them to think we *expect* trouble from them.

Many parents have shared with me that when they think of the teen years their initial thought is, "I wouldn't want to go through that time again!" I worry that if parents feel that way, it will harm their ability to support their teens through their bumps and bruises. Teens count on us to maintain perspective and even borrow our "calm" as they experience stress. When our own adolescent moments of discomfort rise to mind when our children experience challenges, it becomes difficult for us to avoid going down that rabbit hole of catastrophic thinking. I am not naively suggesting that you move past your own pain to parent well. Instead, I want to reassure you that history does not always repeat itself and you are better positioned to guide your teen when you listen more and react less (much more about this in Chapters 17 and 18). In fact, trust me when I tell you the experiences you've had—even the painful ones—position you to be a particularly useful guide.

Productive Thoughts

If the stereotyped thoughts in the left column of the following table come to mind when you think of adolescence, work to replace them with the productive thoughts in the right column. The time they are living through is not a time to get past, it is a time where your involvement matters. Remember: your teen may not be perfect, but your child needs you to expect the best of them!

Catch yourself when you have these thoughts about adolescence...	Work to replace them with these productive thoughts!
A period teens survive	An opportunity to grow and develop
A time parents survive	An opportunity for parents to engage with and shape their teens
A time to get past	A time to gain lessons
A time of rebellion	A time of working to gain increased independence
A time of high and unpredictable emotions	A period where sensitivity is developing and empathy is growing
A time of so many changes!	A time of profound development!

(continued)

Catch yourself when you have these thoughts about adolescence...	Work to replace them with these productive thoughts!
A painful time	A time to learn from challenges
A time where teens only care about friends	A time where teens are learning to relate to people outside the family
A time where adults are rejected	A time where adults are carefully observed and serve as role models
A risky time	A time for teens to test and expand limits and for adults to set protective boundaries

Worthwhile Changes Require Self-reflection

It's not easy to create a new internal script about adolescence (or anything really!) until you shift from the one you currently have. This takes conscious and reflective work. You may have been exposed to people who roll their eyes when they speak of teens. You may have turned to experts who put the word "survival" in their book titles. You may go through tough moments with your own teen and, as you do, you may think that what others say about teens is true. All of these forces may have created a bias in your own mind against adolescents.

Biases can be unlearned but only when we confront them and choose to be better. Let's think through how you can get to a place where you genuinely see adolescence as an opportunity.

- When you understand development and its tremendous potential, it is hard not to see the opportunity in front of you. I hope that this book will reinforce in you the belief that adults can and do shape teens' positive development.

- When your teen has challenging moments, it is important to not automatically put their behavior into the "teens being teens" bucket. If you do, it will reinforce your biases. Instead, understand behaviors in a larger context. If you take this approach, your relationship can grow stronger through even the most difficult times. **Note:** Always remember we are hurt most by the ones we care most about. You are not struggling because your child is a teen, you are hurting because of how deeply you love them.

- Keep your sensors open for destructive messages and biases coming from others about adolescents. Hear them. Catch them. Choose to say to yourself, "This person has an inaccurate view of teens or may have had a bad personal experience. I choose not to let their view become my own because my teen deserves my high expectations."

- Finally, catch your own thoughts. If you find yourself repeating a myth or undermining message about teens, take a step back and notice that. Remind yourself that you must never lower the expectations for your own teen. Reframe your thoughts and move forward with the truth about teens. Remind yourself of all that is good and right about your child (see Chapter 4)!

Let's be clear here. This strategy will not prevent your teen from experiencing challenging moments. They're people. They'll mess up. If your child (or your relationship) experiences trouble, that does not make you a bad parent. Good parents are those who seize the opportunity to support their child in any way they can, including seeking professional guidance.

Stand by your child during good and difficult times along their journey and always maintain high expectations. That is the best strategy to guide your teen to become their very best self. And join with others to take advantage of the opportunity that nurturing the next generation brings to all of us.

CHAPTER 2

Recognizing and Nurturing the Adult Coming Into Focus

Perhaps the most exciting thing about parenting adolescents is seeing the adult coming into focus. Of course, they metamorphose in size and shape, but the most breathtaking changes are those that can't be seen. Your child will change from being someone who sees things concretely—just as they appear—into someone who understands complexity, nuance, and possibility. They will develop wisdom based on earned experiences. They will wrestle with values until they find their own and sometimes form opinions different from those you may hold. All of this together will form the identity of a person who will ultimately be able to navigate the world independently. It is an astonishing process to witness.

You spend the first couple decades of parenthood nurturing your child and preparing them for adulthood. Ultimately, they will learn to be independent from you, but hopefully they choose to be *inter*dependent with you. This means that the longer span of your relationship will be as adults who mutually care for and about each other. This is powerful, if not mind-blowing! As I write this, I am in this very stage with my daughters. I am a kid person and, on some level, I mourned as they left the child and adolescent years behind. But having a mutually meaningful adult relationship with your children is WONDERFUL!

As you see this adult forming, it is important to keep your role in perspective. You certainly are an indispensable guide. And you can and should invest heavily in shaping your relationship. Ultimately, though, your child is going to become the person they are destined to be. It is possible that this person will surprise you in some ways. Your job is to love without condition and to learn to take pride in the person who is developing without taking either full credit (you do get partial credit!) or responsibility. The person who stands in front of you is part of you but fully themselves. Seeing them as independent is a critical strategy to keeping your relationship strong both now as they are learning they can stand on their own *and* far into the future because they will better trust they can both remain close with you and lead their own lives (see Chapter 13).

Stay focused on long-term *inter*dependence and a healthy lifelong relationship. Your adult child's sense of security will be heavily influenced by knowing that they are loved by you. Their desire to stay close in a mutually fulfilling way will be tightly tied to knowing they are fully accepted by you.

Parenting for the Future

Recognizing that adolescence is fundamentally about our child transforming into an adult is at the heart of how we choose to parent. When we stay focused on the future, our vision on how to parent today sharpens. Our understanding of what a successful adolescence looks like broadens. It allows us to pinpoint which strengths we need to fortify within our child.

Before we briefly discuss the strengths you hope to foster in your soon-to-be adult, I'd like to suggest a bit of caution. First, bear in mind that not *every* person needs *every* strength. Perfection is not an option for anybody; we are choosing to have *thriving* as a goal instead. Second, even as we consider parenting for adulthood, we shouldn't make this the centerpiece of our daily interactions with our adolescents. Always talking with our teens about the FUTURE is just...too...much...pressure on them. They'll worry so much about how their every action affects them that they might forget to enjoy the present. Furthermore, they may develop anxiety about the future, and that can interfere with their ability to make the thoughtful decisions that will shape their path. Instead, I want this to remain mostly unspoken as you hone your guidance. When you do talk with your teen about their future, use supportive, loving language such as, "I care about this in you because I want you to be the kind of person you are capable of becoming."

We can parent the child in front of us and thereby focus only on whether they are smiling or frowning. We can gauge their success by the grades or scores they are receiving now OR we can parent to build the strengths an adult will need to thrive throughout life. I've long referred to this as parenting for the 35-year-old. This topic is thoroughly discussed in my book, *Building Resilience in Children and Teens: Giving Kids Roots and Wings,* but I want to introduce it briefly here so you can parent with an eye toward *recognizing* the adult you are building.

Strengths a 35-Year-Old Needs to THRIVE

Let's think about those strengths we hope to see in our developing adult. Some strengths you will recognize as existing ones; other strengths you'll realize you may want to fortify. Forgive me for my idealism; if we are building future adults, let's build those who have both satisfying and meaningful lives and hold a commitment to repairing the world.

- **Purpose:** Adults thrive when they have a sense of meaning and purpose, when they know they matter. They are satisfied when driven by passion and grounded in relationships. They understand work is important, but family is central to their well-being, and friendships enrich them. They have supportive relationships they can lean on. They practice self-compassion, so they have the energy to care for others.

- **Wonder:** The happiest adults never lose their sense of wonder. They continue to celebrate the child within them and remain unabashedly playful. They embrace their creativity and seek opportunities to color outside the lines. They love the growth that follows lifelong learning.

- **Morality:** Adults need to be grounded in morality out of concern for the earth and humanity. They need an inner compass that guides them to always consider how their actions affect others.

- **Compassion:** The 35-year-olds we hope to raise are generous and compassionate. They will not avert their eyes to human suffering. They must be committed to solving problems by reaching across our differences rather than stoking division. The future must belong to those who understand that solutions are built by well-worn paths between neighbors.

- **Flexibility:** Adults thrive when they are flexible and creative, committed to innovation, and open to new ideas. They experience and view failure as a correctable misstep and seek guidance on how to do better.

- **Tenacity:** Hardworking adults succeed. They have tenacity and can delay gratification. They learn to move past or over obstacles rather than give up. They have grit, as described fully through Dr Angela Duckworth's work and summarized in her superb book, *Grit: The Power of Passion and Perseverance.*

- **Growth:** Successful adults have a growth mindset as described by Dr Carol Dweck. They see constructive criticism as needed for growth rather than experiencing it as a personal attack. They know both intelligence and skills are built through hard work and experience. They believe in trial and error and savor and respond to feedback.

- **Respect:** Adults who have social and emotional intelligence can be the most respectful (and therefore best) collaborators. They listen, observe, and then share their own thoughts and experiences. They never dominate or belittle others.

- **Collaboration:** Adults thrive when they are able to harness pooled intelligence, meaning they grasp that only collaborative thought will solve unyielding problems. Rather than highlight others' shortcomings, they harness complementary skill sets as the foundation for a shared optimal outcome. They listen to those closest to the problem because they know they have earned the wisdom to find the most fitting solutions.

- **Diversity:** Adults poised to make a difference don't "tolerate" differences, they *honor* diverse thought. They recognize that they themselves will grow only when exposed to people from different backgrounds and experiences than their own.

- **Resilience:** The 35-year-olds who thrive will do so largely because they are resilient. We can't predict the future or protect people we love from its challenges. But we can prepare them to bounce back and use adversity and the recovery process to build their strength. Rather than crumbling after challenges, they regroup and try again. (Resilience is covered in Chapter 24, and *Building Resilience in Children and Teens: Giving Kids Roots and Wings* offers a deep dive.)

Recognizing and Reinforcing Strengths

Our job as parents is not to force these strengths on our children but, rather, to recognize the strengths they possess and reinforce them. We should guide them in a way that will build the skill sets they need fortified. Above all, we model how to be an adult who lives with our own imperfections but always seeks to build on our existing strengths, overcome our challenges, and live each day with the goal of learning something. Remember this: when your adolescent thinks about what it means to be an adult, they will look first to you.

CHAPTER 3

Recognizing and Reaffirming How Much You Matter

"**D**o I still matter?" That's the question many parents face as their children head into their teen years. The answer is YES! Parents matter to their adolescents—as much as, and maybe more than, ever!

You matter more than anybody or anything else in your teen's life. Too many parents minimize the impact they have in their tweens' and teens' lives. It is critical that you understand your influence; otherwise, you may miss the opportunity to optimize your child's development, solidify their values, keep them safe today, and guide them to thrive tomorrow and far into the future.

Why Are We Even Having This Discussion?

So, why do we even question our value? We didn't do this when our children were toddlers or even 8 years old. Why, during such a vital phase of development, do parents of teens question their worth?

Too often, teens are painted with a broad brush and receive a collective eye roll. Books and blogs intended to "support" parents take a sky-is-falling approach that may sell books and earn online clicks but undermine the parent-teen relationship. As we have discussed, these inaccurate and misleading portrayals take an incalculable toll on our understanding of the opportunity we have to actively guide our adolescents.

Parenting teens isn't always easy. Teens often push parents away as they test their independence. In Chapter 13, we'll discuss why this is a temporary

13

response to the internal conflict they have over how much they need us. Nevertheless, it doesn't feel nice to be moved to the side, and it feels worse when our children can sometimes list for us the reasons we have become unnecessary. That takes a toll too, as parents can become caught in the trap of believing the hurtful words their children say.

Teens transition from being family-focused to being peer-focused. This is partly because they spend most of their daytime in school and often go straight into extracurricular activities. A major developmental task during adolescence is learning to navigate the peer world. This prepares them to land a job, navigate the workplace, maintain adult friendships, and pursue romantic relationships. These life milestones may seem far off, but preparing for them is practically what defines adolescence. As our children spend more time with friends and less time talking to us, it is reasonable to imagine they care less about what we think or say. But it is not true.

"But I heard..."

Your teen genuinely cares what you think, say, and do. That's true no matter what you've heard. Don't let myths guide your thinking.

Myth: Adolescents don't care what adults think and dislike their parents.

Myth: Teens prefer to figure things out on their own. Because they are inherently rebellious, they are uninterested in what their parents think, say, or do.

These myths have been around for more than a century and have made far too many parents think they didn't matter. Books, movies, and TV shows have pushed this narrative for years as well. It's a myth that's reinforced whenever parents have a heated disagreement with their teens—they can easily blame it on their "raging hormones" or their age. Conflicts happen in all human relationships. And adolescents sometimes do need to temporarily push their parents away in the journey toward independence. But don't think this means they don't care about you!

In the 1990s, Ellen Galinsky conducted a landmark study called *Ask the Children: The Breakthrough Study That Reveals How to Succeed at Work and Parenting,* where she surveyed more than 1,000 young people on their thoughts about their working parents. She found that teens cherish spending time with their parents, care about their well-being, and want their guidance on how the world works. Similar findings were reported in a 2004 Child Trends research brief, "Parent-Teen Relationships and Interactions: Far More Positive Than Not." In that study, the vast majority of teens said they think highly of their parents, want to be like them, and enjoy spending time with them.

Take comfort in **the Truth:** Adults are the most important people in the lives of young people, and teens like adults. In fact, adolescents care more about what their parents think than they care about anybody else's opinion.

A Few of the Ways You Matter

This entire book is about making the most of all the ways you matter. Just for kicks, let's name a few.

- Teens need support as they develop their decision-making skills. Contrary to the myth of invulnerability, they worry about their safety and want guidance from adults. They don't want to be controlled, but they do want to be protected. They desire wisdom gained through life experience and that they know comes from a place of genuine caring.

- Adolescents care deeply about their parents' opinions and values. Although your teen may increasingly be driven to fit in with peers, you remain the most influential force in their life. Adolescents seek guidance from us on what it means to be a good person.

- Your adolescent wants to please you as much as they did when they were 5 years old. When they know what you care about and the expectations you hold for them, they will try to meet them.

- Young people rely on parents to learn the rules of society. This was true when you taught them how to take turns and share when they were 3 years old and is true in the teen years when you teach them the rules of the road and prepare them for their first job interview.

- Your teen will rely on you to set the boundaries around safety. They will still need to test their limits, but they'll appreciate being able to do so within clearly set boundaries.

- Teens are more likely to make unwise decisions when in the company of peers who expect them to do so. They are safer with peers who encourage safe behaviors. You can't pick their friends, but you should guide them to understand healthy versus unhealthy relationships.

- Adolescents want to know their parents' opinions about substance use and healthy sexuality and value those opinions more than they do that of their friends. "Whaaaat?!" you ask. Yes, we've learned this from long-term scientific research. You are your teen's most valuable and desired teacher. You. Not peers. Not the media. You. Become motivated to teach them accurate information while sharing your desire to keep them safe. Hint: Listen to their views first. (More on why listening is your best strategy is in Chapters 16–18.)

- Ready for a good cry? Your teen wants to look to you to see a healthy, responsible adult. In fact, more than anything, our children want us to be well and happy. Adolescents are most secure when they know their parents are OK. So, you want to know how to best influence your child? Be the person you want to see as a reflection in their eyes. Be the kind of well-balanced, self-compassionate adult you hope your child will grow into.

- Teens are "super learners." They seek out opportunities that allow them to push boundaries past what they've learned—and sometimes past our comfort level. But they want to be safe and value your desire to protect them. They seek your input as they are forming their own opinions. They are passionate, thoughtful, and idealistic. As such, they want to know how you feel about things they care about.

Your Vital Role in Your Teen's Life

Remember how you held your breath when your toddler skinned their knee? In the teen years, more of your teen's pain will be grappling with big questions, especially the largest of all: "Who am I?" The feedback they receive as they strive to answer it creates the opportunity for profound growth. But it also offers the possibility for deep self-doubt if they receive destructive messages about their capabilities or even their worth. Bullying is an extreme example here because it explicitly devalues a person. Most teens, however, have experiences where they receive subtle messages that question their value. They must launch into adulthood knowing they are good at their very core and are worthy of love—just as they are.

Your unconditional love and unwavering presence during these years is the immutable foundation of lifelong security and self-worth. Do you still matter? What could matter more than the person who knows you the best fully accepting you? What could be more protective than someone seeing you as good to your core? That is what gives them strength to resist outside noise about them. They'll know how the person who knows them best sees them.

You matter. Now go talk to your teen about what matters.

CHAPTER 4

Continue Recognizing All That Is Good and Right in Your Child

N o words can capture the depth or intensity of love you have for your child. It is instinctual. It is biological. It is spiritual.

"Why do we love? Because it makes our children know they are worthy of being loved."* This genuine sense that they are worthy of being cared for and about—exactly as they are—offers the bedrock of security from which they will launch into adulthood. It is the basis of them having the grounding to form meaningful friendships and romantic relationships.

Please forgive the audacity of my attempting to define love: *Love is seeing someone as they really are. As they deserve to be seen. Not based on a behavior they might be displaying in the moment. Not based on what they might be producing or achieving and not based on a label someone else has assigned to them. Just as they really are.*

This definition doesn't capture the feelings; rather, it is meant to guide you how to express your love. Your teen has to *know* how deeply they are cherished for your love to have its greatest power. They will gain the most protection from you when they know what you actually see in them. This involves noticing who they really are and reflecting it back to them. To love in this way, you must observe more than you direct and listen more than you talk. You must be authentically present. That presence—that

---

* I was inspired by this phrase describing the connection between the love we offer and how young people gain their sense of worthiness when Kevin Ryan, president of Covenant House International, described why we must serve youth with unconditional love.

unwavering presence—is what offers them security. The fact that you adore them while knowing both their strengths and their challenges means that they can build their sense of self from the way *you* view them, not from the input they might gain from negative forces in their lives. This will become the root of their resilience.

Loving fully does not mean you have to like completely. It is OK to dislike a behavior. Loving means still caring despite the behavior. In fact, there may be no better way of demonstrating that you care than by rejecting a behavior while fully embracing the person.

Real-world Protection

The world can be unpredictable at times, and teens withstand pressures from many directions as they "find" themselves. They may try on different "hats" as they explore who they are. Because how we see them forms the foundation of how they see themselves, we must see them in the best light. Why? So that they will see what we see.

Our world is full of people who measure others' value based only on how they behave or what they produce. This can harm teens by making them anxious, thinking their worthiness is determined by the scores they earn or the grades they achieve. They begin to see themselves as products. It is particularly harmful for adolescents whose challenging behaviors are used to depict them as "troubled" or troublesome. Your knowledge of who your teen is, and has always been, can counteract these negative forces. You can set the standard of your teen's knowledge of who they are capable of being—their very best self.

Knowing Who Your Child Really Is and Always Has Been

We take much for granted as our children grow into teens. Sometimes we stop noticing the very things that gave us joy earlier in their lives. This could be because we share less of our day with them than we did when they were toddlers. Or it could be that, in their journey toward independence, they choose to show us less of what is happening in their lives. But I think the greatest factor is that when young people become more adult-sized, we stop appreciating the miracles of development or mistakenly believe teens need our feedback less.

We must be more intentional in continuing to see their strengths. Teens crave your attention as much as they did when they were little, and their desire to please you remains strong. I concede that many teens will deny this because their inner struggle toward independence forces them to feel as though they need you less. Deny it or not, they benefit from being celebrated.

In searching for who your teen is, a good first step is to recall who they always have been. Draw from the memories of earlier years. When our children were little, we were delighted by their antics as their little personalities revealed themselves. We were impressed when they first showed signed of mental toughness, such as tenacity and even stubbornness. We were amazed as their core values took shape. Their sense of fairness showed the first time they chose to share—even if it was hard for them. Their concern for others was expressed when they ran to you asking for a bandage for another child. Their desire to protect the vulnerable might have first come to light when they insisted you help the bird that fell from its nest.

My girls have grown into deeply compassionate and caring people, and the seeds of these strengths showed when they were 3-year-olds. I recall the day they asked for a family meeting so my wife and I would understand the urgency of keeping the lights on in the house at night. We assumed they were scared of the dark and we found it adorable that they thought this was a high enough priority item to call for a meeting. It turned out they had noticed the moths fluttering around the lights in the living room and were worried that the moths would get lost if we turned the lights off. We strategized a solution with our preschoolers. We turned on the porch light before turning off the living room light. Then, the girls patiently used flashlights to walk the insects out to be reunited with their moth grandmas. Really! Good to their core. Committed to protecting the vulnerable. It's who they were when they were 3 years old, and it's who they still are at 25 years old.

Think about noticing and elevating your teen's existing strengths. Consider taking a break before reading on and reminisce with your spouse or another adult about your child as a toddler and as a school-aged child. Laugh a little. Cry. Be amazed again. Reexperience the joy and the pride. Think about their greatest strengths over the years. I'll bet your teen possesses many of the same strengths—now more fully developed. It'll fill you with particular pride to also notice the new strengths that have risen.

Recognizing and Elevating Their Strengths

Recognizing who teens can become—based on who they already are—gives them the sense of self and confidence needed to launch into a successful adulthood. These strengths are starting points to much of what they will be able to accomplish in their life. As I prepare professionals to seek these strengths in their work with young people, I describe them as "behaviorally operational strengths." These are skill sets and attributes that can be built on to strengthen resilience, influence future success, and connect more deeply to other people.

Strength Recognition Is Not Simply About Praise

Too often, people think that the goal of strength-based communication is simply to praise. This can lead to the trap of highlighting superficial characteristics, such as how someone looks or dresses. Praise for certain behaviors, on the other hand, may be useful. Certainly, if you show your appreciation for helping around the house, your teen will be more likely to complete their chores. Here, however, we are speaking of something much more basic and ultimately meaningful. To shape your teens' best self, you must notice and be able to describe what defines them as a person.

Recognizing strengths does more than help teens feel good about themselves. It elevates, solidifies, and magnifies those strengths. It positions your teen to understand they possess the capacity to do the right thing, to move beyond temporary setbacks, and to correct mistaken decisions. Recognize these inherent strengths and point them out when you see them. This will show your teen that you really see and value who they *are*. They need to hear this.

The following are examples of strengths worthy of notice. Your teen likely has some in abundance; others may require fortification. Nobody possesses all these strengths. Your goal is to see your child as their very own best self—not to imagine a superhuman.

- **Wisdom:** Is your child a thinker? Contemplative? Wise beyond their years? When people are thoughtful, they tend to be open to gaining wisdom from others.

- **Wonder:** Does your teen still get excited about the little things others take for granted? Are they always looking for new opportunities to stretch? People who maintain a sense of awe will continue to appreciate life's simple and grand pleasures and never stop learning.

- **Gratitude:** Does your teen stop to thank others for what they are given? Are they prayerful? People who appreciate what they have will experience joy in living. They also may be more generous with others as they realize we all have much to share.

- **Sensitivity:** Does your teen care deeply—sometimes so much it pains them? Some people feel more richly and fully than others. They are destined to impact many lives because people will turn to them for support. This is an important strength to recognize in the teen years because sometimes the journey through adolescence can be tougher for these sensors.

- **Compassion:** Does your child care for, and about, others? People who care for others will more easily find a sense of meaning and purpose. They may more easily connect to others because judgment will not get in their way.

They will not avert their eyes to human tragedy and instead will seek to address others' needs.

- **Fairness:** Was your child the one who always cared that they got the goodies or rewards they thought they deserved *and* that others did too? People committed to fairness will work toward justice by ensuring that all people have adequate resources.

- **Respect:** Does your teen remember to listen to others? To really hear them? To honor their presence? Some people have the innate ability to know what it means to treat someone else well. It includes seeing others as the experts in their own lives and honoring their earned wisdom.

- **Humor:** Does your teen make you laugh? Even when things are all too serious? People with finely tuned humor can enable others to more easily access their emotions and get through the bumps and bruises of life.

- **Loyalty:** Does your child stand up for friends and others they care about, including you? A strength of many young people is their loyalty to each other. This strength will transfer to family, friends, colleagues, and community later.

- **Protectiveness:** Is your teen someone who is sensitized to the presence of danger and steers others away from it? When people are driven to protect others, they are essential members of our communities. We hope they will also commit to protecting themselves.

- **Perseverance:** Does your child refuse to give up? Look and listen for the remarkable baby steps that demonstrate perseverance when others would have given up. People are more likely to succeed when they set their minds to complete a task.

- **Drive:** Does your child remain focused on the endgame, even when it means pushing themself? When people are goal oriented, they are better able to keep the long-term goal in mind and resist short-term distractions.

- **Resourcefulness:** Does your child figure things out? Earn what they need for themself? It is sometimes remarkable how a young person can stretch their resources or make things work out for them.

- **Honesty:** Does your teen speak their truth, even if it sometimes makes others uncomfortable? Some people are gifted with the ability to share their story in a way that engages others while remaining faithful to themselves and their own values.

- **Insight:** Does your teen tend to explain why they do what they do? Do they understand the feelings behind their actions? If an adolescent is able to describe to you the "whys" behind their behaviors, they may possess insight beyond their years. This strength can be used to help them develop plans that will work for them. When people can see within themselves, they are likely to see solutions others may not.

- **Resilience:** Does your child seem to be able to bounce? Do they tend to grow instead of being defeated? Have they been through hardship but still remain exceptionally loving? When people have proven the ability to recover from hard times, they can imagine overcoming future challenges. Resilient people are more likely to get through difficult times, but they also will use their skill sets to gain the most out of life in the best of times.

Active Noticing Will Pay Off

Our goal is to recognize, elevate, and fortify strengths, not to beat our kids over the head with strength-based communication. It's important your adolescent knows you are observing and appreciating what you see, but don't make this process feel like a whole new level of **pressure**. You don't want them to feel that they will disappoint you if they don't live up to your expectations every moment. Instead, they should take comfort and pride in what you see and feel happy that these strengths are not going unnoticed. Don't make pointing out strengths the centerpiece of your conversations. Rather, you might say "You know what I see in you when I noticed _____. That makes me proud." Then, at some later time when you see it again, you simply say, "There it is again, your _____ coming through. You've really got something there."

Your teen's awareness of their own strengths and their understanding that you see them through this positive lens will pay off in myriad ways. It will give them a source of pride and increase their motivation to build on that strength. It will be key in helping them to steer toward positive behaviors and choices. In challenging times, it will give them a source of strength from which they can overcome an obstacle. In the most challenging times, your understanding of who they are will be the kernel of the strategy that brings them back to being their best self. Your knowledge of all that is good and right about them will become their North Star. They may feel lost but will always have something they can find to guide them back.

Reinforcing the Good and Right

Remember when our 2- or 3-year-olds wanted our attention more than anything? When the mainstay of effective discipline was to catch them being good and redirect them when they were not? It worked in shaping their behavior because we focused our attention on them when they were behaving well. It also worked because they felt good when they pleased us. Our teens want and need our focused attention and to please us every bit as much as they did when they were toddlers.

It's Not About Performance

Too many parents focus their energies either on how their adolescents are performing (grades, trophies, and scores) or behaving. When parents focus on performance, their children might deliver but also may feel insecure about whether their parents approve. Our strongest reactions and most focused attention are typically on unacceptable behaviors. Our children subconsciously learn to repeat the worrisome behaviors that we focus on most.

Similar to their toddler years, "catch them being good, and redirect them when they're not" still holds true throughout adolescence. When we genuinely recognize our teens' greatest attributes, it reinforces the ongoing display of their strengths. And it lowers their performance anxiety because they know they please us as they are.

Recognizing Their Own "Ruby Slippers"

We must surround teens with messages that we see them as good people and expect them to rise to their personal heights. But ultimately, we must help them recognize that *they* possess the strengths and skill sets they can build on. We must not make them reliant on our affirmations for them to access those strengths. In their journey toward leading independent lives, they must become reliant on themselves for the reinforcement of their strengths. The goal here is to have each young person recognize and celebrate their own "ruby slippers," much as Dorothy realized at the end of *The Wizard of Oz* that she never really needed the Scarecrow or even the Wizard himself; she only needed to access what was already in her possession. That is perhaps the key point here: you are noticing something valuable about your teen. It is fully their strength to access; you are just celebrating it.

The North Star

Adolescence is a period of tremendous opportunity when tweens and teens open themselves up to the possibilities of the world. However, as they imagine where they fit, they can be vulnerable to how others view them. While others may too narrowly define their worth, families serve as the anchor that reminds them of their goodness. Families are also well aware of faults. This makes our positive feelings even more powerful. When we offer that essential security, it solidifies and strengthens our relationships.

It is the accountability we have for our children that buffers them against undermining forces in their lives. When peer pressure poses a danger, our high expectations become critical. When young people have to navigate forces of discrimination and low expectation, it is our unwavering high expectations that can give them the drive to push forward. If other people communicate that they think there is only so much our children can achieve, our knowledge that they can do better is deeply protective. If other people see our children through the lens of a mistake they may have made or an unwise behavior in which they might be engaging, our knowledge of all of their goodness and potential is what can bring them back to being their better selves.

Key to Steering Away From Negative Behaviors

As you observe strengths, don't always just be looking at what is going well in your teen's life. Sometimes a problem is rooted in something that is actually a strength that the teen has not yet learned how to manage. A useful example here is sensitivity. Sensitivity and caring predict that, in the long run, a young person will foster deep and rich relationships. But it can be overwhelming to be sensitive early in adolescence. As a result, some young people try to dampen their sensitivity rather than experience the depth of their feelings. They might pretend they don't feel at all or even drink alcohol or do drugs to numb their feelings. In this case, we help the adolescent move away from unhealthy behaviors not by condemning their actions but by recognizing their strengths. Let me be clear: we can condemn alcohol and drugs and point out the obvious dangers, but we don't shame the teen for having made that poor choice. Instead, we celebrate our children's sensitivity as a starting point to help them find other ways to handle the intensity of emotions with which they've been blessed. The goal is to build on the point of strength and hope for a ripple effect that will diminish the teen's need to continue engaging in the undermining behavior. It allows us to deal with problems without instilling the shame that pushes our teens away from us and more deeply into the problem behavior.

Point out how the behavior you dislike is not in keeping with who you know your teen really is. Your words can be relatively simple: "I know you can _____, because you have always _____." For example, "I know you can be kinder to your brother. You are the same young man who kept us from killing any bugs when we went camping. You've always been compassionate and protective. Your brother needs that side of you now."

Heart-Belly-Head-Hands Approach

I want to share an approach I teach professionals that allows us to connect respectfully with youth who need to return to healthier, wiser behaviors. It invites teens to problem-solve, while you serve as the guide along the journey.

I describe this as the "heart-belly-head-hands" approach. Your heart sends you real feelings when you care. Your stomach often tightens when you are worried.

Your head solves problems. And your hands represent your support and unwavering presence. Your parental love—and worry—makes you a real expert here. Allow yourself to trust your instincts and share what you feel with your teens.

- **Heart:** Share all that you know about your teen that makes you care so deeply. Leave them with no doubt that your caring is more than your "job" as a parent. It is rooted in the special things you know about them.
  - **Reflect:** Take a deep breath. Show that you are pausing to reflect before you share. Gather your thoughts.
- **Belly:** Explain why you are worried. Despite their strengths, you fear that some of their choices may undermine the possibilities that life holds.
- **Head:** Brainstorm a plan together. Recognize that your teen is the expert in their own life. Stay thoughtful and calm because that will enable them to think.
- **Hands:** Ask your teen how you can best be supportive to them. While they may be the expert in their own life, you are their guide and come prepared with wisdom and experience.

The fact that you are a key support doesn't mean you should act alone. In fact, a strength-based approach can help guide teens toward the professional help they might need and deserve (see Chapter 39).

The following is a fleshed-out scenario using the case of the youth with substance misuse to mask sensitivity described previously:

- **Heart:** "One of the greatest things about you is how deeply you feel and how intensely you care. It predicts a wonderful future for you with deep relationships. I couldn't be prouder of the person you are."
  - **Reflect:** Pause. Let the power of your statement sink in.
- **Belly:** "I understand you are smoking weed to get away from those feelings because they can be overwhelming at times. But you might give away your greatest strength in the process if you give up your ability to care so deeply. I worry because marijuana can take away your motivation and even your ability to care."
- **Head:** "Let's come up with a plan that will help you learn to manage your sensitivity, including how much it can hurt to feel, OK? We have to think about how you can feel better without the marijuana, so you don't lose your motivation or caring. I have some thoughts, but I'd like to hear from you what you think would work."
- **Hands:** "I'll help make the calls with you, but I'll trust the professional to give you the support I may not know how to give. You'll get through this because you're strong and because I will always remain by your side."

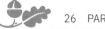

Bringing Your Child Back From Challenging Times

The love we have for our children is wired so deeply within us that it defies explanation. Having a child is like having your heart on the outside of your body. Your love serves a dual purpose: as the essence of what you can offer to propel young people to become their best selves and the strongest tool in our toolbox to bring them back from the brink of disaster.

In challenging times, your memories will ground them in their true selves. They'll remember who they really are and who they want to be. They'll recall how much they want to please you. If we remind them of the strengths they have to succeed, we energize them to transform failure into a learning experience from which they can rebound. We dive into this concept much more deeply in Chapters 36 and 37 as we consider how to restore our relationships after challenging times and our teens to being their best selves after they have strayed into worrisome behaviors. Don't worry, you won't be alone. You'll work with a professional, because both you and your teen deserve the support, but you'll start the process on the right foot because you will be rooted in a strength-based approach.

Seeing the Strengths Within ALL Teens

We can lift this entire generation by advocating for communities and media to recognize what is good and right about teens.

- Notice the acts of generosity and compassion shown by youth and spread these good news stories. Notice the heroic acts but also the everyday acts. Recognize kindness as normal. Then, talk about teens differently in your everyday conversations. It'll catch on.

- Point out the idealism of youth and recognize that societies grow and evolve because our youth imagine something better. Encourage others to hear teens express their thoughts and feelings about issues that concern them.

- Advocate for the recognition of all community youth. We must move away from only celebrating the highest achievers or telling the stories of when teens stray into delinquency. Do your part by speaking to teens and asking them what they care about and how they hope to spend their lives. Every young person must feel seen and valued.

- Give youth opportunities to contribute to our communities. If you know a project in need of person power and ENERGY, ask teens to join in. When they serve others, they'll receive gratitude instead of condemnation. And that will help them rise to be their best selves.

CHAPTER 5

Recognizing Your Own Needs and Those of the Rest of Your Family

Many parents feel pushed and pulled in so many directions that we worry we are not doing right by our children. So, we sacrifice our own well-being and ultimately judge ourselves by how our kids turn out. If they are successful, we determine our self-sacrifice and choices must have paid off. But setting aside our own well-being to give more to our children does not help them. Caring for yourself with the same fidelity with which you care about your children is not selfish—it is a strategic act of good parenting.

Here's why.

- Parents are models of what healthy adults look like.

- Young people learn positive coping strategies from their parents.

- Adolescents care deeply about the well-being of their parents and feel more secure when they know we are OK.

- Relationships between parents and teens benefit when parents are content with themselves.

- Young people talk to adults who are settled and calm. They often withhold information from parents who they think will become overly upset. People who are content will more easily maintain their calm.

- Adolescents whose parents live meaningful and satisfying lives look forward to growing up.

Be Something They Aspire to Become

You might assume from looking at this heading that I am referring to them aspiring to do what you do for a living. But I am talking about who you are, not what you do. How you live your life. How you achieve balance. How you find joy even after what you need to do is accomplished. How you learn to be satisfied with your choices—as imperfect as they are. When we show our teens what healthy, functioning adults look like, they learn how to shape themselves. When we care for ourselves, we make it more likely that they will grow to be adults who care for themselves.

We must show what brings us joy and meaning in addition to caring for our children—having friendships and romantic lives, our working lives and volunteer efforts, our faith, our hobbies. When we demonstrate how wonderful adulthood can be, our teens will invest in growing up well, instead of fearing their development. Teens who fear their development may live only for the moment instead of simultaneously planning for the future. Your hope is to raise children who experience joy in the moment but also consider how their actions impact others today and their future tomorrow.

Earned Self-compassion

Many of us have mixed feelings about the choices we've made. If we've worked long hours, we feel badly there wasn't more time for home. If we've stayed home, we worry we haven't modeled how to build a career. Then, there are so many things we need to "manage" in our teen's lives—school, peers, extracurricular activities, religious involvement. As a result of all of these conflicting feelings and pressures, we apply the efficiencies of the workplace to our child-rearing. This "professionalization of parenting" leads us to judge our choices and evaluate our "management" skills by how our kids turn out—achievements, grades, scores, behaviors. This puts tremendous pressure on our children to produce and can backfire badly. They need to know that we value them for who they are, not for what they accomplish.

Take a step back and recognize that it is your relationship that matters. We give our children a gift when we enjoy them and are content with ourselves, including the choices we've made. Give yourself a break. You're juggling the best you can. You've made the best decisions with the choices you've had. Self-care begins with ending self-blame. Your self-compassion is good for you, but it's essential for your teen who can learn this resilience skill through your example. Critically: They are watching you and determining if you have a forgiving nature. If you forgive yourself of your imperfections and limitations, then they'll feel more comfortable coming to you when they've made a mistake because they'll trust you will also be forgiving of them and compassionate toward them.

But How?! There's No Time for Self-care

I hope to have made a convincing case of why taking care of yourself is a strategic act of good parenting. But I am not naive enough to think that makes it easy. There is too much to do, too many hats to wear, and too many things to worry about. It can feel like we are on a treadmill and the best we can do is run fast enough to prevent ourselves from falling off. I've been there and don't want to pretend I always get this right. So, for some transparency here: my first step was constantly reminding myself that being a good parent meant modeling an adult life. It was only by knowing that I was being watched so closely that I quelled my own fears that I wasn't doing enough for my wife and daughters. This reframed it all for me: *caring for myself was caring for them.* Then it was about reminding myself that treadmills have different speed settings—and even a pause button. I made myself—against my nature—push the pause button so people watching me saw that I could. In time, of course, I learned that investing in myself didn't waste time; it created efficiency, clearer thinking patterns, and restored energy. Energy I could put toward my 2 loves—my family *and* my work.

What does hitting the pause button look like? It's an intentional and thoughtful choice. Consider it an obligation. One you owe your family. Schedule time into your day if you have to. If something comes up during that scheduled slot (and it will!), then treat it the way you would a missed work assignment or a friend you let down. Reschedule; don't cancel.

Yoga at 5:30 pm?

So, what should you do with this self-care time? Workplace programs suggest that the "Yoga at 5:30 pm" class will ease our stress. It may. But that is only one way to achieve self-care. A workout class is not the only answer; rather, we need self-care to be a lifestyle. Let's briefly cover some of the things you might do as self-care. You can expect these same topics to come up in Chapter 24 when we talk about how you build your child's resilience. Get it? You are not just practicing self-care; you're modeling for your teen how they'll care for themselves as well.

I can't give you an exact recipe because I don't know you, but consider these key ingredients and season to your taste.

- **Exercise:** Working out releases endorphins and other calming chemicals in the brain. Exercise also reduces the hormone of chronic stress called cortisol. Too much cortisol leads to weight gain, high blood pressure, and heart disease. Simply put, stress and anxiety make us feel like we are being chased by tigers or always wondering whether they are lurking in the grass. Exercise makes us feel like we have escaped the tigers by running away from them.

- **Sleep:** If you're exhausted, you can't mount the clear thinking that helps you problem-solve or maintain the even temperament needed to navigate challenges. Try these suggestions.
  - Change cell phones and other screens to nighttime brightness settings a few hours before going to sleep.
  - Don't drink caffeinated drinks or foods within 6 hours of bedtime. Choose water, herbal teas, or warm milk instead.
  - Take a relaxing bath or shower an hour or so before lights out.
  - Release your emotions and the to-do lists swirling around your mind before bedtime. Take the active step of setting them aside and saying, "I'm done."
- **Nutrition:** What we eat influences how we feel and how we behave. You want an even-keeled temperament to better handle stress. Avoid sugary foods and drinks that deliver a spike in energy followed by rapidly bottoming out. Instead, choose foods that deliver a consistent supply of energy to the brain. These foods include complex carbohydrates such as fruits, vegetables, and whole grains.
- **Relaxation:** Give yourself the instant vacations that come from relaxation. Here's where yoga or meditation come in. A starting point is learning the power of deep breathing to transform your body into a relaxed state. The internet is full of applications that can build your relaxation skills.
- **Connection:** The term *self-care* does not imply that you should do it on your own. In fact, there is no better way to care for yourself than to reach out to others for support. When we realize we are not alone, even in the most stressful times, we gain the strength to navigate our challenges.
- **Reflection:** The best problem-solving can occur when you least expect a brilliant idea to pop into your mind. Create the space to just think about your day or what has been burdening you when you are not in the thick of it. Sometimes that is all that is needed to engage your thinking powers.
- **Organize your thoughts and feelings and let them go:** We sometimes try to "contain" feelings in hopes they'll disappear or with the intention of processing them later. The problem is that when we keep adding to that "container," rather than deal with what we put in it, the walls of that container need to thicken to keep all that we feel inside. Our container can become so thick that it becomes practically impenetrable. Then we can't even access our emotions, thoughts, or feelings, and we shut down. While we often do not have the luxury of fully experiencing our emotions in the moment, self-care involves making time to do so at some other point. Otherwise, our feelings escape in ways that we can't control—like when we want to support our teens but instead have a meltdown when they

come to us with a problem. In Chapter 10, I'll prepare you to support your teen's healthy emotional development by helping them to organize and then express their thoughts and feelings; please realize that every point applies to you as well.

- **Time for yourself...to do nothing:** So much of self-care is intentional, taking active steps to stay physically healthy, or even to organize, process, and release emotions. Sometimes, though, self-care is about literally doing nothing. Just being. Try being bored. Take a nap. Jump in the shower. Take a hike, not for stress reduction or physical health, but... just...for...fun. Escape.

Planning for Your Child(ren) to Be "in Flight"

Perhaps the strangest truth about parenting is that we work ourselves out of a job; we raise our children to leave us. I refer to the concept of *inter*-dependence throughout this book because I believe fostering our teens' independence is a wise step on the road toward our teens *choosing* to remain deeply connected to us throughout life. However, no matter how tight our lifelong connection, our children will still fly from our nests to create their own. I reject the phrase "empty nest." It makes us fear our children's growth because emptiness is not a feeling we aspire toward. Instead, use the term "in flight." It speaks the truth: our children are no longer living in our nest but are welcome to stop in for the safety and security we will always provide. (And we wouldn't mind being asked to visit their nests every once in a while!)

Aspirations aside, the reality is that raising our children remains a small portion in the timeline of our lives. We must put our entire hearts and souls into it. But we have to have lives beyond the ones that define us as parents. Otherwise, what will we do when they're gone? As your children enter adolescence, don't lament their eventual leaving. See this instead as an *opportunity* to build a strong and compassionate individual who will launch safely and securely into adulthood. This is also an opportunity to realize you are becoming closer to the point when your daily life no longer revolves around parenting. Recognize yourself as deserving of a rich and full life separate from also being an engaged and active parent. Prepare for a sense of fulfillment regardless of whether your nest has children in it.

This means that if you have a life partner, recognize them as the person who will share that nest with you for many years to come. Too many parents become so child focused that they forget to remain partner focused. Because you want to have a good life yourself and because you want to model a healthy adulthood for your teen, celebrate your life partner and continue to nurture your own growth as you plan for a long, satisfying life.

To drive this point home: do you want your teen to grow up and focus all their energies on caring for their children and lose themself in the process? I didn't think so. Demonstrate that good parents are child-centered but maintain an adult existence as well.

Recognize the Needs of Others in the Home

Although most young people make it through the teen years with relatively few bumps and bruises, some adolescents have a more difficult time. It is easy to focus on the person in crisis needing your urgent focus. It is critically important, however, to continue to pay as much attention to those members of the family who are not forcing you to pay attention. Say clearly, "Right now I am focused on helping your brother/sister resolve a problem, but you matter to me just as much. We have to make time together very soon so I can hear what is going on with you." When we forget to do so, children will figure out how to get our attention. And if they've learned that their parents focus most of their energies on the teen or tween making the most noise or generating the most distress, they may learn to become louder themselves. Alternatively, they may choose to become "the perfect child"—one who never causes waves and always works to please others. "Good children" or perfectionists don't ask for the attention they deserve and may tuck away emotions needing to be expressed, thereby depriving themselves of needed guidance.

For these reasons, we must never forget to recognize the needs of ourselves, our life partners and spouses, and each and every member of our household. In doing so, we will create a healthier and more functioning household for everyone, including our teen. By focusing on everyone in the family system, we create a better environment for all. Above all, we model for them how to become a healthy adult who is part of a strong and functioning family.

PART 2

Honoring

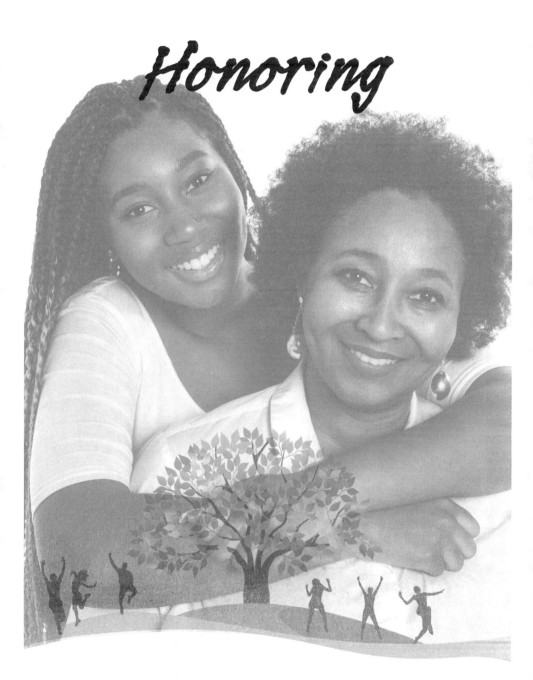

Our goal is not just to understand our adolescent's development—it is to honor *it. When we authentically appreciate the ways in which our children are transforming into young adults, we will more likely nurture those changes. That includes marking off safe territory within which they can freely stretch their wings. When your teen knows that you recognize their increasing capabilities and support their growing independence but remain a protective force in their lives, they'll welcome you as an irreplaceable guide in their journey toward adulthood.*

CHAPTER 6

Honoring the Many Moving Pieces of Development

My favorite thing about being a pediatrician is that I can foster unique relationships with each and every one of my patients. I know in my heart that I have connected with them if each one knows that I strive to be a supportive resource for them. The goal is to enhance their lifelong well-being, but my relationship pays off most dramatically when I can support tweens, teens, and their families through challenging times. To form effective partnerships, I had to learn to communicate to ensure an 11-year-old understood my thoughts, while communicating a different health-promoting message to the 17-year-old down the hall. It's not as simple as having a different script for each age, because no 2 young people are alike. Each is uneven in their development; they might have an adult-sized body but still be thinking not much differently than a younger child.

I enjoy the challenge of shifting my communication strategies with each patient in a way that strives to engage each young person's highest thinking powers. As a parent, you don't have to shift your approach to communication a couple of times an hour because you only have to focus on your own child or children. But you do need to evolve the way you engage your teen's thoughtfulness as their ability to consider issues and problem-solve advances. You'll also need to be prepared to address new issues as their emotions take on a new intensity and bodies change.

Seeing growth in your own child is always a bit shocking because we never actually watch our children grow. Most growth is the kind you couldn't see even with a time-lapse video anyway. The breathtaking growth is on the inside—how your child thinks and understands ideas differently, how they feel more fully and intensely, how their sense of morality and justice sharpens, how they view the world, and how they begin to imagine who they will be and how they will contribute to the world.

The challenge (and thrill!) of parenting tweens and teens is that the moment you sense you've mastered the current stage of development, nature's timeline ensures that your teen's continued growth will require you to build new communication skills and strategies.

The Many Facets of Adolescent Development

Adolescents are doing a *lot* of work to maintain their footing while so much is changing within and around them. Each moving piece of development influences the others, and each aspect of development proceeds at its own pace. Because our children are undergoing so many simultaneous changes, we must remain a stabilizing force for them. First, we need to support their understanding that growth is a lifelong journey. Their job now is to learn about themselves—to keep asking the important questions—not to have all of the answers. Second, we reassure them that we will stand beside them supporting, not defining, their journey. Above all, we offer them the security that comes with the certainty that we will always love them completely.

We'll touch on some of the elements of development here, but we dive deeper into these topics in Chapters 7 through 11.

Physical Development

One has only to look at a seventh-grade class to be astounded at the range of heights and physical maturity. Physical development involves growth in size and shape as well as the development of reproductive organs into an adult state. It is initiated by several hormones and activates a cascade of additional hormones. As adolescents ask, "Am I normal?" their rapidly changing bodies can leave them feeling uncomfortable and even isolated. We provide an important stabilizing force during this time to help our children navigate the wide range and uneven pace of typical adolescent physical development.

Brain Development

There are 2 windows of extraordinarily rapid brain growth for humans: from birth through age 3 and adolescence. The brain is the operating system for thinking, for experiencing and regulating emotions, and for moral reasoning. Understanding the uneven way in which the brain develops informs you how to better communicate with your teen, how to effectively guide them through challenging emotional and behavioral moments, and how to build their wise decision-making skills.

Emotional Development

Emotional experiences such as those with their close peers expose your teens to new opportunities for learning and growth. Adolescence is a critical time to increase social learning. It is their ability to feel fully and be affected by others' feelings that prepares them for future relationships with colleagues and family members. In fact, the emotional nature of adolescents is a sign of increasing maturity, *not* immaturity.

Cognitive Development: Thinking on Whole New Levels

Cognitive development is how your child's thinking will change over time. It involves how teens change from children who see things rather simplistically into adults who can manage complexity, grasp nuance, make judgments, and plan for the future. Understanding cognitive development teaches us key communication strategies that will support teens to reason things out wisely for themselves.

Moral Development: Building Character

Think of character or morality as choosing to do the right thing even if nobody is watching. Like other aspects of development, morality can be uneven and is a process, not a single event. Human morality promotes our well-being and human flourishing. Adolescents journey from seeing things as good or bad to understanding complexity and a higher level of morality. We rely on this development in young people because it drives them to dream of building and living in a better world. Understanding how teens develop an increasing moral compass enables you to appreciate this inspirational time and to support the building of that bridge to a better world.

Identity Development

Identity development is the glue that ties all the other aspects of development together. This involves how one sees themself. The way we learn to see ourselves is shaped by the way we look physically, how we feel, how complex our thinking is, and the consideration of how we impact those around us. The overarching question of adolescence—"Who am I?"—is likely the hardest question humans tackle. We adults have the benefit of understanding that the search for personal meaning and a unique identity is a lifelong quest. Unfortunately, too many adolescents believe they have to answer the question in time to write their college essay or build their work résumé. We can support identity development by reminding youth that finding ourselves is a marathon, not a sprint. Understanding the imperative of our teens developing a heathy sense of self underscores one of our greatest roles in their life—to accept them.

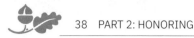

Development Is on Your Side

Adolescence can be challenging for the entire family. Understanding development can help to explain why. Your child is experiencing many physical and emotional changes, all while trying to figure out who they are. Your teen may look at the world and become frustrated by the problems they can't solve. They're trying to fit in and have so many questions. So, while it is absolutely a time of great opportunity, it also can be a time of unknowns, anxiety, and stress.

It can particularly be frustrating—or maddening—when your teen doesn't seem to grasp something you think they need to understand for their own safety or well-being. You cut them slack when they were younger and even managed your frustration and expectations when they were in middle school. But it does become more difficult to understand when someone becomes more adultlike but may still think like a child. Development is uneven. It progresses along stages, so a teen might be fully developed physically and still have quite a bit of growth left emotionally. They might be able to perform or execute a complex math problem but aren't yet able to work through a moral dilemma.

Take a breath. The brain is maturing, thinking skills are solidifying, and your teen will become more comfortable with their emotional self. Your job is to keep them safe within protective boundaries while they are exposed to new experiences that promote healthy development. Stay stable and supportive. Development is on your side. Give it time.

Nourishing Development

You knew I wasn't going to end this chapter with that passive statement, "Give it time." While that is solid advice and a meaningful perspective, it's not adequate when it comes to development. It is true that development will proceed with or without you, but optimal development needs your active involvement and support. When we *honor* development and treat it as something that needs nourishment, we support our teens to thrive to their potential.

CHAPTER 7

The Largest Questions Life Offers
Identity Development

It was an honor to cowrite this chapter with a respected colleague and valued friend, Joanna Lee Williams, PhD. Dr Williams is a developmental psychologist and associate professor in the School Psychology Program at Rutgers University.She is a leading thinker in understanding the role of race and ethnicity in identity development. She is also a core faculty member of the Center for Parent and Teen Communication.

I t is during adolescence that people begin to explore the fundamental question about their identity, "Who am I?" Teens (mistakenly) believe they must answer the question quickly and definitively. In fact, there is no more loaded question to ask nor one more difficult to answer. It is a question that has many parts.

- Who am I, separate from my parents? Different from my siblings?
- Am I someone people enjoy being with? How do I fit in with my friends?
- How do I maintain my own values, while still having others like me?
- Who am I attracted to?
- Will anybody ever be attracted to me?
- What am I good at?
- What are my strengths, and how do I compensate for my limitations?
- How will I choose to earn a living?
- How will I contribute to the world?
- What do I believe?

Two other major questions accompany "Who am I?" with all its subparts. "Am I normal?" and, "Do I fit in?" When we as parents understand these associated questions, we grasp why peers matter so much to our teens. Peers are the people they are trying to fit in with and with whom they measure themselves as "normal" against.

These foundational questions offer a framework you can consider as you think about what your teen is experiencing. Ask yourself which of the 3 questions is driving a behavior or best explains the emotional work your child is experiencing. Are they struggling with their role in the world? Their attractions? Their sense of fitting in? Both the dreams we want to nurture in our teen and the risks we want them to avoid are at the root of these questions. On the one hand, we hope to expose them to opportunities that allow for self-discovery. This includes the chance to experiment, to try on different hats to find ones that fit, and to develop healthy peer relationships. On the other hand, we must guide them away from testing out ideas that expose them to danger or being heavily influenced by peers with whom "fitting in" threatens their well-being. One of the hardest things we do as parents is sometimes hold our breath knowing that because our children sometimes learn best from mistakes, we can't and shouldn't prevent them entirely from learning through uncomfortable experiences. We hope to find that balance between protection from danger and acknowledging that people sometimes learn best from experience. We'll discuss this more in Chapter 28.

Weaving a Tapestry of Many Threads

None of us are simply defined. Think about how different you are in various settings. In your home, you likely see yourself primarily as a parent or life partner. At a family reunion, you might suddenly be the baby sibling or the oldest cousin and find yourself playing out roles that haven't defined you since childhood. At work, you see yourself as a colleague with particular skills. In a spiritual or cultural setting, your dominant identity may be that part of you shared with others in the group (race, religion, ethnicity, or national background). It is our diverse and intersecting identities that add to the richness of our lives.

It is during the tween and teen years that adolescents discover that people can be many different things simultaneously and enriched by the sum of our parts. As your teen explores their identities, some categories may change across time and settings. But similar to adults, adolescents are whole persons—they do not experience their identities in silos.

Adolescence is also the time when identity development must be nurtured because external forces, such as bullying, racism, or low expectations, may undermine the development of a healthy sense of self. We'll discuss this in Chapter 30.

Let's briefly consider some of the forces that contribute to the various elements of identity development.

Changing Bodies

Teens' bodies are changing rapidly as they progress through puberty. Therefore, the question, "Am I normal?" may take a leading role in identity exploration. Adolescents may become self-conscious of their bodies and, therefore, more sensitive to input from others, especially peers. This can be magnified when peers describe people in terms that reflect their size, shape, or sexual development. This can have lasting effects. You can protect your teen from tightly linking their identity to their physical characteristics by reinforcing the wide range of healthy developing bodies. But more critically, you can engage with your teen's inner world so they have the opportunity to shift their focus away from their outward appearance and toward their developing thoughts, feelings, and values that more genuinely define who they are becoming.

Personal and Social Identity

Teens can imagine the person they want to be and become aware of precisely who they do *not* want to be. They can purposefully build their self-narratives with their own values, motives, and hopes. They may try on different images, each time evaluating how they felt about themselves when they behaved in a certain way or presented themselves in a particular manner. Over time, they see which images feel most natural to them and begin to weave these different self-presentations into a single narrative—one that fits them—their story of themselves. That is their *personal identity*.

While society often emphasizes individuality, many teens thoughtfully consider *social identity*—what *connects* us to others. Social identity categories include demographic boxes, such as race, ethnicity, and gender, that your teen will learn to check on a census or standardized test, but social identity includes so much more that shapes them, including their sexuality and faith. Furthermore, their social identities include the spaces teens find themselves most comfortable within, such as academics, athletics, or extracurricular activities. Each of these social identities creates a sense of connection to something beyond their individual selves.

Gender and Sexuality

Questions about gender and sexuality intensify in adolescence. Many parents avoid in-depth discussions on these topics, knowing the fundamentals are often covered in schools. Remember, though, that the mechanics may be covered elsewhere but only caring adults can speak to the values of self-regard and respect for others that are essential to healthy sexuality and serve as the foundation of meaningful relationships.

A teen may have an experience such as a first crush that prompts them to explore what "womanhood" or "manhood" means. For some teens, understanding their "maleness" or "femaleness" comes at a time when peers start defining the boundaries and setting expectations about gender-typical behavior. This is an opportunity to prevent your children from boxing themselves into behaviors that may not match their best selves. For example, typical notions of masculinity can prevent young men from believing they can express their emotions or sensitivities. So too, societal expectations for young women can create a sense that expressing their views assertively is somehow not feminine. It is our role to help our children understand that they should be their whole selves, not squeeze themselves into a mold of society's design. We do this by being an active counterforce against these notions. We discuss this further in Chapter 10.

Despite growing acceptance, lesbian, gay, bisexual, transgender, queer (questioning), intersex, asexual (agender) (LGBTQIA+) youth may have additional challenges in identity development. They are more likely to be victimized by bullying and to experience depression and even suicidal thoughts. However, research and experience has repeatedly demonstrated that LGBTQIA+ youth thrive when they have relationships with caring adults and supportive settings. LGBTQIA+ teens in schools with gay-straight alliances (GSAs) have better health and a greater sense of belonging. In this digital age, the internet can also provide identity-affirming spaces for teens who may otherwise feel ostracized or alone. Most critically, having parents and other family members who fully accept a teen for who they are is essential. Many families benefit from support from other families who have traveled this journey before them. Several excellent resources exist, but a starting point is PFLAG (https://pflag.org).

Racial-Ethnic Identity

For some youth, identity is shaped by deep connections to family and cultural traditions—"I am proud to call myself [fill in the blank] because I come from a long history of others who did the same." For other youth, the process may contain more twists, turns, and bumps as they balance new passions with the expectations of family and friends. How a teen understands and feels about their racial or cultural heritage often becomes a central focus in adolescence. Race and culture are often particularly important for youth of Color and immigrant youth—they may be viewed by others in "racial" terms.

All teens are exposed to messages about different racial-ethnic groups; these messages can shape both how they make meaning of their own heritage and how they view people from different backgrounds. You can help your teen critically sort through these messages so they understand that stereotypes and generalizations do not define their identity and should not define how they see people from other groups. (See Chapter 30. In this chapter, Drs Maria Veronica Svetaz and Tamera Coyne-Beasley offer guidance on how to support positive racial-ethnic identity in the context of discrimination.)

Give your teen the space to ask questions about race and provide them with language and information to keep such conversations going. If we *all* teach pride in our own cultures and genuine respect for other cultures, we will build a better world. If we choose to stay silent about the ways in which race influences our society instead, it will leave our teens to draw their own conclusions, which leaves them vulnerable to misinformation or susceptible to believing stereotypes.

Younger adolescents may start noticing race and racial dynamics more frequently, and specific encounters (eg, comments by a teacher, a post on social media, events in the news, through peers) may prompt self-reflection about race. School transitions, such as from elementary into middle school, may also increase the visibility of race, especially as social cliques become more central. During this time, youth may start spending more time with others who share the same racial background, which can help support identity exploration. Older teens become more capable of reflecting on what their race or ethnicity means to them and how it fits into their broader self-narrative. They may relate more strongly to the collective experiences and needs of their group and seek opportunities to build connections with teens with similar racial backgrounds or identities. As older adolescents become more confident in what their race means to them, they may actively seek opportunities to interact with people from racial backgrounds different than their own.

Developing a Healthy Racial–Ethnic Identity for Teens of Color

Tragically, we live in a society that still devalues or holds negative stereotypes about certain racial groups. This means that some teens, as they explore their racial identity, can become vulnerable to "stereotype threat" when concerns about living up or down to group stereotypes interfere with performance. Research has demonstrated, for example, that if an individual repeatedly hears falsehoods about a gender or racial-ethnic groups' abilities in an academic area, their scores will be lower when they are tested in that area and reminded of their identity. The critical point is that this has *nothing* to do with ability or talent; it is about the confidence one loses when faced with biases. As sophisticated thinkers, teens will become more aware of and sensitive to racial discrimination. This is where supportive adults can play a critical role, by helping teens affirm the importance of their race while also affirming other valuable parts of their identity.

For youth of Color, when they have a strong and positive sense of racial-ethnic identity, they can thrive academically, socially, emotionally, and even physically. This powerful self-confidence can also protect our youth from the damaging effects of discrimination.

Although we know a healthy racial-ethnic identity is beneficial for youth of Color, White teens also draw conclusions about race and what it means to them based on what you do—or do not—say and do. Silence about race can send a message that it is something White youth can ignore or that only "other" people have a racial-ethnic identity. In some White families, identity support may come through rich discussions and shared stories about ethnic and cultural heritage. In others it may involve conversations to help teens learn how to recognize and respond to racial injustice.

Feeling connected to one's racial-ethnic heritage can be a source of strength as teens reflect on who they are and who they are becoming. Making space for teens to share their thoughts and questions lets them know that it is OK to talk about race, even if we do not have all the answers. Ongoing conversations make it more likely that their developing identities are a source of pride and that they can envision themselves as self-advocates and allies.

Ages and Stages of Development

Each stage of identity development builds on the last. In the following list, we offer *approximate* ages and descriptions of the processes that generally occur during these ages. There is a wide range of typical development, and you'll notice that your child may be more advanced in some areas and need additional time to grow in others.

Early Adolescents (Ages 11–13)

- Have a desire to identify themselves in multiple ways outside of their role in the family.
- Have an increased awareness of themselves as part of a peer group. For some, this includes navigating where they fit into the social landscape, which may take time and involve multiple attempts.
- Develop flexibility in how they present themselves in different situations.
- Prioritize personal values and decisions to reflect how they see themselves.
- Experience greater sensitivity to feedback from others, particularly peers.

Middle Adolescents (Ages 14–17)

- Begin to imagine their own identity and role in the larger world.
- Actively explore identity alternatives. These may include trying on the personalities or testing out the behaviors that would fit in with various peer groups.
- Consider themselves and their beliefs in relation to broader social or cultural groups, such as gender, race, and religion.
- Take stronger stances on social, ethical, or moral issues, and begin to see their identity as linked to their stances on these issues.
- Increase their sense of stability as they see themselves across different places (eg, school, religious or cultural settings, extracurricular activities) and social groups.

Late Adolescents/Young Adults (Ages 18–24)

- Give deeper consideration of self in terms of adult roles or career goals.
- Think about who they are in terms of intimate relationships.
- Begin to balance idealistic views of who they may become with a more nuanced understanding of reality.
- Can make strong commitments to personal and social group identities (gender, race, religion), but new experiences can result in further exploration and change.

Supporting Healthy Identity Development

Stand in your child's shoes for a moment and relate to the excitement and possibilities associated with figuring out who you are and what you can be. Add the anxiety and confusion that identity formation can also generate. Experience the pushes and pulls of friendships that come and go—that feeling of being judged too often. Taken to the extreme, imagine the potential damaging impact bullying or low expectations can have on a person's developing identity. As they ask, "Who am I?" the message they receive is that they may be someone of little value who is not normal and doesn't fit in. You are both the catalyst toward positive growth and the antidote to unsettling feelings.

Sometimes the best way to support our children is to temper our parental instincts. We are driven to want to protect our kids and make things easier for them. But, if they are to gain their own identity, they have to trust that they have ultimately navigated the journey on their own. So, avoid being a fixer, even when your child is struggling. When you fix a problem, the message they'll receive is, "I didn't think you could do this on your own." Second, avoid supplying them with your vision of their identity, and don't judge the hats they're trying on (as long as they are remaining safe). Part of developing one's identity is gaining a sense of independence and asserting individuality, and, when teens feel overly directed or judged by their parents, they may make choices *precisely* because they are uniquely their own. In other words, being overly controlling or passing judgment backfires. Finally, refrain from using the well-intentioned statement, "Just be yourself," to a teen struggling to fit in. This phrase may increase your teen's frustration because they don't yet know what it means to be themselves; it underscores precisely the struggle they've not yet surmounted.

Say This (to support healthy identity development)	Not That
You'll figure out what is most important to you.	Just be yourself.
You'll find the kind of friends who will share your values and who will support you when you need to turn to them.	Those friends aren't the kind of people you want influencing you.
Life is a journey. It takes a long time to figure out what matters most to you.	It is important to tell people who you are so they'll admit you into (college/the program).
You are a vital part of the family and our community. And you enrich us all with your values and beliefs.	We have always believed this or done it this way.
Each person can possess many strengths. We learn about our strengths over time when we behave in a way that allows us to be our best and truest selves.	Men do... Men think... Women do... Women think... People think...

Throughout this book, you'll often see the phrase, "Preparation is protection." The only way that you'll be able to override your parental instincts to fix your child's discomfort is if you remember that the best way to protect your child is to allow them to develop the thought processes and skill sets they need to use now and throughout their lifetime. Each of the following ideas builds your child's ability to figure things out independently and solve problems themself—that's long-standing protection!

BE A SOUNDING BOARD. The question, "Who am I?" can only be answered by the person asking the question. Listen. Let them try out their ideas on you, and if they share something that you've long understood, remember it is still new for them. Sometimes just saying things out loud helps them to hone their thoughts and form their opinions. You can ask questions in response to what they are saying to move them to the next step. "That was a really interesting thought. What would you think if _____?" You may also ask clarifying questions such as, "I hear you saying _____. Does that mean _____ to you?" Share solutions only when asked.

PARENT THE 35-YEAR-OLD. Define success wisely. Adolescence is difficult enough without your child thinking they have achieved success, or not, by 18 years of age. Understand you are raising someone to be successful as a 35-, 40-, and 50-year-old. This will give you a broader view of the character strengths you should nourish, while taking the pressure off your child today.

CREATE BOUNDARIES. The drive to experience new things is ingrained in adolescence. Taking risks (albeit safe ones) is critical to figuring out one's place in the world. Adolescents need to experiment a bit. Maybe too much at times. If we outlaw our teens' ability to take chances, we stifle their development. Instead, parents need to focus on creating safe boundaries beyond which our teens cannot stray. Then, we let them push against those boundaries and try new things all within the safe territory we have marked off.

ENCOURAGE BEING REFLECTIVE. Thoughtfulness is a luxury young people operating at a quick pace don't believe they have. Explain that the best decisions come when you think them through, engage others, consider options, and weigh alternatives. Better yet, invite your teen to help you think through a big decision you need to make.

EMPHASIZE THE LIFELONG PROCESS. Figuring out who you are during the teenage years is part of a lifelong process. All people have opportunities for self-improvement—even reinvention—throughout our lives. Over time, we learn that the measure of our character is how we make amends and grow from our experiences. By demonstrating that life offers us second chances, you'll diminish the pressure they are experiencing to get it "right."

MODEL WHAT A HEALTHY ADULT LOOKS LIKE. Identity development involves imagining the adult you hope to become. But it is hard to imagine oneself as an adult during the teen years. It really helps to have a role model who lives a life they could hope to achieve. You can model values for your child to measure themself against. If your child has an interest you don't share, introduce them to other adult role models.

MODEL THAT ADULTHOOD CAN BE FUN. You don't want your teen thinking they must be in a rush to live now because the future consists only of self-sacrifice and hard work. Maintaining a rich social life, making time for pleasure, and committing to your romantic relationship helps them imagine a future they hope to attain.

MODEL LIFELONG LEARNING. It is important that teens do not think their only opportunity to experiment and test boundaries is while they are young. Spontaneity adds excitement to our lives. Let them see how you continue to enjoy new adventures, even those you haven't planned. Next, show them that lessons are everywhere so long as we remain open to seeing them.

The Most Important Thing You Can Do

Your unconditional love is the bedrock of your teen's security, now and far into the future. "Who am I?" your teen asks. "You are you. And I couldn't imagine wishing you were anyone different," you answer with your unwavering presence.

....

Recommended Resource

PFLAG (https://pflag.org). PFLAG's mission is to build on a foundation of loving families united with LGBTQIA+ people and allies who support one another.

CHAPTER 8

The Amazing Developing Teen Brain

How we interact with our world and each other is embedded in the structures and pathways of our brains. The more we understand about brain development, the more we recognize we can nurture optimal development and shape our neural pathways. There are 2 windows of astoundingly rapid brain development—the first 3 years after birth and adolescence. The tween and teen years are a critical window when young people must absorb as much information and know-how as possible.

Unfortunately, brain science is often misinterpreted, making some adults believe teens are inherently irrational or overly emotional. This pushes adults away precisely when we need to engage most fully. It causes some parents to wrongly conclude the best way to parent a teen is to protect them from their risky self rather than partner with them to build the skill sets needed to make wise and thoughtful decisions.

In the introduction, we listed 7 essential truths and 7 undermining myths of adolescence. A misinterpretation of brain science has contributed to 2 of the myths:

- **Myth:** Adolescents think they are invincible and are wired for risk.
- **Myth:** Adolescents are driven by emotion, and it is hard to talk sense into them.

In welcomed contrast, a more accurate understanding of teen brain development is offered throughout this chapter, which will enable you to better understand 4 of the essential truths about adolescence.

- **Truth:** Adolescence is a time of astoundingly rapid brain development, and we can shape our children's future far into adulthood by nurturing that development.

- **Truth:** Adolescents are super learners, and they will learn more during this period of their life than at any other time that follows.

- **Truth:** Young people care deeply about safety and want to avoid danger but need guidance as they learn about risk. Because adolescents are super learners, they are also driven to explore (and sometimes push!) limits and to engage in experimentation. This makes sense because new knowledge is gained by expanding limits and peeking beyond the edges of what is already known.

- **Truth:** Teens can be as rational and thoughtful as adults. To take advantage of this capability, we need to talk to them calmly, in a manner that acknowledges their intelligence and recognizes that they are the experts in their own lives.

Brain science teaches us the power adult engagement holds during adolescence. It informs us of the opportunity we are given to help shape our tweens and teens when we learn how to best connect with and advise them, during both calm and challenging moments. Understanding how the teen brain functions will give you a solid foundation to effectively communicate with teens, especially during emotionally charged moments. This foundation is essential as we dive into *guiding* your teen in Part 4.

The Developing Adolescent Brain and Behavior

Emerging science allows us to understand adolescent brain development as we never have before. In the following paragraphs, we highlight what drives teens' behavior and their thirst for knowledge gained through new experiences.

Developing Brain Pathways

The brain consists of many different parts, which communicate with each other through connections known as *neural pathways*. These connections allow us to integrate thoughts, feelings, sights, sounds, tastes, and experiences into action now and solidify knowledge and wisdom into our memories to be accessed later.

Brain development is essentially the brain learning to become more efficient in its communication. In infancy, the brain is wired inefficiently—information travels from one place to the other slowly, as if the pathways were unpaved roads. The developing brain replaces these unpaved roads over time with "superhighways"—pathways that transport information rapidly and efficiently. Ask yourself, "Where are superhighways built?" They are not placed randomly but are constructed between towns. When it relates to the brain, think of these "towns" as our exposures and experiences. What happens to us—for better or worse—determines how and where these towns are built. A superhighway forms for ease and efficiency to travel to that town in the future. This efficiency allows us to both access our intelligence stored as memory and to avoid dangers by enabling us to act rapidly without needing to think through every step along the way. In fact, learning is about laying down the brain pathways that allow us to retrieve knowledge as needed.

Young people who have grown up in nurturing homes and safe communities have brains constructed for a world that is predictable and safe. Furthermore, enriching educational exposures and challenging and satisfying extracurricular opportunities each create their own towns. We must use the adolescent years to lay down the kind of towns that will enable our teens to be emotionally healthy and to be equipped with the knowledge that will serve them over a lifetime.

Tragically, if our teens are exposed to trauma early in life, their brain pathways may become highly developed in those areas that enable them to react quickly to danger. Their brains may develop to be hypervigilant, constantly scanning for potential danger and remaining on an alert mode poised to quickly react to ensure safety. This constant state of alertness can harm their physical and emotional well-being. Critically, young people who have endured hardships but who *also* had nurturant adults in their lives are less likely to have developed vigilant brain pathways and are more likely to comfortably turn to others for security.

Now, let's use the technical terms so you will better understand the science as it continues to emerge. The brain is going through a process called *myelination* throughout adolescence. Myelin can be thought of as insulation. It ensures that electrical signals that run through our nerves travel efficiently and quickly. The myelinating processes create the superhighways of the brain. The myelinated brain is what is known as *white matter,* and the brain increasingly consists of white matter as it matures.

We also lose many connections between brain cells during adolescence. (Don't worry!) This process, called *pruning,* ensures that the remaining connections are efficient. Another way of thinking about this is if you don't use it, you *should* lose it. After all, if you are developing superhighways, there is no reason to continue to maintain the unpaved roads. It is tragic, however, if a young person is not given enriching educational opportunities and their chances to make new brain connections—learning—is wasted, and, instead, the potential connections are pruned away.

Pulling this together: the developing brain is increasingly myelinated for efficiency and capacity to quickly access information while older, less used, pathways are being pruned away. This leads to a critical point: adolescence is not only a time of astounding brain growth; it also offers an opportunity to reshape the brain as part of healing processes. In other words, if some of those brain pathways were laid down because of adverse experiences, we must make adolescence a time for genuine healing. We must offer young people who have experienced hardship nurturant and safe relationships for their brains to reshape themselves to learn to trust again. We can lay down new towns that make the world look different. This is uplifting news to us all because it speaks to human resilience. It tells us that adolescence offers more than an opportunity to build; it offers an opportunity to heal.

Emotional Brilliance and Reasoning Capacity

When we speak of knowledge, we might first refer to what can be learned in a book. In fact, the capacity to form human relationships might be the most important kind of knowledge we need both to survive and to thrive. This knowledge allows us to work with others toward a common goal and to develop romantic relationships. It is also our ability to understand human relationships that enable us to remain safe from many potential perils. We have to know how to connect with people to grow stronger as a unit and be able to quickly judge when another person is dangerous. This ability might explain why our emotional centers develop earlier than our rational or reasoning centers. Put simply, we may have to know how to react and connect more urgently than we need to solidify our thinking capacities.

The emotional centers of the brain, found in the limbic system and amygdala, develop rapidly during early adolescence. This may explain tweens' sometimes overwhelming need to connect with others. They are learning to read people and the environment and to react quickly in response to observed cues. At times, their ability to fine-tune what they observe is not yet mature, and they may overreact to spoken or unspoken signals or over-read social cues. This partially explains why adolescents can have both the exuberance we envy and the uncomfortable heightened emotions we need to support them through.

The reasoning center of the brain, known as the prefrontal cortex, is also developing rapidly during those years but at a slower pace relative to the brilliant emotional centers. This part of the brain stores our knowledge, helps us plan for the future, and helps us solve problems. The prefrontal cortex is often described as the keeper of our *executive functions*—those abilities we have to organize ourselves and prioritize our actions amid competing demands. It also is the part of the brain that helps us think through or interpret (and sometimes calm) our emotions. This part of our brain continues to catch up to the part that drives emotions but won't be evenly matched until about age 25 years. Knowing how to engage the prefrontal cortex, even in stressful moments, is key to effective communication.

Reward Centers That Drive Learning and Behavior

Our brains have "reward centers" that contain "feel-good" chemicals called neurotransmitters. These chemicals, such as dopamine, are involved in the recognition and anticipation of pleasure. Reward centers respond to exciting experiences and can drive people toward repeating these experiences or seeking new ones. In fact, just having a new experience is itself a thrill, thereby reinforcing a person's desire to stretch into uncharted territories. Teens' reward centers generate pleasure when they are with peers and, therefore, teens are driven to build peer relationships. Dopamine is also heavily involved in those pathways that help people focus and pay attention. This suggests that dopamine activation drives teens toward new experiences while simultaneously helping them learn from those experiences. Teens are *super learners*—there will never be a period of life following adolescence where learning is as rapid or efficient.

Why Adolescents Need to Experiment

Brain development ensures that teens gain as much knowledge as possible before they launch into adulthood. Their brains are shaped by the lessons offered by life, as well as exposures to lessons in our homes and schools. By the end of adolescence, young people should be (relatively) ready to become independent and (somewhat) ready to have meaningful relationships. Achieving success in these critical areas requires practice, failure and recovery, and willingness to take some risks. It also involves being able to connect with people in a highly personal way. It is not surprising, therefore, that adolescents are wired to seek sensations—new experiences—and to feel most lively when with peers. They are experimenters by design to maximize their social skills and general know-how.

Sensation seeking—the desire to have pleasurable, exciting, and new experiences—peaks during the teen years. Nevertheless, most adolescents do *not* engage in highly risky activities and make it through adolescence just fine. They weigh risks and benefits and do not believe they are invincible. Although some youth may test their limits to experience pleasure, they also absorb feedback and pay attention to negative consequences in a way that alters their future behaviors—reigning in their pleasure seeking. Your reasoned advice and shared wisdom counts. It is important to note, however, that young people may have increased risk-taking in the presence of peers who expect them to take risks. The great news: if peers do not expect risk-taking, their influence can be protective against negative peer pressure.

There is a subgroup of adolescents who behave impulsively and are less likely to curb their urges or consider potential consequences. There are a

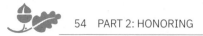

few key points to pull away from the distinction between sensation seeking and impulsive action.

1. Sensation seeking is a normal, healthy, perhaps even necessary part of adolescent development. It drives teens to experiences from which they will learn.

2. A subset of individuals is impulsive from childhood through adulthood. You may hear about impulsive adolescents more because their sometimes dangerous behaviors can drive the news, but they do not represent most teens.

3. You know your own child best. If your teen has a history of impulsive actions or behaviors, without regard to consequence, it is important you set protective boundaries.

Enriching Opportunities for Super Learners

Development is happening before your eyes, and the brains our teens build will predict and sustain their future success. Adolescents take in what we teach them formally and informally. They learn what is expected from them. We should expose them to intelligence-building knowledge and to experiences enabling them to reach their potential. This should *not* be interpreted as a call to pressure your child in school or to expose them to every possible activity. **Rather, it is about creating an enriching, nurturing environment.**

We also need to support healthy sensation seeking and experimenting. Brain science suggests that they are driven to find thrilling new experiences both as a means to expand their knowledge and to learn lifelong lessons. Our job is to guide our teens toward thrills they will grow from and away from those that may harm them. Life is full of opportunities to test our limits and even to take our breath away. Trying out for a school play or a sports team. Asking another teen out for a date. Running a marathon. Diving from the high dive. Expressing deep emotions in a poetry slam. These healthy opportunities fill their neurobiological need, making it less likely they will seek thrills elsewhere. When we encourage golden opportunities at the very edge of current experience and existing knowledge but within safe boundaries, teen brains will be satisfied. When we do not set appropriate boundaries and fail to create satisfying and safe thrills at the edges of what they already know, our teens may stray (or push!) into risky territory. Let's bring this point home: negative risk-taking is more likely to occur when we adults do not honor adolescent development and fail to create enriching opportunities for our super learners.

Experimentation Within Clear Boundaries

We can shape, support, and protect teens' development. The science confirms what common sense and experience tells us is true: we adults play a critical protective role in the lives of our tweens and teens. Daniel Romer,

PhD, a leading health and developmental psychologist at the Annenberg School for Communication at the University of Pennsylvania, proposes the Life-span Wisdom Model. It recognizes adolescence as a time where experiences needed for lifelong learning must be maximized. It recognizes that some of those experiences may involve risk and that while changes going on in the body and brain promote risk-taking, positive and meaningful social influencers (such as parents!) can promote risk avoidance.

To support healthy brain development, indeed development in general, we must

1. Provide a protective, nurturing environment.
2. Engage our adolescents in meaningful discussions in which they will learn and grow.
3. Provide safe opportunities for exploration and experimentation.
4. Help them develop calm, rational decision-making skills. Modeling these skill sets is a critical starting point.
5. Encourage proper sleep, good nutrition, and healthy exercise.

Our children will be best able to begin answering those multilayered developmental questions ("Who am I?" "Am I normal?" "Do I fit in?") when, as parents, we create the environments necessary for optimal development. Brain science tells us that children will most successfully grow when we create calm settings, allowing them to do their best thinking ,and when we promote safe and appropriate experimentation.

Parents play a crucial role in setting the boundaries that will allow for necessary trial and error within safe territory. If your teen is in a peer group that puts them at risk, your rules have to be firmer because brain science (and human history) tells us that people behave more impulsively in groups than as individuals. So too, that subset of young people who are truly impulsive will need firmer boundaries since they are less likely to learn quickly from consequences. For example, you should ensure your teen is not in a home without trusted adult supervision if their friends act impulsively or engage in risky behaviors such as drinking alcohol. As you set these boundaries, your teens must know they exist because you care for them, not because you are trying to control them. This will be explained fully in Chapter 24.

Protect the Brain From Harmful Substances

It is important that teens understand we are against them using drugs or other harmful substances. We want to keep them safe and poised to make wise, responsible decisions. It's also because we know that these substances are harmful to the developing brain. Teens are strongly receptive to pleasure-inducing neurotransmitters because they have an abundance of reward centers as part of the design that encourages learning through new experiences and relationships. Drugs also load the brain with dopamine, causing intense pleasure. Teens have extra dopamine sensitivity and, therefore, are particularly susceptible to want to continue using. Substance use disorder is not a behavior of choice or a sign of moral weakness. It is biologically driven and can happen to anyone after repeated exposures to substances.

Protect the Brain From Injury

Parents insist on helmets when their children ride bicycles, but some let their guard down as their children grow in the teen years. Brain injury can have lifelong implications. Insist on helmet use when teens are biking or skateboarding. As your teens enter driving age, reinforce the urgency of consistent seat belt use, speak about the dangers of distracted driving, and take advantage of the proven benefits of graduated driver licensing programs. Finally, if your teen participates in athletic activities, make sure that their coaches know how to minimize concussion risk and how to react if your child does sustain a sports-related head injury. Use the Center for Injury Research and Prevention as a valued resource (https://injury.research.chop.edu).

Brain Science Offers the Foundation for Effective Communication

If you know how to communicate effectively with your teen, you will be impressed by how rational and thoughtful they can be. Too often, people have depicted the reasoning part of the brain as practically absent during the teen years. This incorrectly implies that teens are driven entirely by emotions and can't be reasoned with. In fact, the key to elevating your teen's thinking powers is to use calm communication strategies that avoid the reasoning centers from being flooded by emotional responses. This is described as "cold communication" rather than "hot communication."

When we use "cold communication," we are calm and thoughtful. Our presence makes the teen feel safe; we should be emotionally warm and nurturing. We should be careful not to create a heightened emotional state. When using "cold communication," you are talking to your child's rational brain. In sharp contrast, if you are angry or condescending you are using "hot communication," and your teen's brilliant emotional centers will dominate, hijacking the ability for their rational centers to operate effectively.

It is on us to guide our teens in ways they can hear and understand. Young people understand and consider risk. They want adults to share their wisdom. By the age of 16 years (earlier for some), they can problem-solve at essentially the same level as adults, *if* we can help them do so in calm settings. Their emotional centers are designed to take in information rapidly and react to it. This is a great strength of the adolescent brain; the problem is that adolescents' emotional centers are so well-developed that stress can easily activate them, thereby dominating their rational centers. That may prevent emotionally charged teens from being able to problem-solve. This is not a problem unique to teens; stressful situations also activate adults' emotional centers, making it harder for us to think when feeling unsafe or challenged. The difference is that our thinking centers are more firmly developed, and our experience and wisdom can (usually) tamp down our initial emotional responses.

When you want to address a topic and need your teen to bring their most thoughtful self to the conversation, consider the following:

BE CALM. It is easier said than done, but it is critical. If you are unable to be calm, give yourself a time-out. Practice this line: "I need a bit of space and time to think this through. I'll get back to you. We'll get through this together." Model the active steps you take to regain composure.

BE SINCERE. One of the greatest traits our tweens and teens possess is their ability to read people. It is an exciting developmental process, central to building empathy and meaningful relationships. Their ability to do this is remarkable but is not yet fully sophisticated. This means they sometimes overread our body language or tone of voice. (Think: "Why are you making that face?!") Work through your own thoughts before you offer advice. Usually, some deep breaths and a bit of time will help you "de-catastrophize" a situation and approach it sincerely in a more even-keeled, reassuring manner.

DON'T LECTURE. When a young person is upset, it is hard for them to problem-solve. When you deliver your advice by lecturing, your child will grasp your disappointment, understand your anger, and absorb your fear, but likely miss the true message. Talk with them, not at them. Give them time to process what you are saying.

BE WARM. Teens who are nurtured (ie, *know* they are loved) develop better reasoning abilities and less reactive emotional centers.

You've Got This!

To support healthy adolescent development, and brain development in particular, we must

1. Provide a protective, nurturing environment.

2. Engage teens in discussions in which they will learn and grow.

3. Provide safe opportunities for exploration and experimentation.

4. Help them develop calm, rational decision-making skills. We start by modeling these skill sets.

How Brain Science Guides Us to Bring Out the Best in Our Teens	
The Truth About Teens	**Actions We Take to Optimize That Truth**
Adolescence is a time of astoundingly rapid brain development, and we can shape our children's future far into adulthood by nurturing that development.	Adolescents (and their brains) develop best when nourished by protective relationships.
	Use nurturant relationships to help young people heal from childhood hardships.
	Honor the fact that teens are super learners and need opportunities to maximize their exposure to new knowledge (see next topic).
Adolescents are super learners, and they will learn more during this period of their life than at any other time that follows.	Help your teen to gain exposure to a variety of settings where they can gain new knowledge.
	Understand that knowledge is gained when adolescents stretch into new, safe territory and gain new experiences.
	Know that knowledge is also gained through failure and recovery.
	Know that school is only one place to learn. Athletic fields and extracurricular activities offer endless learning. Elders can share wisdom, mentors can generate experiences, and peers can share growth experiences.
	Knowledge is solidified when we help our teens nurture their brains with the right combination of exercise, nutrition, relaxation, and proper sleep.

How Brain Science Guides Us to Bring Out the Best in Our Teens (*continued*)

The Truth About Teens	Actions We Take to Optimize That Truth
Young people care deeply about safety but need guidance as they learn about risk.	Speak clearly about risks. Make it clear you set rules and make boundaries because you care about safety, *not* because you aim to be controlling.
	Help your teen satisfy their (brain-driven) need to explore new territory by helping them find exciting new experiences.
	Set clear boundaries around safety that your teen knows they cannot stray beyond.
	Help your teen think through potential consequences of different actions before they have chosen a path.
Teens can be as rational and thoughtful as adults.	Learn how to activate the prefrontal cortex rather than emotional centers.
	Use the following cold communication skills: • Talk calmly; give yourself a time-out if you need that to get to calm. • Express your love; show warmth. • Acknowledge their intelligence. • Recognize them as the expert in their own lives.
	Avoid the following pitfalls of hot communication: • Don't lecture; it makes teens feel belittled. • Don't approach an issue while angry. • Don't act like you know more than your teen does about their own world. • Don't suggest that a mistake will inevitably lead to catastrophic consequences.

(*continued*)

How Brain Science Guides Us to Bring Out the Best in Our Teens (*continued*)	
The Truth About Teens	**Actions We Take to Optimize That Truth**
Teens can be as rational and thoughtful as adults (*continued*).	Be a sounding board as teens express their own thoughts.
	Share your appreciation of their thoughtfulness and recognize their growing maturity.

I'll bet you already intuitively knew a lot of this. Maybe you didn't know the neuroscience or jargon, but your experience has shown you that tweens and teens are often emotional. You've witnessed teens taking chances and pushing boundaries. You've noticed their remarkable ability to learn and adapt. And you are reading this book in the first place because you know that adult guidance shapes and protects teens. You've got this!

....

Recommended Resource

The Center for Injury Research and Prevention (https://injury.research.chop.edu). This center pursues innovative solutions to prevent injury in children, youth, and young adults and offers guidance to caregivers.

CHAPTER 9

Changing Bodies and Developing Sexuality

From as early as I can remember, I filed into the classroom first after recess and, during school performances, stood in the front row. In junior high, I was still very much a child when my peers entered puberty. I was lucky enough to get a lot of attention from the girls—in the same way a puppy would have. I was "Little Doll." That's *really* what they called me. Would you like to know one of the highlights of my high school years? It is the day a 411 information operator said to me, "I have that number for you, sir." Did you hear it?!? *Sir!*

What's My Role in My Child's Physical Changes?

Some adolescents feel so insecure about their bodies that they focus on how they look and imagine everyone else who sees them is also focused on their appearance. This is not self-centeredness or self-involvement; it is self-consciousness, which is quite different. If one believed it was self-centeredness, one reaction might be to minimize their feelings: "Nobody cares about what you look like." But if we understand their behavior should be framed as self-consciousness instead, then we grasp that our role should be supportive.

Be reassuring about the range of normal-developing bodies and the uneven pace of physical changes. Provide straightforward explanations about physical changes. Remind them that each person will have their own unique shape or size. Help them understand there is no physical ideal, only the goal of being healthy, confident, and secure in who we are. If your child is physically advancing more quickly or more slowly than most of their peers, they may need extra reassurance. This includes both the early developing girl who receives more attention than she desires and the late developing boy getting less attention than he'd hope.

Because your child may be uncomfortable holding these conversations, your approach should vary depending on their nature. If they are comfortable with their curiosity, then you can offer opportunities for them to ask you questions. If they feel awkward about these topics, casually offer information starting with the point, "All young people need to learn about this, and parents should teach about this." Still other teens want to explore on their own or seek out friends or trusted adults other than parents. For these (and all) teens, having reference books available works, as does having routine health appointments where professionals cover these topics and create a comfortable space for questions. Finally, be a sounding board. When your teen knows you will listen without judgment and give them space to talk, cry, or blow off steam, they'll let you know what they need.

The best thing you may do for your teen is to focus on something else! Your child may genuinely believe everyone else cares most about their imperfections. Your critical role here is to not focus on their bodies or their appearance. Recognize your teen's unique strengths, such as being compassionate, insightful, idealistic, hardworking, or creative—all the stuff that really matters is completely unrelated to their appearance. In parallel, encourage your child's friendships with lifelong peers who also see your teen in ways that have nothing to do with their appearance.

Supporting Healthy Sexual Development

Sexual thoughts and feelings accompany the hormonal changes of puberty. This can be overwhelming for tweens, teens, and parents alike. A healthy sexuality is a critical part of one's identity, and we cover it in Chapter 7. I want to underscore that there is nothing you can say or do that will shape someone's attractions or identity. However, your importance in your child accepting themselves and the complexity of their own feelings and attractions is immeasurable. And you helping them to have a healthy view of sexuality and relationships is irreplaceable.

If you don't discuss sexuality with your teen, who will? I'll give you the answer. Schools will address the mechanics and hopefully the safety issues. The more nuanced issues will be handled by the media, the internet, and their peers. And you may not like what any of them say because they may lack accuracy or values, or both. You can best speak to the values around healthy relationships that mean so much more than the mechanics. Only you can tailor guidance to match the temperament and needs of your teen. Perhaps most importantly, only you will guide your teen to think things through for themself. Media talks at you. The internet has fabulous information but only if you find a reputable website. Search terms can easily lead you to sites with inaccurate information or worse. And the internet is designed to earn more clicks. You want your child to do the opposite, to take the time for reflection. To slow down. To learn at the pace that matches their development. Peers can be very helpful or quite harmful. They might be more interested in how they are viewed than in being a sounding board and, therefore, may give misinformation or exaggerate their own experiences. You can't prevent your child from seeking out other sources, but you can steer them toward good sources, including yourself.

Sexuality may be uncomfortable to talk about with anybody, let alone our children. (I am dictating this on a word program and the word sexuality comes up as *********. This program won't even let me dictate the word! So how do we get our kids comfortable talking about this subject when my computer program isn't even comfortable with it?) Become comfortable with the subject before you address it. Don't force it. Don't make this THE TALK. These conversations should be ongoing, not an EVENT. That's just too much pressure on you. If you're feeling pressure, just imagine what your teen is thinking when they see you being nervous or stuttering. If you approach this instead as an ongoing discussion, it allows you to be responsive to your teen's questions and discuss only as much as they want to handle in a single sit-down. These ongoing conversations ideally should begin before your teen is dating, which will allow you to discuss topics without them feeling as personal to your teen ("Why don't you trust me?"; "Why do you hate my girlfriend!?!"), or as imminent to you ("Sweetheart, I know you have a big date tonight."). If your teen is already in a relationship, then the best time to have this conversation is NOW. Speak generally about feelings, respect, and safety, rather than about a specific relationship or event. It will be easier for your teen to hear without becoming defensive of themself or their partner. If your teen does want to speak about a particular relation-ship, count yourself as blessed, but remember to act more as a sounding board than an interrogator.

Don't be surprised if your tween or teen doesn't want to talk about this with you...or anybody. Fun story: when my girls were in fifth grade, they told me their school needed to collect parental signatures for a special class. I assumed it was a permission slip to learn about *** in school. (My computer program is still too shy to say it!) My girls stood shoulder to shoulder, handed me a pen, and directed me to sign. Never wasting the opportunity to elevate the mundane into a life lesson, I said it was good policy to read everything before signing it. My eyes widened when I realized it was an opt-out form. I said to the girls, "This is for the parents who don't believe sexuality should be taught in schools." My girls said, "Exactly! Sign it!" (I did not. ☺) For context, these are *my* girls, and I support young people to develop healthy sexuality for a living! Knowing that we may not be the desired source of knowledge for our own children, ensure that there are other trusted adults who can discuss these topics with your children, such as an aunt, coach, counselor, or health professional.

My close colleague, Susan Sugerman, MD, MPH, of Girls to Women Health and Wellness and Young Men's Health and Wellness practice in Dallas, TX, created the following tips for parents looking to keep the lines of communication open with their children about sexual health:

PARENTS MATTER. It is the privilege, right, and responsibility of parents to facilitate the development of healthy sexuality in their children. It is their job to be a source of information and wisdom about sexual issues, to support healthy sexuality, to recognize and respond to unhealthy or unsafe sexual experiences, and, most importantly, to monitor and defend the safety of their children.

DON'T BLAME TEENS FOR BEING NORMAL. Our children live in a highly sexualized society where they are exposed to sexual language, images, and behaviors before they are developmentally prepared to handle them. Kids didn't "ask" for hormones but are stuck learning how to handle their changing bodies and urges in a society that shows them "yes" but tells them "not now."

DON'T DISCREDIT LOVE. Understand the importance of romantic attachments in a teenager's life and the intense, strong feelings they generate, even if your definition and perspective of love differ from your child's.

DON'T ABSTAIN FROM EDUCATING YOUR OWN CHILDREN. If you don't educate them, someone else will. They learn from behaviors and attitudes modeled by other adults, from the media and popular culture, and certainly from their peers. Stand up and let your own views be counted as part of their sex education.

TALK ABOUT SEX EARLY AND OFTEN. They don't always hear you. They may not always believe you. They often don't remember, especially if they weren't ready to hear you. (But they are often listening when they are pretending not to be.)

AVOID SEXUALITY CONVERSATIONS THAT ARE ALL *"DON'TS."* Parents often recount that they speak to their teens often about sex. Yet, generally, those conversations are all about the *"don'ts."*

- *Don't* have sex.
- *Don't* get pregnant.
- *Don't* get a sexually transmitted infection.

It's *don't, don't, don't.* But what is left out are the *"dos."* What can they *do* to be sexually healthy with a partner that they care about? How can they decide whether a partner is interested in them as a person? What ways can they address peer or partner pressure to be sexual when they don't feel they are ready?

RIGHT TIME, RIGHT PLACE. Meet them where they are. A young child asking, *"What does sex mean?"* may wonder what the teacher meant when she said, *"line up by sex"* for recess. Find out exactly what the question is, then try to give an honest answer that meets that need.

BE REAL. Dispel myths and rumors. Provide accurate information. Use simple language but respect their intelligence and curiosity. Above all, avoid talking down to teens about sex.

EMPOWER YOUR CHILDREN. Let them know they deserve to feel honored in their relationships, to have their own space, to keep their friends, to include their family, and to feel good about who they are. Teach them to expect a give-and-take but that, in the end, a good relationship helps you to be more of who you already are and feel even better about it.

SET POSITIVE EXPECTATIONS. Discussing what's good about sex will help them to have positive standards by which to judge sexual experiences. Help your kids know *why* sex is worth waiting for and give them realistic guidance about how they will know when it might be worth moving forward.

USE THE MEDIA (THE GOOD, THE BAD, AND THE UGLY). Use topics presented in daily media sources and popular teen culture as springboards for conversations about sex and relationships. Avoid proclamations and judgments, even about fictional characters; your children will anticipate you reacting to them in the same way should they ever be in that situation. Consider role-playing through a situation presented on TV as collaborative, nonjudgmental thought processing; it will provide insight into your child's view of the world and give you the opportunity to offer your ideas for them to reflect on.

LIVE BY EXAMPLE. If you have a good relationship with your partner or spouse, let your children know about some of the ups and downs. Let them witness you and your partner having a disagreement and working it out, and let them see you kiss and make up.

TEACHING KIDS ABOUT SEX DOESN'T MEAN PARENTING WITHOUT VALUES. Acknowledging sexuality is not the same as condoning or giving permission to have sex. Helping your children understand that sexual thoughts and feelings are normal gives you the opportunity to follow up with conversations about *how* (and from *what*) to be abstinent as well as how to regulate your teen's impulses and urges. It opens the door to continued conversation about how to be safe and responsible when they begin to engage in intimate physical or sexual activities.

ASK, DON'T TELL. Find out what your child is thinking when talking about their relationships or sexual experiences. What does it mean to have a boyfriend or girlfriend at what age? Listen to what it means to your teen at that time. Your teen's level of understanding and participation may actually be appropriate for their developmental level. Understand; don't judge. It is also helpful to talk about their friends and relationships. Teens can be chattier about their friends than about themselves, and listening to what their friends are doing will offer insight into how your teen feels.

DON'T ASK TOO MANY QUESTIONS, or you won't get any information at all. Provide a respectful place for sharing what they are willing to share, such as excitement of first love and feeling valued, wanted, and desired by someone else in a very different, intensely intimate way.

KEEP IT GENERIC. Being willing to speak in generalities allows conversations about difficult subjects such as sex to move forward without making anyone feel too uncomfortable. Let your children know that you know of people that had uncomfortable experiences when they were younger, that you have been in difficult situations or know others who have been, and that you're not afraid to discuss those things. Avoid interrogating your teen about what exactly they did or didn't do sexually; you don't want them to demand details about your love life, either.

ADOLESCENCE IS FOR PRACTICE. The teenage years are great for learning about relationships. What is the difference between a crush and real love? Between a "boyfriend" or "girlfriend" and a friend who is a boy or a girl? What belongs on social media and what doesn't? How does he treat you when you're alone compared to when your friends or parents are around? Does she keep a confidence or tell all her friends about it the next day? Without a few battle scars, how will we know a good relationship when we see it? On the other hand, major situations that change our lives (such as a sexually transmitted infection or unintended pregnancy) must be avoided.

THINGS THAT ARE HARD ARE NOT WITHOUT VALUE. Help your teen learn from their mistakes. The goal is to learn to develop and maintain healthy relationship skills. If you protect them from every discomfort, they may never learn the lessons that come from experiencing a broken heart.

BEWARE OF THE "D" WORD. Children fear *disappointing* their parents more than just about anything else in the world. While you should let your children know when their behavior is dangerous or wrong, be clear there is nothing they could ever do that would make you stop loving them. Reassure them that, after you calm down and process the situation, you still want what's best for them and you will find help when they need it. Avoid falling into situations where their fear of your disappointment or anger keeps them from coming to you when they need you the most.

BE CLEAR THAT SAFETY IS NONNEGOTIABLE. Think about your bottom-line priorities for your children. Chances are that nothing matters more to you than their safety. Be very clear, and repeat often, that nothing matters more than knowing that they are going to be OK. Establish a code word or phrase (see "Code Words" in Chapter 12) they can use to get your attention and help when they need to get out of a potentially dangerous or uncomfortable situation. Set a standard for protecting themselves from a sexually transmitted infection and unwanted pregnancy regardless of whether you agree with their decision-making about sex.

FIND A SURROGATE. Talking about sex is difficult. When necessary, identify and encourage them to ask for help from other trusted adults; it doesn't always have to be you.

BUILD YOUR OWN TOOLKIT. Create a list of web resources you believe offer sound information and advice. Consider keeping books at home that support your values about sexuality while providing accurate information. Find resources in your community, such as clinics, hotlines, therapeutic specialists, and support groups, in case you or your children need more support.

Preparation Is Protection

Although we've focused on developing healthy relationships, we must also prepare teens to prevent, recognize, and respond to unhealthy relationships. They need clear examples of the differences between healthy versus controlling and abusive relationships. For example, teens often view jealousy as a sign of caring when, in actuality, it is the first sign of control. Be willing to explore with teenagers why they think their relationships may or may not be good for them, and have resources to provide support if they find themselves (or a friend) needing help to get out of an unhealthy relationship. As Dr Sugerman says, name their power to give them power—their voice, their choice. Just telling teens that they have the right to set limits and that they deserve to be taken seriously may be enough to change how they handle themselves in relationships.

• •

Recommended Resource

Relationships 101. One Love Foundation is committed to ending relationship abuse. It offers primers for young people on signs of healthy and unhealthy relationships (https://www.joinonelove.org).

CHAPTER 10

Celebrating, Elevating, and Experiencing Emotions

We are inspired by our teens' exuberance and capacity to experience life to the fullest. Their positive energy and joyful dispositions can be enviable. Their sensitivity, passion, and compassion make them reliable, committed friends. On the other hand, heightened adolescent emotions can also lead to excessive worry or mental health challenges such as anxiety or depression. Furthermore, teens with uncomfortable feelings can engage in risky behaviors, such as drug use, to numb their thoughts or escape their feelings. As parents, we want to support our children to benefit from the richness of their emotions while learning to manage emotional discomfort in healthy and productive ways.

Pulling from our knowledge of brain development: (1) Adolescents' emotional intensity is a sign of advancing development, even though their emotional regulation is not yet fully matured, and (2) how we communicate can help teens regulate their emotions and access their rational selves.

An Opportunity to Create Lifelong Emotional and Mental Health

Precisely because our tweens and teens have palpable emotions, we are given an opportunity to lay the foundation for the relationship they will have with their emotions over their lifetime. Will they learn that emotions should be suppressed or expressed? Will they have pride in their joyful emotions, but experience shame with their uncomfortable feelings? Will they grow to believe their uncomfortable emotions are handled best alone or with support from others? Will they view seeking help as an act of strength or a display of weakness? When we stand by our teens through their emotional highs and lows, we can support them to view the range of their feelings in a heathy way—now and in the future.

Why Are Adolescent Emotions Heightened?

Humans have a range of emotions, and some of us are apt to experience them more fully or become distressed more easily. There are a few reasons, however, why the teen years can be a time of more extreme emotional highs and lows. Teens face more responsibilities at both school and at home than they did in earlier years, and it takes time to adjust to these changes. Furthermore, some of them internalize the pressure they feel to figure out those big "Who am I?" life questions thrown at them as they search for their identity. Critically, peer interactions hold a lot of power over their mood because of how much teens want to fit in.

Let's revisit how their brain circuitry and chemical reward systems also explain the emotional high and lows. Remember, the adolescent brain is wired to encourage situations in which to gain new knowledge. The brain has reward centers that generate pleasure with new experiences. This drives youth to stretch even further to reach for new opportunities for learning and growth. Also, the part of their brain that initiates and processes emotions develops rapidly during adolescence, giving them what could be described as emotional brilliance. They are highly sensitive to emotional content as they are learning to interpret subtle interpersonal cues. But, in the process of this emotional development, they can be overly sensitive to those cues. Recall also that adolescents are wired to grow socially, and their brain reward centers give them intense positive feedback in the presence of peers. Tying this together, they are more likely to be thrilled in the presence of peers (the highs) but to also be crushed when they sense rejection (the lows, often driven by an overly sensitive interpretation of peer feedback or social cues). Finally, the reasoning part of the brain, which processes emotions and helps stabilize our reactions to them, is also developing but lags a bit behind the emotional centers.

Ages and Stages of Emotional Development

Because emotional development is something young people progress through in stages based on the interplay of brain maturity, life experience, and adult support, the following ages are approximations:

11 TO 12 YEARS: As tweens react to their developing bodies, they may feel uncomfortable or self-conscious. Therefore, they tend to focus on themselves, wondering if the rapid physical changes they are experiencing are normal. To figure that out, they may compare themselves to peers, investing a lot of emotional energy thinking about where they fit in with friends.

13 TO 14 YEARS: As teens begin to establish their independence, parents may feel distancing from them. Their teens may have a need for privacy one moment but reach out for support during another. They continue to build relationships with their peers and may feel sensitized to social stress or exclusion. They become highly sensitive to emotional and social cues and find it harder to self-regulate than they will later, as their brains mature.

15 TO 16 YEARS: Teens in this age group may become increasingly stressed about grades and set high expectations for themselves. Others may react to stress by feigning indifference or behaving as though they were lazy. As teens begin to intensify their development of a sense of self, they may question their identities, which can lead to dysregulated emotions. They may have a range of emotions from seeming to know it all to insecurity. Their increasing desire for independence can lead to rebelliousness. They may begin to test their limits, and some may begin to engage in risky behaviors. However, because they are moving from concrete thinking to thinking more abstractly (see Chapter 11), they better understand the long-term consequences of their actions and better grasp the unspoken intentions of others' behaviors.

17 TO 21 YEARS (AND BEYOND!): By this age, most young people are fully physically developed. These late teens and young adults can more easily access their thinking powers even in emotional contexts and, therefore, better avoid emotional risk-taking. They can plan ahead using creative and well-thought-out strategies and problem-solving. They value peer groups but may focus more on individual deeper friendships and romantic relationships. They may prioritize future goals and worry about their next steps. While future orientation is protective, some older teens and young adults may continue to push their limits and engage in risky behaviors.

Supporting Emotional Development

The most important thing we can do in supporting emotional development is to make it OK for our children to have and experience their emotions. If we raise them to understand that no emotion is wrong, then their relationship with their emotional self will be healthier throughout their lifetime.

Saying that no emotion is wrong does not deny that some are uncomfortable and need to be managed or addressed. Rather, it is about removing judgment from what a person is feeling to create room to learn how to manage emotions in a healthy way. It is the judgment of our thoughts and feelings that can make teens suppress or hide them. Suppressed emotions only delay the pain. Suppressed emotions can lead teens to feel numb because they cannot access what is driving so many of their thoughts, feelings, and behaviors. Suppressed emotions prevent them from reaching out and benefiting from the power human connection has to heal and to strengthen us.

In fact, we need to elevate our emotions. I do not mean we need to increase the intensity of what we feel. Elevating our emotions enables us instead to regulate what we feel. It allows us to be aware of what we feel, thereby allowing us to express ourselves, and adjust our reactions to those feelings. Elevating emotions allows us to take advantage of all the ways we can feel better when uncomfortable or stressed. In some cases, elevating emotions is about celebrating them. Of course, we all want to celebrate the moments where we are feeling pleasure. But celebrating emotions takes it a step further and includes a wider range of emotions. It is about valuing the very fact that we can feel. Emotions are what enable us to get the most out of life, to connect with others, and, ultimately, to have deep satisfaction. The price we pay to live life richly in this way is the presence of our feelings, including those that are not always pleasant. If you have a teen who is a bit more anxious than most and who experiences intense feelings such as sadness, then I extend congratulations. Your teen is a feeler and a sensor. Our goal is not to help them deny or suppress their emotions; it is to enable them to express them and, ultimately, to leverage their intensity to lead them to the most satisfying life.

As your teen develops their emotional maturity, you'll try different approaches at different times, depending both on their mood and their receptivity. They may face issues they do not want to discuss with you. The need for privacy, combined with their need to develop their independence, may cause your teen to appear distant and uncommunicative at times. If you push too hard at these moments, your teen may pull further away. On the other hand, if you give too much space, they may drift away. It is a bit like dancing. In this case, it is about striking the balance between offering privacy at times and your wisdom at others. And remember that you may not have all the right moves. In fact, the very fact that your teen cares so much about what you think and worries about disappointing you—even if they'd deny that—means they may be more comfortable talking to someone other than you, depending on the situation. Let them know it's OK to talk it out with someone else they trust, including professionals.

Strive to be the kind of parent your teen chooses to talk to on their own timeline. This is about being a good listener, not reacting or judging, and supporting them to solve their own problems. Especially during difficult times, never forget that your teen remains the expert on their own life, and you are their guide. This is why listening and being a sounding board is often the best strategy. Listening sends a critical message: you comfort but do not control or dictate, you trust in their ability to get through this, but you'll be by their side as an unwavering support. It is also about being mindful of the time and place you choose to have important conversations to set the tone for calm, comfortable, and private discussions. This might mean doing some self-calming yourself before you enter a conversation.

Support for the Ages and Stages

The type of support you offer should vary to meet the challenge your teen is encountering and must pay attention to their developmental ability to think things through for themself.

11 TO 12 YEARS: In this stage, parents can help address self-consciousness. Reassure your teen that their emotions are common and that everyone their age is going through changes and feels self-conscious at times.

13 TO 14 YEARS: Be a sounding board for your teens on the struggles they are having trying to fit into their peer group. Support them to interpret social cues in different contexts. Recognize they may need more time alone and with their peers, and don't become defensive about the occasional rejection you might feel. Know that even if they are pushing you away, it is harder for them than it is for you. Model what open and safe communication and mutual respect looks like.

15 TO 16 YEARS: Maintain open communication and be aware that peers can be positive or negative forces in your child's life. Know that teens who maintain close relationships with adults such as parents, family members, coaches, or counselors at this age are less likely to engage in high risk-taking and that the key to those close relationships is to be unconditional in your loving and to create a judgment-free zone. At the same time, set safe boundaries and provide information about the danger of risky behaviors to keep them safe. Being nonjudgmental does not mean you accept every behavior; it means that you know that your child's behaviors do not define them. Remain calm so you can lend that calm to your teen. Talk in a way that is developmentally appropriate; this means not lecturing and allowing teens more time to process and to come up with their own solutions.

17 TO 21 YEARS (AND BEYOND!): Our goal as parents is to encourage reflective thinking and wise decision-making. During this age range, your teen will have solidified their ability to think abstractly and that means they can have insight into the thoughts and feelings that drive their behaviors. Once that insight is achieved, they can learn to "catch" those thoughts and feelings at early stages to prevent themself from repeating behavioral mistakes or reliving circumstances that inflict emotional pain. Remind them of your presence and help (when asked!) as they work to recover from their missteps.

Our Journey Into Emotional Development Has Only Begun

How you *honor* your teen's emotional development is critical to how you *shape* your relationship and *guide* your children to become their very best selves. Therefore, the points that we've discussed so far will be further developed throughout this book. The following is a preview of chapters that prepare you to support your teen emotionally. Feel free to read them in whatever order fits your situation.

— In Chapter 15, The Root of Lifelong Security: Your Unwavering Presence, we underscore how you can help your child better manage their emotions precisely because they know they could never lose you.

— Chapter 16, Make the Most of Living With an Expert, discusses why supporting youth to leverage their own internal wisdom is the most effective way to ensure that you, as their parent, will continue to be welcomed by them as they process what they are feeling.

— Chapter 17, Listen More, Judge Less, offers a deeper dive into the concept of listening. As previously stated, this is the key to knowing what is going on in your teen's life and them inviting you to guide them.

— Chapter 18, Talk Wisely, Learn More, covers how to communicate with a stressed or highly emotional teen while engaging their thinking capacity and helping them make good decisions.

— Chapter 19, Mind Your Body, reveals that most of what we communicate remains unspoken. This is a vital lesson to understand because teens are particularly sensitive to subtle social cues sent through body signals.

— Chapter 20, Like a Duck on the Water, is a pivotal chapter as you consider the "how-tos" of supporting your teen's emotional development. It is about you lending your calm (co-regulation) so your teen can build their emotional stability (self-regulation).

— Chapter 23, Preparation Is Protection, speaks to the reality that the world is not predictable but that every emotion that is not denied or set aside offers an opportunity to build a resilience skill.

— Chapter 25, Building Resilience in Difficult and Uncertain Times, will introduce you to an approach that will enable your teen to manage their stress. Resilience is about so much more than "management," though; it is about thriving during both challenging times and good times.

Healthy Emotional Management

When our emotions are riding high, there are 2 very different things people can do to manage their feelings. One is to escape from them, and the other is to deal with them. Both involve active and thoughtful steps even if, at first glance, the word "escape" might be misinterpreted as ignoring the problem.

Escape as Emotional Management

It is OK to set aside the intensity of our feelings for a bit and to take an "instant vacation." The best kind of vacations are ones that don't allow for our worries to intrude into our thoughts. For this reason, reading a book for pleasure is one of the best instant vacations. When we read, we have to imagine the sights and sounds and even the smells and tastes. Most importantly, we experience the feelings. Because we are immersed in another world, there's no room for our problems. Other instant vacations include going for hikes or practicing mindfulness. Escaping emotions in healthy ways is a key element of drug use prevention. Think about it for a minute: substance use disorder is about escaping our thoughts and feelings, but this is only a temporary escape and extremely dangerous. We must encourage teens to use healthier, safer strategies.

Dealing With Emotions Directly

There are many ways that we can deal with our emotions. The first is to pinpoint what problems may be driving our emotions and, when possible, address those problems directly. Second, the power of human connection cannot be overstated and really is the reason you are reading this book. You know that your presence is undeniably the most protective thing in your child's life. However, your teen's emotional health also benefits from other positive connections. When we join with other people, we gain strength to manage our emotions. As importantly we also lend strength to others, just as a stick, by standing alone, is fragile and can bend in the wind but when joined together with another stick becomes harder to bend and when part of a bundle of sticks becomes impossible to break. For a reason that has something to do with physics and everything to do with spirituality, together we are more powerful than the sum of our individual parts. Third, we manage our emotions when we are able to name and express them in a productive manner, as subsequently described.

Name and Express Thoughts and Feelings

When stressful emotions rise above manageable levels, it's normal to set them aside—to try to "contain" feelings in the hope they will disappear or be processed later. The downside to placing those feelings away is that oftentimes those feelings are added to the "container" indefinitely, rather than dealing with them head-on. Ultimately, the walls of the container need to thicken to keep it all in. The walls may become impenetrable to the point we can no longer access what is contained within. We become numb, shut down, and hold our feelings inside. In some ways, that's worse than feeling stressed.

It's OK to place emotions into a safe container. Sometimes it enables us to function. But they must be processed at some other point. Otherwise, they may come out in odd ways through anger or sadness. We can help our teens learn to name what they are feeling and to create a safe space for their feelings. Just naming feelings brings a sense of control, making emotions feel less chaotic. We can create the safe spaces for teens to learn to speak their truths, to say out loud what they are feeling. "I'm feeling confused, frustrated, sad, angry, hurt, jealous about _____." Whatever it is, name it.

Then the hard work begins. Processing emotions is not as simple as naming them. But letting them out is key. One way to express stressful or emotional experiences is to find the action that fits your temperament that can complete the following sentence: "I _____(ed) it out!" Strategies may include actions such as wrote, talked, prayed, laughed, cried, drew, sung, danced, rapped, and screamed. Following are some examples:

- "I wrote it out." Writing offers many opportunities for expression. Developing stories takes creative energy. Journaling creates a safe space to let go of emotions while clarifying and controlling them at the same time.

- "I talked it out." Sharing thoughts and feelings with someone who cares reminds us that we matter to others. Being heard is healing.

- "I prayed it out." Being connected to something bigger can serve as a reminder of the greater meaning and purpose of life.

- "I laughed it out." With a sense of humor, you can get through almost anything. It creates a "reset"—a chance to start fresh.

- "I cried it out." There are tears of joy, tears of pain, and tears of grief. The deep release that accompanies sobbing also offers a "reset."

- "I danced/sang/rapped/sculpted/drew it out." Creative expression can be powerful for anybody but may be particularly useful for people who have a harder time finding the right words.

- "I screamed it out." Sometimes what's needed to release feelings is basic and raw. Screaming offers a release from the depths of emotions. Scream in the shower, into a pillow, or into the "void."

Avoiding Being Boxed in by Gender Stereotypes

We are all harmed by stereotypical views of "gender-appropriate" emotional expression. We must discard associations of specific emotions with masculinity or femininity and instead see possessing a range of emotions as our birthright as humans. My bias: I want *all* people to be both strong and compassionate, to be assertive when necessary, emboldened when needed to advocate for their needs, and sensitive to the feelings and needs of others.

Supporting Our Boys to Be Their Full, Rich Selves

Imagine a boy with earbuds, who, when asked a question, says, "Huh, what happened?" Everyone wants to know what is going on in teens' heads, and we don't always know, but it's definitely *not* nothing. In fact, those earbuds shutting out the sound, or short expressions of feigned indifference that perpetuates the illusion of not hearing—"Wha-a-t?"—may be strategies to avoid the depth of their feelings. They've been told feelings are a luxury they've grown past as young men and are certainly something men should not show.

This is deeply personal for me. I am *now* thankful for my sensitivity. As an adolescent, however, I felt deeply and fully but didn't know what to do with all those feelings. In fact, when those feelings peaked at about 17 years of age, it led me into a depression. There were a lot of factors involved, but the biggest one is that I didn't feel normal for being so full of emotions. I didn't feel as if my sensitivity was an acceptable male trait. I felt ashamed of the very best part of me. And I never reached for help because I was shackled by the belief that showing vulnerability was a sign of weakness. Being caring and compassionate is precisely why I have been a good father and why I strive to be a good husband and are the strengths that make me a good doctor. I could have avoided a lot of suffering if I celebrated those parts of myself earlier on rather than trying to suppress them to be more like everyone else. If only someone had guided me instead to appreciate all of myself in that way.

Consider the following: *Young men have rich inner lives.* Reflect for a moment on how rarely you have heard that sentence. The way young men are portrayed by society damages their sense of selves and their expectations of normal behaviors. It makes them not be able to access their emotions because they tuck them away out of sight. They become disconnected from the very best part of themselves. Little regard is given to the complexity of their hopes, thoughts, dreams, and fears. They are not seen often enough as individuals capable of complex thoughts and as people who desire meaningful, intimate relationships. *We can and must do better.*

We must reinforce that masculinity isn't about being tough and silent, but it *is* about being caring, loving, and demonstrative. We also must commit to not raising boys to think intimacy is feminine. They need to know that strong men address feelings, attend to the feelings and needs of their partners, and are involved, engaged fathers, brothers, sons, and friends.

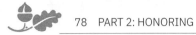

Supporting Our Girls to Be Their Full, Rich Selves

Whereas our men are told sensitivity is not in their domain, young women have been told they must uniformly display sensitivity to others, even at the expense of their own needs. Women who are effective self-advocates or assertive receive messages that their femininity is in question. Their advocacy is interpreted as selfishness and their assertiveness as aggression. Here, too, we can and must do better.

This is also personal to me, but, in this case, it's not through my own experience; rather, I see friends and colleagues who have had to struggle against stifling stereotypes to fully display their brilliance and potential. I also flatly refuse to allow my daughters to diminish their personal strengths.

My wife, Celia, possesses both deep sensitivity and tireless passion for speaking truths. Celia ensured our girls grew up with clear messages about the strengths they gained both from their sensitivity *and* from the power of their voices. Every time our daughters entered their bedroom, they passed a door with carefully chosen bumper stickers. The one strategically placed at tween eye level stated, "Well-behaved women seldom make history." This quote, attributed to Laurel Thatcher Ulrich, said it all.

****

When we speak of emotions, we rarely talk about the emotions of self-worth that drive our assertiveness and self-advocacy. *All* young people, regardless of gender identity, need to hear the following:

- "Show people how you feel."
- "Strong people care about love and friendships."
- "Brave people talk about their feelings."
- "Good parents show affection to their children and let them know how much they are loved."
- "Strong people reach to others for support."
- "I am so proud of you when I hear how you feel, especially when you stand up and ask for what you need from others."
- "I appreciate your thoughts and feelings on this matter and am proud that you are able to state them clearly."

CHAPTER 11

Thinking, Dreaming, and Caring at a Whole New Level

S ome developmental changes are hard to miss, such as when you turn around and notice that your child has grown a head taller. The most miraculous changes, however, cannot be measured. The transformations in how your adolescent can think (cognitive development) and care (moral development) enable them to live a richer, fuller life. Cognitive development prepares young people to be able to manage complexity, make judgments, and plan for the future. Moral development ensures that the future they plan for will be one rooted in values—one in which they care for and about others.

Our teens' rapidly developing thinking skills, coupled with their heightened levels of caring, can create uncomfortable moments for us. To get to the point where they can learn to navigate the world safely and independently, they must learn not to take everything at face value. They likely will practice having questioning attitudes in our own homes. Further, as they imagine a better world, they may challenge things we have grown accustomed to but that ought to change. You have the opportunity to support your teen as they reflect on issues of morality and celebrate them as a dreamer.

Cognitive Development

Cognitive development is about learning to think in more complex ways. As adolescents mature, they can better reason through problems, increasingly make decisions, and suddenly interpret underlying meanings. Puberty and the experiences life offer both play a role in the way the brain and body develop together to rapidly increase teens' abilities to more accurately interpret the world around them. It's not as though teens wake up one day with philosophical thoughts, the desire to comprehend algebra, or to understand nuanced human behavior. Rather, they build on newfound understandings, which often takes their questioning to new levels, which, in turn, leads them to the answers that allow them to further stretch their thinking capacities.

Concrete Versus Abstract Thinking

One central cognitive transition in adolescence is moving from concrete to abstract thinking. Tweens around the ages of 11 or 12 years tend to think in concrete ways, meaning they see things as they are. Not too complicated. They may be avid listeners and learners, but they learn based on what they can see, touch, and manipulate. The type of math they are able to do illustrates this well. A concrete thinker can add, subtract, or change objects from one form (2 nickels) to another (a dime). They can be thoughtful, but mostly about things they can easily describe or imagine experiencing here and now. While they have close, loving relationships, they are largely focused on what people do for them. They do not look far into the future, imagine nuance, or grasp complex motivations that sometimes drive behavior.

As cognitive development progresses in adolescence, teens begin to be able to think in more abstract ways. They imagine possibilities far into the future and may think about the concept of thinking itself. Teens may be intrigued by philosophy and other intellectual pursuits and they begin to appreciate symbolism. It is this ability to imagine what they cannot see or directly manipulate that enables them to take on new mathematical concepts, such as those in algebra and beyond. When they interact with others, they understand that actions may not represent true thoughts or intentions. As they move further into adulthood, they begin to more fully figure out and embrace their role in the world and plan for the future.

It is worth noting that we can't draw on our abstract thinking skills when we are highly stressed; in fight-or-flight mode, we are thinking about survival, not nuance. After all, you are not supposed to look at an attacking tiger and say, "Can we think this through?" As we discussed in Chapter 8 on brain development, "hot communication" activates the stressed system and people's emotional centers dominate over their thinking (or cognitive) centers. Understanding this will be key as we discuss guiding your teen in Part 4. We can't bestow wise decision-making skills, and we can't just explain them to our teens. Instead, we nurture young people's increasing cognitive skills so they can draw from their developing capacity to think things through and make wise decisions.

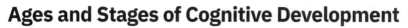

Ages and Stages of Cognitive Development

While cognitive development is tied to physical development, we cannot assume just because a teen's body has matured that their brain has caught up yet. The ability to think can also differ by setting. For example, teens may use improvements in memory or selective attention in school but not at home. They may not apply the same thinking skills with friends as they would use in the home because their emotions are more likely to dominate in peer settings.

You can't see cognitive development, so the following are some clues that changes in the brain are taking place. As always, the ages offered are approximate ranges.

Early Adolescents (11–13 Years)

- Begin to tell you why they are thinking what they are thinking and doing what they're doing.
- Focus on personal decisions as they start understanding that parental authority is not absolute.
- Question parental authority, why rules are made, and why rules of society exist.

Middle Adolescents (14–17 Years)

- May question authority, as they can better distinguish between issues that authority figures have the right to regulate and issues that are their personal choices.
- Can better link current behaviors to future consequences.
- Begin to imagine their own identity and role in the world.
- Have a need to make their own plans, including what they are doing today and considering for the future.
- Can increasingly consider complexity.
- Begin to see higher ethical and moral standards as a result of their questioning of rules.

Late Adolescents/Young Adults (18–24 Years)

- Make early career decisions and plan for their role in the adult world.
- Can apply their views to global concepts such as justice and equity, and their views may grow increasingly idealistic.
- Begin to balance their idealism with reality-based constraints. They learn that not all dreams can be realized as quickly as they'd hoped because they must attend to other tasks first or work to surmount barriers to change.
- Become more comfortable debating their ideas and opposing authority.

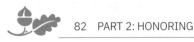

Supporting Your Teen's Growing Thinking Capacity

We honor cognitive development when we give our teens the opportunity to flex and develop their thinking muscles. Following are some ways to do that:

Encourage Them to Think About...Thinking

Thinking about thinking is exhilarating. The fact that questions drive more questions is at the root of creativity and innovation. Let your teen know their ideas are valued. Even if you know the answers, sit with your teen and enjoy conversations about complexity so you can nurture their ability to think and solve problems. When those abilities are new, young people enjoy playing with this skill often. Don't shut down thinking by giving them the answers. Learn to say, "What do you think? I'm here to listen," and to catch yourself before saying, "I think...." And always set the tone with, "Tell me what you understand," and never say or imply, "You're too young to understand." Let's circle back to what we learned about cold communication in Chapter 8. When we calmly listen and then guide adolescents to think things through, while offering information in age-appropriate language, their prefrontal cortex is activated and thoughtfulness is engaged.

Support Decision-making

We should encourage decision-making, including letting teens follow through on their decisions and learning from the consequences. This powerful strategy reinforces wise and well-thought-out decisions and helps them learn how to make better ones. Help your teen solidify the positive lessons from thoughtful plans and help them reconsider their mistakes. Encourage them to imagine how consequences could have been avoided. As your teen grows older, they will begin thinking about plans for their future. Encourage them to find themself over time, explaining that big decisions needn't be rushed.

Let Them Test Limits

As teens become increasingly independent, they must learn about possibilities beyond the limitation of current constraints. It is, therefore, a young person's cognitive task to push boundaries and imagine what is beyond set limits. "Imagining" sometimes translates into action, as teens will *occasionally* sidestep a rule just to see what happens. "Will I really get hurt?" "How will my parent(s) react?" "Will I have more fun or learn more if I take this chance?" Remember, though, that it is your job to prevent them from making poor decisions in territory that could harm their safety or compromise their morality. Continue to set clear boundaries and model desirable behaviors. Exercise their cognitive muscles by helping them understand why rules and limits exist.

Appreciate the Return of "No" and "Why?"

Remember when your children were 2 years old? Their favorite word probably was, "No!" That was both annoying and endearing, but it was their first time dipping their toe into the idea that they had the capacity to make choices. The next stage of development was questioning, "Why?" to everything you said. A bit maddening but also enthralling as you watched their understanding of the universe take shape—you answered all of their questions because you wanted them to be bright and inquisitive, even as you grew exhausted. Well, "no" and "why" are back. The fact that teens question authority is a critical step in their control over their choices. To understand how and why things work, they must demand explanations rather than blindly accept our rules or society's standards and expectations. What may seem like your teen being argumentative is actually a sign of cognitive growth. And the ability to make an effective argument is important in the long run! Also, engage your teen in discussions about current events and ask them to consider their own thoughts and opinions about local or global issues.

Honor Teen Intelligence by Turning Off the Lecture

We want to honor our teens' intelligence and help them to problem-solve. We do so by facilitating their thought processes so they can develop and, ultimately, execute their solutions. Lectures undermine teens' intelligence by stifling their ability to solve their own problems. The lecture is essentially a top-down approach to parenting. It tends to be very abstract and makes assumptions about future behavior and consequences, which some adolescents may have difficulty understanding. Lectures are also usually delivered during a stressful time, and when we talk to them using this "hot communication" approach, they may end up paying more attention to our anger than to the message being conveyed. We'll cover this concept fully in Chapter 27.

Be a Model

Adults are used to our ability to think abstractly. It's not a shiny new toy to us. So, we may not talk very much about why we think what we think. With teens, it's important to share how we actively think through problems, value thoughtfulness in others, consider complexity and consequences, and plan for the future. The more they understand how we do these things, the easier it will be for teens to develop their own cognitive skills.

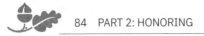

Moral and Character Development

Being moral is about choosing to do the right thing—even when nobody is watching. The last phrase, *even when nobody is watching,* suggests morality is fully ingrained—an inviolable part of us. It is not so simple. Rather, being moral is something we strive to be—it takes work. We might wrestle within ourselves as our innermost thoughts and feelings sometimes conflict. Our desire for immediate pleasure or instant gratification may be in opposition to our hope to be our best selves, our sense of duty to consider others' needs, or our dream to contribute to the greater good. It is the character strengths we possess, such as commitment to kindness and willingness to exhibit self-control, that make us more likely to live up to our moral values.

Supporting your teen's moral and character development is about preparing for the endgame—shaping your teen to be their very best self. The character strengths they possess and the moral values they live by will define them. In fact, this subject is so important that this book has an entire section on building character strengths and moral values in your teen (see Part 5).

In this chapter, I hope only to have underscored that character strengths and moral values build as developmental processes, just like the other moving pieces of development we've discussed. Most importantly, I highlighted the critical nature of your involvement. You've been working on moral and character development from the beginning. Your feedback helped transform your child from being that loveable self-centered 2-year-old—"Mine!"—into a person who understood that they had to share as a matter of fairness to those around them. If you look back at some of your most meaningful (and likely most distressing) moments of parenting, I will bet it was when your child strayed from being the good person you knew they were to when they were being hurtful to others, or seemingly thoughtless in their actions. Now as you consider parenting to shape who your teen *really* is—and who they will be at age 35 years—this topic is critical. You'll influence not through dictates but through allowing your teen to clarify their own values while guiding them with core values important to you.

Development is on your side because your teen is evolving from being someone who, as a child, made decisions to stay out of trouble into someone who holds the potential of caring about doing things precisely because they are right. The teen years are those in which we humans begin caring more deeply about what is consistent with our values and during which we begin dreaming about making the world better. It is an honor to witness this aspect of development and to play a meaningful role in supporting our teens to shape themselves.

CHAPTER 12

External Pressures Can Support or Undermine Development

uring adolescence, your tween or teen is highly sensitized to how they are viewed by others and how they might fit in. A critical role for you in *honoring* their development is to work to ensure others' input into their developing sense of self is a *constructive* rather than *destructive* force. This chapter covers 2 critical points: (1) how parents influence teens' sense of worthiness and (2) how teens' peers can affect their well-being. As you read it, reflect on the many other important influencers that also shape your teen's development, including their siblings, extended family members, teachers, coaches, cultural leaders, community role models, and clergy. The ways in which their academic lives can foster a love of learning versus impose undue pressures will be covered in Chapter 22. The unrelenting pressures from low expectations, including racism, are covered in Chapter 30.

What Will the Voice in Their Head That Represents You Sound Like?

What does your teen think they need to do to please you? The answer to that question likely translates into a script they hear in their head that sounds a lot like you, their parent. If your child knows that all they have to do to please you is to be their best self (not perfect, just a good version of themselves), then their internal script will sound like, "The world may be confusing, but I am a good person, worth caring about." That message will support their development now and help them remain resilient throughout their lives.

With the best of intentions, caring parents can inadvertently implant a very different internal script that says, "I'm not good enough unless...." In my experience from decades of practice, that script may be created when parents narrowly define success. Those parents worry how their children will measure up in the college or job market and therefore overfocus on grades, performance, and scores. This, in turn, feeds into a teen developing performance anxiety and self-doubt, which can sharply undermine many of the very strengths they need to thrive.

Resilience isn't only about overcoming external challenges. Sometimes it's about overcoming voices from within our own heads that tell us we are unacceptable unless we consistently perform at the standards that please everybody. Striving for perfection is no way to live, because it is not possible to both be your authentic self and perfect. And there is no such thing as perfection. Chapter 22 dives more deeply into how to raise children to be authentically successful—true to being their best selves.

Could Their Internal Voice Be Telling Them to Spare You?

Teens care deeply about our well-being, especially in cases where they've seen us suffer because of an illness, divorce, or stress at work. Some teens choose to be quiet or "perfect" to spare their parents more pain. This worsens if frustrated parents make statements such as, "Do you think I need to deal with your problem right now with everything that's already on my mind?" But those statements are rare and usually parents needn't say a word for some teens to worry about adding to a parent's burden. They strive to achieve good grades to make their parents proud and keep their worries a tightly held secret, always showing their best face. The voice in their head says, "I'll figure this out myself. I need to protect my parent." The irony is that they haven't spared their parents at all because they've excluded them from the most meaningful moments of parenting.

If this hits home for you, help your teen understand that nothing matters more to you than being a good parent. Tell them they do you no favors by protecting you. Say something like, "I'm going through a lot, but you're always the most important thing to me. Please don't try to protect me by holding back the details of your life. Give me the chance to do what I care about most—being your parent."

Peers for Better or Worse

Most teens end up not too different from their parents, but rarely does anybody want to be *exactly* like their parent. Until teens get to that sweet spot of being fully themselves and similar enough to you, they may go through a period of trying on hats that look different from any you'd wear.

The need for your teen to relate to their peers is more than a stepping-stone toward independence. It is a biological necessity, representing the first steps toward adult social, romantic, and professional workplace relationships. Your teen's peer interactions help them develop essential life skills, such as being able to grow from constructive feedback and develop leadership and collaborative strategies. For these reasons, it is important to view teens separating from adults, adopting their own subculture, and focusing on their peers as a sign of developmental progress.

Too often, we assume peer influence looks like a mean teen pushing your sweet child into doing something dangerous. In fact, most influence has nothing to do with taunts, threats, or even spoken words; it is about your teen *choosing* to do what it takes to fit in. Remember those nagging questions, "Am I normal?" and "Do I fit in?" Well, your adolescent is trying desperately to answer those questions by looking around them. This raises 2 points. First, when your child is keenly observing other teens to compare themself to, it matters which peers they are seeing. Second, peer influence can be positive as easily as it can be negative.

Supporting Positive Peer Relationships

Peers can positively impact motivation, willingness to work hard, and healthy decision-making. Friends can also help your teen find the courage and confidence to try new things. Friends who make healthy choices for themselves likely will encourage your teen to do the same. For example, if a group of friends takes part in a volunteer project, it may inspire others to join in. Other times, friends may inspire your teen to give up established bad habits and begin new, healthier ones. Friends can support each other through hardships and ultimately celebrate their resilience and fortitude together.

You shouldn't try to pick your teen's friends. That will backfire when your teen is testing their independence. (That's a polite way of saying feeling rebellious.) Instead, follow these tips to increase the chances your teen will be surrounded by positive peers.

ENCOURAGE A VARIETY OF ACTIVITIES. Adolescents that participate in structured extracurricular programs show improved academic performance, better physical health, and less involvement in risky behaviors.

ENCOURAGE MULTIPLE PEER GROUPS. Your tween or teen should have friends from many circles (eg, neighborhood, clubs, school, sports, religious activities). This increases the likelihood of exposure to positive peers and enables your teen to still have friends to turn to when peer groups shift. Because "in one week and out the next" is an unfortunate hallmark of early adolescence, no one should be fully reliant on one set of friends.

CHECK IN ON YOUR TEEN'S FRIENDSHIPS WITHOUT HOVERING. Show interest in what your teen does with their friends. If you don't ask too many details, your teen will likely share what they are most enjoying. Knowing what your teen is up to and who they're spending time with offers you insight into their life without being overly intrusive. And when you are interested in the positive activities they are doing with their friends, they will know your approval of these activities suggests they are good for them.

DON'T JUDGE YOUR TEEN'S FRIENDS FOR HUMAN ERRORS. Even positive peers will make mistakes. This is an opportunity to help your teen think both about how they might handle a situation differently themself and to practice how to restore and maintain relationships that hit a bump in the road. On the other hand, if you harshly judge your teen's friends for missteps, your teen may resent your judgment or move on to a new set of peers who haven't had a history of positive influence.

MODEL HEALTHY RELATIONSHIPS. Meaningful friendships are a stepping-stone toward healthy future professional, family, and romantic relationships. Relationships within your home are a model for relationships outside the home. Ensure that your teen learns to expect kindness, empathy, flexibility, and respect in all relationships.

Making It Easier on Teens to Do the Right Thing

Teens are less likely to reject rules if they are the same rules their friends follow. First, support them to be in environments where positive peer models abound. You can also connect with their friends' parents to arrive at reasonable common rules. Your collective goal is to have all of your teenagers feel "normal" living within your shared protective boundaries. For example, you could all agree on adult supervision at parties and curfews on weeknights. You might also agree that all households place personal electronic devices in chargers outside of bedrooms overnight so teens actually get the sleep they need. When peers follow the same rules, your teen will see these protective boundaries as expected and will less likely question their purpose.

Minimizing Negative Peer Influences

Many teens fear feeling like an outsider. Some choose risky or unwise behaviors to look mature, feel normal, or attempt to fit in with a new group. A first step to helping teens navigate peer culture is to help them clarify their values and think through what they want for themselves. This is best done through calm and thoughtful conversations not linked directly to a BIG decision. Our hope is for them to have a solid sense of what matters to them so that in heated moments with peers they are less likely to be making decisions in the moment.

Many adults live by the mantra, "Kids need to work it out themselves," but rarely do people learn the fine art of human relations without some support or role modeling. Adolescents with different social skills will require different types of coaching. The shy teen will need to learn to not respond to peer conflict with fear, worry, and increased isolation. An aggressive or assertive teen will need to be coached to take a breath, pause, and filter their thoughts before being too direct or harsh and to avoid physical confrontation when frustrated.

Adolescents at different ages also require different levels of support. Phyllis Fagell is a middle school counselor and journalist who explains in her book, *Middle School Matters,* that middle schoolers are "operating in a world where their friendships are both intense and fragile." *Intense* because friendships fill a developmental urge to find a "family" outside of the home as tweens and early teens dip their toes into independent waters. *Fragile* because their relationships shift so rapidly and sometimes unpredictably. A best friend from 6 months ago may wonder why your child expects them to continue hanging out just because they spent so much time together last year. A friend who always loved to play make-believe may decide that it is immature and roll their eyes at your tween who may still enjoy that kind of play. A group of tweens who always played outside may now choose to stay indoors immersed in video games. Your middle schooler needs your stability during these changes and your support to have multiple circles of friends. In high school, friends may become involved in different activities and friendship groups change according to those interests, but close friends might be more tightly matched in terms of values or interests than in earlier years. You may have to support your older teen through the sense of loss they feel as friends with new romantic partners seem to disappear.

It will be hard for you to guide your child fully if you don't have an idea of the world they are trying to navigate. If possible, observe in that world a bit. Create a home where their friends feel welcomed and your teens want to have them over. Attend events at school or sports or club activities. Whether or not you can directly observe, you can always ask your teen to help you understand their world. This shouldn't be with ominous or probing questions; just ask your teen what they like about their friend group and if there's anything that would make them happier within the group. They will hear that you are open to listening to their frustrations about friends or about themself. Then, you can begin to understand the role they feel they need to play to fit into their peer group. For example, if your teen is popular among their friends, they may feel pressure to maintain their social status and take risks to do so.

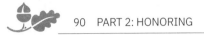

Developing Peer Navigation Skills

Sometimes peer pressure is similar to the way it is portrayed in TV shows or movies; therefore, our tweens and teens should be ready to handle taunts and stated pressures. Sometimes it is internally driven to try to fit into an existing crowd or be accepted by a new one. Rather than blaming teens for "not being able to stand up" to others or admonish them for not having solidified their internal strengths, it is helpful to support them to build their skills. Following are 3 skill sets to prepare your teen to navigate negative peer influence:

1. Recognize manipulation and successfully navigate around it.

2. Learn to say "No!" effectively.

3. Shift the blame to "save face."

Successfully Navigating Around Manipulation

Often, words are not even exchanged when peer pressure is at play. Rather, the pressure is internally driven, responding to one's own need to feel part of a crowd: "If I do this, I'll fit in," or "If I do it just once, I'll earn my way into the popular crowd."

Peer pressure, however, can be directed toward a young person from another adolescent who is trying to influence them. These direct messages can be blatant, "Do this or..." or, more often, be subtle yet manipulative, "It's just that we...." To be able to respond to manipulative messages, your teen has to first recognize that they are being manipulated. Then, they need the vocabulary to respond when they are receiving subtle or blatant pressure.

In a perfect world, we would have conversations about these topics and even conduct role-play sessions. If your teen is not open to this, look for teachable moments instead. For example, you might be driving and pass a group of young smokers. You might casually say, "Why do you think that boy is smoking? How do you think he started smoking?" Your younger teen may respond with, "He was forced into it, or some kids tricked him." This enables you to agree that while some kids might be teased or goaded into doing something, others might do it just to fit in or look older. And then follow up with, "What could he have said if he didn't want to smoke?" or "Could he have fit in some other way? Or hung out with other friends who weren't smoking?" These low-pressure teachable moments help your teen think situations through and even develop scripts they can use in real-life high-pressure situations.

If you tell your teens to respond to manipulative messages by calling them out and unequivocally stating their values, they may dismiss that advice because of their fear of becoming an outsider. Instead, prepare your teen to control their own actions without having to forcefully challenge their friends. The technique has 3 stages.

1. Your teen needs to be able to recognize a line. For your teen to comfortably learn this, keep the discussion away from personal situations. You might use a commercial manipulating an audience while watching TV or do it while driving around and witnessing teen behaviors.

2. Your teen needs to be taught how to firmly state their positions with no ambivalence and without being argumentative, accusatory, or condescending. *("I'm not getting drunk." "I'm not cheating.")*

3. Your teen should offer an alternative that allows them to continue the relationship on their terms but doesn't challenge the friendship. *("I won't get drunk, but I'll shoot hoops with you later." "I won't cheat, but I do pretty well in biology. So, if you want, I'll help you catch up.")*

Learning to Say "No!" Effectively

When the word "no" is used in a wishy-washy way, it loses its power. When "no" is said with a smile or giggle, it is interpreted as, "Keep asking." Too often, adolescents explain that they don't like to say "no" because "It sounds mean." You are not asking them to be mean, just to be clear. In fact, suggest that, when they mean "yes," they should also just say "yes" and then take steps to ensure they are safe.

Shifting the Blame to "Save Face"

Teens may know what they should do, but, if that choice doesn't play well in peer culture, they may decide against following their own common sense. Help your teen get out of difficult situations without losing face or compromising their standing with peers. The following 2 techniques offer adolescents a way out while still fitting in by shifting the blame to you:

The Check-in Rule

The check-in rule is a bedtime routine that has to be used every time, no exceptions. No matter what time your adolescent arrives home, they must say goodnight even if it means waking you. You'll find that this is often the time when your teen feels most vulnerable and could use a listening ear or a shoulder to lean on. Having a nightly "check-in rule" also helps adolescents shift blame to you. Teens have a face-saving reason to avoid drinking (aside from it being illegal) or staying out too late: "Are you kidding? My mom/dad smells me!" Your teen also may be more likely to do the right thing just because they know you're paying attention.

Code Words

Choose a code word or phrase to be used when your teen needs to leave a risky social situation and feels uncomfortable or unable to get home safely on their own. When they call or text you in front of their friends, your teen presumably asks permission for something, but casually inserts the code: "Yeah, I won't be home so I can't walk Sparky." ("Sparky" is the code word you both agreed on.) Alerted to a difficult situation, you demand your teen comes home. If they can get home safely, they leave grumbling about how overbearing you are. If they can't leave on their own, your teen should reject your instructions in a feigned act of rebellion. If this happens, demand they meet you outside and arrange a pickup. If you want your teen to use this potentially lifesaving tool, agree that you will never punish them as long as they reach out to you for help.

Negative Peer Influence to the Extreme

While negative peer influence can lead to danger, I would argue that bullying causes the most harm to development because it impacts how someone sees themself. A poor self-image can severely impact emotional and mental health during the teen years and harm the self-narrative one carries throughout life. If we think of bullying as an unpleasant, expected rite of childhood—"kids being kids"—it is hard to grasp why it can be so scarring for teens. Simply, when the answer to "Who am I?" is "Someone others belittle," it can have profound implications on self-esteem and well-being.

Here's the critical news: bullying can be addressed successfully. It is beyond the scope of this book to detail anti-bullying strategies, but my goal here is for you to insist the community in which the bullying is occurring (schools, clubs, etc) adopts a "no bullying" standard. No strategy eliminates bullying entirely, but peer-based interventions work.

If you encounter resistance from other parents and they offer the "kids will be kids" argument, help them understand the difference between playful teasing and bullying. Teasing is fun for all involved, and all members of the group receive a dose of teasing. Healthy behaviors *never* involve emotional abuse or aggression. Bullying, on the other hand, is intended to harm or disturb, occurs repeatedly over time, and involves an imbalance of power (eg, physical appearance, size or strength, social status, access to personal or embarrassing information).

Bullying can be physical, but, more often, people who bully attack with words and relational aggression. This can be in person or through cyberbullying. To be crystal clear: nonphysical bullying can still be deeply damaging to a developing teen's emotional health.

People who bully need to be identified, held accountable, and given help. Victims need the emotional support that will enable them to heal. It is important, however, to understand that bullying likely would not exist if there were only people who bully and victims. Those who bully thrive on others knowing about their aggression; the audience is integral to bullying. The audience can be part of the problem or be the solution. Similar to most peer cultures, there are several types of people within the audience. Followers like the experience and may even play an active role but do not take the lead. Supporters may excitedly draw attention to the bullying but don't join in. Bystanders aren't involved but watch what happens. We are better able to understand audience members in the context of development. The followers and supporters want to feel "normal," and, unfortunately, one way to achieve this is by declaring someone else as "abnormal." Bystanders don't challenge the person who bullies because it might draw attention to themselves, and their own insecurities prefer them to be off center stage.

The champions are the defenders who dislike the act and help the victim. When others stand by and do nothing or become caught up in some way, they essentially give the go-ahead. The best bullying prevention programs are those where all youth are encouraged to be the champions and to make clear that it is unacceptable for anyone to be victimized. School or community cultures can be created that say, "This place has to be safe for everyone and bullying is never acceptable." When these cultures are promoted by adults and celebrated by young people, bullying decreases—allowing all young people to develop safely.

Parenting Matters

Once again, let's underscore your vital role. Your influence over your teen is not in competition with peer influence. It exists on its own right. Your unconditional love for them remains the most positive external influence that shapes their internal narratives. And your ability to build their skills remains the most effective way for them to learn to navigate the other external forces in their lives, including their peers.

Recommended Resource

Stopbullying.gov provides information from various government agencies on what bullying is, what cyberbullying is, who is at risk, and how you can prevent and respond to bullying.

CHAPTER 13

Honoring Your Teen's Need to Stand on Their Own

People enter adolescence as little more than a child but leave it (somewhat) prepared to navigate the world as an adult. During these few short years, your child will transform from being fully taken care of to being able to care for themself and others. The moving pieces of teen development, ranging from changes in their bodies and brains to how they think and feel, are designed to prepare our children for independence.

Being independent means that you *can* stand on your own. It doesn't mean you *should* stand on your own. We, as adults, know that we are stronger together and that the happiest people have *inter*dependent lives with others they *choose* to hold near. But a person will most comfortably choose to reach out to others if they are confident; they don't need to be fully dependent on anyone but themself. Your teen hasn't gained that confidence yet.

The very best advice I can offer is to *honor* your teen's need to develop independence and to prepare them to do so. Although the next group of chapters (Part 3) is about *shaping* your relationship with your teen, it is this chapter that really sets the tone not just for your relationship now but for the relationship that you're going to have with your adult child. If you honor your teen's growing independence during adolescence—the station on the way to adulthood—they will choose to be *inter*dependent with you later. If, on the other hand, they see you as too controlling now, they may push you away.

Remember this: you can do everything right and your teen may still temporarily push you away. Find comfort in the word *temporarily*. When your teen is confidently standing on their own, they will then seek that loving *inter*dependence we all need to flourish in this complicated, fast-moving, and all too often impersonal world.

Honoring Independence: One Step at a Time

Everyday challenges can trigger a parent-teen struggle but also offer the opportunity for you to partner with your adolescent to foster their independence. Your teenager might think they should be able to do something just because they've reached a certain age or their friends are doing it but might lack the needed skills to handle the situation. If you partner with and prepare your adolescent, you'll turn potential sources of conflict and rebellion into opportunities for them to master new skill sets and to demonstrate the responsibility that will build their own confidence in their increasing levels of *earned* independence.

Your commitment to honoring independence does not mean you just trust things will go well. Put into place the supports and circumstances that make it more likely things will go as planned, but step back and give enough space so your child never questions whether the journey is their own. The road to independence is rarely without bumps and bruises. We hope, however, that each time our child falls down, they will learn to get back up and discover that their legs are just a bit stronger.

Preparation is protection. Let's think first about moving those pieces into place to increase the chances for success. If you do so, your answer to your 11-year-old's request to have their own cell phone won't hinge solely on whether they are old enough. Instead, it will be about whether you can ensure they know the dangers of online communications AND the irreplaceable importance and pleasures of in-person communications. The day your teen begins to drive won't be as terrifying if you've modeled safe driving behaviors and they've agreed that you will continue to monitor their progress and build their skills even after they're licensed. You won't be overwhelmed when they start dating if you have raised them to have respect for themself and others, the skills to recognize and respond to pressure, and the know-how to protect their physical and emotional safety.

Almost every new experience requires a set of skills, but they are not cookie-cutter ready to be taught or applied. Your first step in thinking about needed skills is to observe. Think back to when you childproofed your home. You moved around on your knees to see the room at toddler eye level. Once you did that, you knew to turn the pot handle inward on the stove and to cover the electric sockets. Now, having a "teen's-eye view" will heighten your awareness about the challenges your teen may encounter. Then you'll be better prepared to consider what kinds of supports and monitoring need to be in place.

Next, listen. Remember your teen may not have a lot of experience, but they are the expert on their own life. Ask them to give you a tour of their lives, which can bring your observation skills to a new level. Then, once you understand what they hope to achieve, respectfully ask what they think they can handle now and what guidance or support they seek. Invite them to develop a plan with you. Don't be surprised when you learn that boundaries are actually appreciated. It is the boundaries that allow them to test their limits safely. We will dive further into this topic in Chapter 26.

Finally, sit down with them and construct a road map of the steps that need to be mastered to gain the skills and confidence that will prepare them to succeed. Help them understand that more independence and privileges will continue to be earned as long as they continue to demonstrate responsibility. When teens know that our goal is to help them ultimately find their way to independence, they'll be much more likely to appreciate your involvement, including your need to monitor for safety. Critically, they will feel supported rather than controlled.

Why Teens (Temporarily) Reject Parents

There may be painful moments during the teen years when it feels as if your tween or teen is rejecting you. Those are the "What happened to my little girl?" moments when our teens behave disrespectfully, subtly push us away, or actively shun us. The same child who loved snuggling a year ago may now seem embarrassed by your presence. You, similar to many parents of teens, may have to learn the magical act of turning invisible in public. If you have the foundation of a strong relationship, trust that this is a bump in the road. Breathe. The reason our teens reject us is because of how much they love us. Really.

Preparing to Leave the Nest

Imagine a young bird in a warm nest lined with fluffy feathers. All the little bird has to do is open their mouth or squeak just a little and the parent birds bring all the juicy worms desired. Life is good and predictable (childhood). Then, the brain during puberty signals that they're going to ultimately leave that nest. After a period of denial, they begin to imagine what it would be like to flap those wings and fly away. They look at that cozy nest and suddenly notice it is actually a bit prickly. They look at the wonderful birds who have met their every need and realize they'd rather feed themselves—and could (darn it!) if only given the proper chance. In fact, they begin to realize that the ways parent birds do things are unnecessary and a bit embarrassing (the tweens and early teens!). The years pass. The flight from the nest draws nearer, they look at the nest and realize that it is more than just prickly. It is uninhabitable (second semester of senior year of high school). But here's the thing to understand— if they thought the nest was still comfortable, they'd never fly.

A Developmental Leap

Flying from the nest—leaving the family home—is one of the greatest developmental challenges of a lifetime. It is jarring. Even foolish. "Why would I leave this security for the unknown?" The only way teens can separate from parents is to move through the phase of believing that they really don't need us. If we react to, rather than understand what is going on, we run the risk of damaging our relationship. If we take it personally, we may react by rejecting our children. If we deny our teens the space they need to stretch their wings, they will push us further away.

Instead, we must be steadfast in our presence without hovering. Stay solidly loving, even if the love feels like it is not returned. Remain available, even if told you are no longer needed. After this phase passes, your relationship will transform into one that is more mutual—a stronger relationship that will last a lifetime.

How do you survive this period of occasional rejection? Understand it. Our children are so deeply connected to us—love us so deeply—that they have to convince themselves it is possible to leave. Trust that your teen is pushing you away so they have the space to more clearly find themselves. Your belief that they will like who they find remains the most positive and influential force in their life.

Support Each Other

At times, it may seem as if children reject one parent more than the other. It may be related to gender or style of parenting—or it may lack any clear explanation. It feels awful to be the parent that is more actively rejected. And although we don't usually say these things out loud, it can feel nice (or at least be somewhat of a relief) to be the favorite one.

Support your partner through this period. It is possible that the favored parent will be the one rejected next week. Stay strong together and remain loving as a unit. It will make it much easier for your teen to return home after they've left. If you no longer share a home with your teen's other parent, this point matters more. Your teen may try to play you against each other. It is always best for the teen when you support each other by agreeing on your parenting or co-parenting strategies.

Avoid Installing Control Buttons

When we overprotect or overcontrol teens, they feel an internal force to keep us at a distance. Constantly reminding them of the importance of staying connected can backfire because it reminds them of their internal struggle of separating from people they care so much about. On the other hand, when we prepare them to navigate the world independently, they see us as a valued source of wisdom to draw from now and throughout their lives.

Imagine how the following thoughts set the tone for a relationship that prioritizes both independence and strong, connected families:

> Parent: "My job is to prepare you to handle the world. I'll give you more responsibilities when I know you are ready for them. In the meantime, I'll watch you carefully to be sure you stay safe. I'll do the best I can to be a good role model and guide you when I should. I'll also let you make most of your own decisions as long as they are within safe boundaries. I'll celebrate your successes and be there to support you to rebound from your mistakes. We all make them. That's how we grow. I love you and always will. It's an honor to watch you become an adult."

A teen told this will not feel controlled and will be more likely to welcome guidance. If you want a healthy relationship with your adult children, be authentically excited by and supportive of your child's growing capabilities, trust them as experts in their own lives, and always be available *when asked*. When young people know our intention is to help them ultimately reach their goals, they'll allow us to monitor the process, even appreciating our protective presence in their lives. Part 4 on *guiding* will dive deeply into how to prepare and protect our teens while always honoring their independence.

"In Flight" and Return Landings

If we think of our children as those young birds reliant on us for their survival, we can view teens as people needing to learn to spread their wings to ultimately fly from the nest. However, don't visualize your home as an empty nest after they've left. If you have the mindset that you will have an "empty nest," your children's growing independence will feel painful, and, at best, the thought of your teen growing will leave you with a lump in your throat.

The term "empty nest" leaves us feeling barren, alone, abandoned. Words matter. They create the tone for our experiences. If we speak of an "empty nest," we will resent our teens spreading their wings in fear of the day they will take flight. In turn, our teens will sense our anxiety and they'll feel guilty for growing. Their worry about us may become a barrier to their developing independence.

We can shift our attitudes, and, therefore, how we experience our children leaving, by shifting the words we use to describe our homes after our teens leave. The next time a well-intentioned friend asks, "Are you getting ready for an empty nest?" respond, "I am preparing for my children to be 'in flight' and will always look forward to their return landings." This chapter was about honoring your teen's independence while putting into place the relationships that will make them more likely to want to return often.

CHAPTER 14

Being Pro-Development

ur children grab our hearts from the very moment they are born. We joyfully celebrate each milestone they achieve. Precisely because of how much we love them, we also experience their pain and are frustrated when things do not go smoothly for them.

There are challenging moments at every stage of our children's growth alongside the joys. Looking back, we have often set aside the challenges and instead recall our positive memories. The "noes" of the 2s were maddening, but we also stood in awe of our children's growing vocabulary and celebrated their efforts at independent thought. The escapes of the 3s sometimes filled us with terror but, when our hearts stopped racing, we felt a touch of pride that our children had the confidence to follow some of their own paths. We appreciated each sign of growth, even though they brought a new set of challenges. **That is what it means to be "pro-development."**

It is critical that we remain pro-development during our child's adolescent years because society has unfairly and incorrectly painted the teen years as a time of storm and stress. These undermining messages about teens are popularized in the media, emphasized in the news, and too often reinforced by well-meaning friends or family members. When our children see us roll our eyes talking about teenagers or note our furrowed brows as we listen to "wisdom" from people who suggest parents prepare to "survive" adolescence, they worry about growing. They fear their development is somehow disappointing us. Whether our children are 4 years old going on 5 years old, or 12 years old going on 13 years old, they *must* know we celebrate their growth.

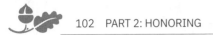

Honoring Development

We honor development when we support it but know better than to attempt to interfere with it. Let's summarize just a few key ways in which we support development in our teens.

- We understand that the question, "Who am I?" may be the toughest any of us struggle to answer. We launch our teens with a secure identity into adulthood by letting them know that we think they are perfect just as they are.

- We know that the brain is wired for optimal learning. This involves a drive to have new experiences and to be surrounded by peers. Knowing that this holds the potential for risk, we set clear boundaries within which they can safely experiment. We also create enriching experiences to maximize their learning.

- We understand that the emotional nature of adolescence is a sign of increasing maturity. We remain stable, calm forces that allow them to feel. We communicate with them in ways that activate the thoughtful parts of their brains so that they can make wise decisions.

- We recognize that as young people ruminate about being normal and fitting in, their rapidly changing bodies give them plenty to worry about. We help them to understand the wide range of typical development and the uneven pace of physical changes. We shift the focus away from appearance and toward developing thoughts, feelings, and values.

- We listen to their feelings and appreciate that we have teens able to express their emotions. We do so knowing that people who can feel fully may become deeply connected and empathetic adults.

- We celebrate adolescence as the second stage of the endless "whys." We understand that their ability to see nuance and consider complexity is a sign of their cognitive development. Answering their questions as best we can and engaging with them respectfully creates thoughtful individuals.

- We appreciate their idealism and respect that they are grappling with the big questions—even if they challenge our passivity or inaction. We know that their idealism and righteous indignation predicts that they will develop a strong set of moral values.

- We recognize the importance of peers in their lives as stepping stones to the relationships they will have in the workplace and with family. We foster opportunities for them to develop healthy peer relationships and prepare them to withstand negative influences.

- We recognize that adolescence is about growing independence. We know that honoring our children's ability to stand on their own is the first step toward the lifelong *inter*dependence we hope to achieve.

Temporary Challenges Unique to Adolescence

Parenting during the adolescent period will lead to many inevitable challenges. These *temporary* bumps in the road are easier to manage when you understand them in the context of your teen's development. Just as you got through sleepless nights during infancy, you'll get through these challenges better because you are grounded in an understanding of why they occur. You'll understand they are phases many children pass through on the journey to adulthood. In fact, because you understand how normal some of these bumps are, you'll be less likely to take challenging behaviors personally. Though easier said than done, learning to take your own feelings of being hurt or rejected out of the equation frees your supportive instincts and enables you to be the stabilizing force your teen needs.

In time, these temporary bumps will be in the past and you can choose to recall all the wonderful parts of parenting adolescents. My girls are 25 years old now, and I genuinely enjoy their company and the rich, deep conversations we share. Honestly, if I want to have fun, they're at the top of my list. During adolescence, however, they didn't need a pal, they needed loving, occasionally firm, guidance. Now, a growing friendship—genuinely mutual enjoyment and sharing of life's wisdom—is right on track with my young adult children. Adolescent challenges—what challenges?!? I don't remember any.

Before we list challenges, remember 2 key points: (1) despite what you may hear, most kids do well during adolescence; and (2) some of the more sensitive young people experience more trials during adolescence but go on to have rich and satisfying lives precisely because of the depth of their emotions. Let's recap a few common challenges you may experience with your teen.

- **Adolescents are often emotional.** This is because the part of their brain that experiences emotions fully is developing rapidly. Ultimately, when fully mature, these same emotions will be critical to generating empathy, displaying passion and compassion, and maintaining healthy relationships.

- **Adolescents may reject their parents and even act as though they hate us.** Leaving a comfortable parental home is sheer craziness, and yet it is something every teen is destined to do. Leaving the home we grew up in to face a world largely on our own may be the biggest developmental risk of our lifetime. The only way to prepare oneself to leave is to begin to imagine that you couldn't stand another moment at home. Our children pull away because they must. When they act as though they can't stand us, they do so because they love us so much it hurts.

- **Adolescents sometimes may seem over-reliant on parents.** Some young people can't imagine preparing to leave the security within our homes.

These adolescents might move more slowly in gaining new responsibilities and may opt to stay within our homes or nearby after high school. We continue to support their development by giving them the security they need while also encouraging them to build their skills in independent decision-making and self-sufficiency (eg, paying bills, doing laundry, preparing meals). We also remind them that increased independence does not mean diminished relationships; even as they learn to stand on their own, we remain caring and involved.

- **Adolescents tend to test—and sometimes push—limits.** Adolescence is designed for seeking out new possibilities. It is the developmental phase where we must learn our strengths and limitations, discover how to fail and recover, and begin to imagine our larger role in the world. It is risk-taking that allows us to do all of this. If we shut down these possibilities, we stifle their growth. To deny exploration is to prevent learning. On the other hand, good parenting involves setting clear limits beyond which our children cannot stray. They may complain, but we aid their growth when we give them well-understood boundaries within which they can be free to try new things and to safely fail and recover.

- **Adolescents are susceptible to peer influence.** Peer influence can be concerning, if not scary, but can also be a positive force in a teen's life. Adolescents' interest and investment in their peer relationships is a critical developmental step toward them being able to build communities, function at work, and possibly settle into a romantic relationship, if desired. No matter what you may hear, peers never replace parents as teens' most trusted sources of information and guidance.

When you understand each of these challenges and others, within the context of development, your child will have less internal conflict over what they are experiencing because they don't need to worry that you do not understand what they are going through. When your presence is reliable, your teen knows you'll always be there to guide them while standing by their side. This is the reassurance needed for them to be able to incorporate a lifelong lesson of resilience—"This may be a tough moment, but I'll get through this. And I'll do so more easily when I reach for support from those who care about me."

The First Step to Shaping Your Relationship and Successfully Guiding Your Teen

This section on *honoring* the many moving pieces of development was written to help you better understand what your teen is experiencing during adolescence. It was meant to empower you to grasp how much your involvement can optimize the opportunities presented during these years. As importantly, it builds the foundation for understanding how you might support your teen through some of the challenges that come with experiencing so many simultaneous changes.

We will draw extensively from your knowledge about development throughout the next parts of this book. Understanding your child's growing emotional intelligence, their evolving capacity to think at new levels, and their desire to engage in moral actions will prepare you to *shape* a healthy relationship with them (see Part 3, Chapters 15–21). It will also help you to better use engaging communication strategies rather than alienating ones. In turn, knowing how to better connect with your teen through effective communication will position you to successfully *guide* them to make wise and safe decisions (see Part 4, Chapters 22–30).

Nurturing an Entire Generation

The entire generation of adolescents will collectively lead us into the future. The best chance we have to build a better world is to nurture the entire generation. This means that we have to be pro-development for the teen(s) in our own homes and advocate for a culture that sees and expects the best from each and every young person. Please start conversations with family, friends, and community members so that we can, together, create the supportive, enriching environment teens need to develop into their best selves.

When you are standing on the sidelines of a sporting event and see a tween leaning their head against a loving parent, choose to make a difference. Tell that parent, "It only gets better and better. You're going to find there's more and more of your child to love. Congratulations."

PART 3

Shaping

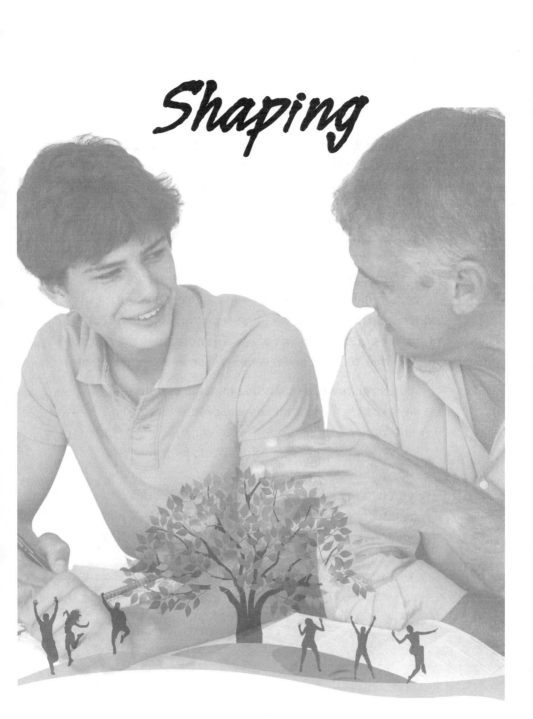

How you manage the good and the challenging moments in these adolescent years can shape your relationship now and throughout your child's life.

To be a guiding force in your teen's life, you have to have the kind of relationship that makes them want to turn to you for wisdom and protection. Healthy relationships are shaped by honest, open, respectful, and supportive communication. They are solidified by you being an undeniable and unwavering presence that remains steady through the ups and downs of life. They are trusted when all parties know that their own views will be heard and valued.

When you are caught in the moments of parenting, it is easy to forget that you will eventually have an adult-adult relationship with your child for longer than you have an adult-child relationship with your teen. People thrive with intergenerational communication and healthy interdependence. Remember this and be intentional about shaping your relationship with your teen: you are making yourself a more effective guide in these years and contributing to your own health and well-being for decades to come.

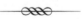

CHAPTER 15

The Root of Lifelong Security
Your Unwavering Presence

After considering the many moving pieces of development, it becomes clearer why teens benefit from the stability parents offer. You can uniquely see all that is good and right in your child, love them without condition, and stand by their side through good and difficult times. Because no one in your teen's life is as well-positioned to do this—and because nobody else doing this would hold as much meaning—your role is undeniable and irreplaceable. Your unwavering presence enables your teen to know that the person who knows them best fully accepts them and views them as good to their core. I want to repeat 2 critical points from Part 1 on "recognizing" here. First, it is the unconditional and steady nature of your love that allows your teen to endure challenges and that launches them into adulthood with a deeply rooted sense of security. Second, the most meaningful and enduring thing about loving your teen so deeply is that it makes them believe that they are worthy of being loved.

I know the kind of consistently loving relationship I am speaking of sounds a bit like poetry and that you live your real life in prose. You want to be unconditional in your love and steadfast in your presence, but it can be hard to rise to those ideals when your teen's behavior is unacceptable or when they seem intent on pushing you away. I am not saying loving without condition is easy, but I am saying it is critical.

I have had many conversations with parents over the years who struggled to live to their idealized vision of themselves. The following are some key points that helped these parents meet this ideal vision and forgive themselves when they fell short. Some will recap points made in previous chapters.

- **Be a sounding board.** The first question that comes to people's minds is, "What do I say to demonstrate that I am reliably present?" It is not about what you say. It is that you're not going anywhere when someone else is talking. It's about being able to hear difficult things while letting the person speaking know you continue to care about them.

- **Presence is also about availability.** It would be lovely if we could set office hours or plan family meetings where teens would willingly and readily express themselves. That is not reality. Often, teens benefit most from our affirmations of who they *really* are after unpleasant and unforeseen experiences in school or social settings. Let your teen know your door is always open. You'll find the same person who pushed you away in the morning, or who spoke in 2 syllables, will pour their heart out to you when they need that home base.

- **Loving is different than liking.** Loving is an active process of choosing to see the best in a person, even when their behaviors are not likeable. You never have to pretend to approve of a behavior to love your child completely. In fact, you dislike it precisely because it pains you to see them doing something harmful. Learn to say, "Because of how much I love you and because of what I know you are capable of, I cannot accept when you _____."

- **Their rejection of you is a passing phase.** Your child rejecting you is a normal and temporary part of growing up. They reject you because they love you so deeply that, on their road to independence, they have to imagine not needing you at all. Do not take it personally. This will prevent you from getting hurt or "taking the bait" and descending into anger. You'll lose your power as the source of stability that your teen needs if you approach a problem with hurt feelings or anger.

- **Parenting is not friendship.** People work hard to please their friends, sometimes even doing so against their own judgment or in contradiction to their values. Especially in difficult times, your child doesn't need a friend; they need guidance. Being a parent is far more important than being a friend, because your teen needn't fear losing you and, therefore, can safely share all that they are feeling.

- **Communicate what really matters to you.** We often think of judgment as the way we react when someone is not behaving well. In fact, judgment is also the spoken messages our words convey and the unspoken messages our bodies send (see Chapter 19) about what will please us. Be sure your teen knows that what pleases you is them working to be their authentic self, not the grades they produce or the scores they attain.

- **Take a breath and create a safe space.** People vent their frustrations in safe spaces where they needn't fear rejection. So, when you are doing your job as a parent really well, you will sometimes see the worst of your teen. Their teachers and coaches will tell you what an angel you've raised. Your teen will be good and supportive to their friends. But you will experience their insecurities, frustration, and anger. Reassure yourself, "I have created a safe space. They must be going through something. I'll learn what it is in time, but, for now, I'll let them feel what they need to feel."

- **Nurture a sense of worthiness.** A child experiencing pain is not a reflection of you and most certainly does not mean you have failed as a parent. You can't make life painless or prevent the bumps and bruises every person endures. You can nurture a deeply rooted sense of self—of worthiness. And while that feeling does not guarantee a life without blemishes, it will make it easier for your child to endure hardships. Furthermore, a sense of worthiness also heightens life's pleasures.

The Lasting Power of Safe Relationships

Every person deserves a safe spot they can turn to—a home base. A space where they can show up feeling awful but know they will be loved. A place where they can have a bad day and not worry about being rejected. A setting where they can vent their frustrations, and even behave badly, but know they will not be judged because there is a person in that safe space who knows who they *really* are. If you serve as this home base in adolescence, your relationship with your child will be forever shaped. Your adult child will still turn to you for the solace and comfort your presence offers. And, having learned how important it is for a person to have this kind of support, they will likely offer it to you, and their own children, in years to come.

The energy from your loving presence will take on a life of its own in ways you cannot yet foresee. Your adult child will pay it forward in their most meaningful relationships within their future families and trusted relationships. They'll have a road map set by your example of what people need during stressful times. They'll learn what it means to really be there for another human being. They'll know that, as the world feels unpredictable, there is nothing more protective than someone who continues to see the best within you and holds you to the standards not of perfection but of being the better you. Perhaps more importantly, it takes a lot of energy to be there for someone else in need. What gives someone the energy to spare? People who see themselves as worthy of being loved despite all their imperfections are secure enough that they can lend their support to others.

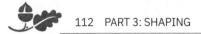

And When You Do Fall Short...

Because you are human, you will have moments in every relationship in your life, including with your children, where you are not behaving to the impossible standard you set for yourself. Be transparent about being so worried/disappointed/angry that you didn't act the way that you wanted to and that you regret it. Apologize. Tell them that sometimes you care so hard that it gets in the way of you thinking wisely. And, most importantly, show them the work you are doing to get back to the calm state that allows you to parent effectively.

Kids don't learn best from perfect people. They learn best from people working to be their better selves.

CHAPTER 16

Make the Most of Living With an Expert

Because adolescence is about learning to navigate the world (somewhat) independently, teens are sensitive about anything that feels controlling. They rebel against dictates. They stop listening when they feel as though they are being talked *at*, instead of talked *with*. They reject advice when they sense they are being told what to do instead of being led to draw their own conclusions. For these reasons, effective parenting in adolescence is about *shaping* the kind of relationships that encourage teens to be receptive to our guidance now and appreciative of our involvement far beyond the teen years. We want them to learn that we are capable of wise counsel but committed to not infringing on their ability to make the important decisions in their lives.

Respect is a cornerstone of any good relationship, and the parent-teen relationship is no exception. We've discussed the importance of recognizing all that is good and right in your teen. This strength-based approach is deeply respectful because teens know they are seen as whole people rather than only through their momentary lapses. We've covered how honoring their development is a critical step toward respecting their increasing skill sets, as well as their need to be able to stretch their wings. Now, we further shape our relationship by taking respect to a whole new level—seeing your teen as the expert on their own life.

Seeing your teen's expertise reinforces that you have confidence in their growing maturity and supports their cognitive development. As discussed in Chapter 11, among the most exciting aspects of your teen's growth is their increasing ability to think through complexity, understand nuance, and plan for the future. To support this development, we help them learn to plan for productive, satisfying futures and to find their own solutions to life's inevitable challenges. How to best act as guides as our teens develop *their* plans and arrive at *their* own solutions is the cornerstone of Chapter 17, which focuses on effective listening, and Chapter 18, which discusses how to talk in a way adolescents can best hear. But, in this chapter, we lay the foundation as we highlight the importance of seeing them as the experts in their own lives.

Your Teen Understands Their World

Your adolescent does not *yet* have the life experience that allows them to solve each problem they confront or to fully plan their future. But they do know what the flow of their life looks like—where they go, who they see, what they do. They have a sense of what they enjoy and what motivates them. They are growing to understand their hopes and dreams. They know their strengths and likely focus too much on their challenges. They know their peers and the pressures they feel to fit in. They know their worries, sensitivities, and insecurities. They know themself.

Recognizing your teen as the expert in their life helps them harness their internal wisdom. It empowers them to understand that the solutions reside within them. It does not belittle your parental wisdom or experience. On the contrary, it enables your teen to draw from your earned experience and apply it to their own lives. For your teen to apply your thoughts, those thoughts must fit their reality. *This has the makings of an effective partnership—you bring the wisdom of experience, and they bring the expertise on the details of their life, including their thoughts and feelings.* For example, your teen may see the end of a romantic relationship as catastrophic, not imagining ever recovering or caring about another person again. You can't know the details of why your teen cared so deeply, but you have the experience and wisdom to share that we can recover from failed relationships even though it doesn't seem possible in the moment. You can respect the depth of their feelings and then share your own experience to serve as a source of comfort.

If your teen has endured hardships growing up, seeing them as an expert in their own life holds even more power. Elevating their expertise recognizes that they have surmounted challenges and learned along the way. It honors them as their own best advocate. That is empowering for all youth but critically therapeutic for young people who have experienced hardships in childhood.

Harnessing Your Teen's Expertise

As teens develop, they'll better understand how the details of their lives fit together. They'll better see how what they do today creates a different tomorrow for them. They'll gain increasing insight into what drives their emotions and how those emotions lead to their behaviors. They'll learn to discern which peers have a sincere interest in their well-being versus those who are manipulating them. These insights and understandings will develop over time as their life experiences interact with their maturing thinking patterns to produce growth. Your role is to facilitate their growth.

A starting point is to ask your teen to guide you about how you can best support them. Sometimes, they just want a listening ear or a shoulder to lean on. Other times, they want detailed advice. Sometimes, they need to try to handle things on their own but they know that you will be there as a guide when called on. Tell your teen that you want to better understand what they are experiencing but that they can decide for themself how much is helpful to share. Delving into their life and asking for details they aren't ready to offer may lead them to shut down.

As we recognize their expertise, this does not mean we are supposed to become passive observers. We guide most effectively when we create the safe space for them to think. Have you noticed that your greatest insights sometimes happen precisely when you aren't working too hard on the problem? Maybe those insights come to mind while in the shower or on a long walk enjoying nature. This is because the thinking parts of our brain do not function well when under stress. Your teen may understand each detail of their life individually but may not have created the space for an "aha experience"—that moment when details come together to paint a larger picture. When we are a sounding board for our children, we create that space. When we ensure that space is a calm one, we enable the adolescent brain to do its most effective work. (This will be covered in more depth in Chapter 20.)

Be Sure They Know You Honor Their Expertise

Let's think through some things to say and not to say to convey your belief that your teen has internal wisdom and holds essential expertise on their own life. But first, recognizing what you don't say may be more important than what you do say. It is about *listening*. You don't have to find words to convince someone that you respect their life experience; you have to commit to saying very little as they share their views and the life they have navigated. Withhold judgment and offer little reaction except for appreciation that they are sharing with you. "Thank you for including me in your life." Hear their strengths even while learning about the complexities they navigate or hardships they have endured. When you listen respectfully and quietly instead of jumping in with solutions or opinions, you send the clear message that you trust their earned wisdom. When you choose to remain calm, cool, and collected, even in the midst of a crisis, you send the message that you trust your teen will harness that wisdom and, with your support, make wise decisions.

Say This (about problem-solving or solution building)	Not That
This is what I think, but you are the expert in your life. What do you think will work best?	I know from experience....
Only you can completely understand your life. Let's think about your experiences and how best to handle this decision.	You are too young to be able to make any of these decisions for yourself.
What do you think about this?	I think....
What's worked for you in the past?	When I was a kid....
What do you think would work best?	I would....
How do you think this would fit into your life?	You need to understand that if you do _____, then _____ will happen.
I might be able to offer you better advice if you offered me some details of what you were going through.	How can I give you advice if you don't tell me what is going on?
I've had experiences that may or may not apply directly to you. It's your job to see how they might.	Because this happened to me, I know _____ will happen to you. (Avoid saying anything that suggests that your story will define what will happen to your teen.)

Choosing to treat teens as experts can be quite a change. It may be different than how you were raised. Try it on for size. Prepare for a shocked reaction—"Who are you, and what happened to my parent?!" But also prepare for a reshaped relationship. You'll end up finding out more about who your teen *really* is. And I'll bet you'll like what you see.

CHAPTER 17

Listen More, Judge Less

Y ou may have heard the expression, "We've been given 2 ears and 1 mouth for a reason." That wisdom is sometimes difficult for parents to apply in their relationship with their teens. We know teens haven't had the life experience that ensures they're ready to take on the world. We want to protect and to guide them. We have so much to say!

Protect them from what? Support them in what way? Guide them to what end? Because you don't have the answers to these questions, you need to heighten your listening skills. Listening will create the space for your teen to choose to share what you need to know to understand their life. And by really hearing your teen, you'll gain a richer understanding of how best to parent them.

There are 2 additional reasons why listening is a critical building block of effective parent-teen relationships. First, our goal is to guide our teens to build their own solutions and plan their own lives. We guide better and more strategically as listeners than we do as talkers. (Stay tuned because, in the next chapter, we're going to cover how to talk effectively!) Second, we better *shape* our relationship now and far into the future when we act as sounding boards than when we reflexively share our opinions. People value guidance throughout their lives but don't appreciate it when others, even family members, impose their views. Rather, adults sustain relationships with people who lend a listening ear while trying to understand their thoughts, feelings, and hopes. Your teen will soon be an adult; set the stage for the kind of respectful, loving relationship that begins with genuine listening.

Listening Is How You Learn What's Going On

Until recently, we encouraged parents to ask lots of questions. Who are you going to be with? Where are you going? When will you be home? The who, what, where, when, and why questions were considered hallmarks of involved parenting. It was assumed parents would monitor their children best when they asked these questions. But this strategy doesn't always work because teens peppered with lots of questions don't always tell the truth. Over time, we've realized that it's not what we *ask*—it's what we *know*. Teens withhold information from parents who demand answers. When we create safe, attentive spaces for teens, they are more likely to fill them with the story of their lives.

But It's So Hard to Say Nothing

Sometimes there just isn't time for listening. You let your 3-year-old make a mess so they could learn to clean up. But you didn't let them put their hands on the stove. Parenting is full of "hands on the stove" moments when your immediate reaction is demanded. These situations involve unsafe driving or extreme risk-taking, including drug use or breaking the law.

Apart from immediately dangerous situations, starting with listening is generally good policy for all human communication. But why does it make us so uncomfortable? First, even though we may know silence is a great strategy to encourage our children to fill the space with their words, we still find it awkward and tend to fill lulls in conversation with our pearls of wisdom. Try instead to fill the space with brief coaching words such as, "Hmm, you're really thinking this through." It's not just silence that makes us uncomfortable but fearing our teens making mistakes. We want to offer course corrections *before* anything gets out of hand. As a father, I've been there. Breathe. If it's dangerous, jump in. Otherwise, remind yourself that your guidance has more staying power when it facilitates teens to figure out for themselves how to make the wiser decision.

Strong Reactions Shut Down Communication

The hard work of truly listening begins by figuring out how to break out of communication habits that prevent real listening. **Critical point:** when we react strongly, people stop sharing what they think will make us uncomfortable or angry. The following are some surprising (and not so surprising) ways in which our reactions too easily give away what we are feeling:

The Alarms

The parent alarm blares, "My teen is in trouble!" Parents jump to the rescue before teens complete their thoughts. "Mom, I met this girl…" may trigger the response, "You're too young to date!" "Dad, what would you say if a friend drinks a lot and asks you to hang out with him?" may be met with, "I knew it; Marcus is a terrible influence. Find other friends." Parents who respond this way miss the opportunity to discuss healthy sexuality, navigating peer pressure, and the dangers of alcohol and drugs. "Mom, Isaiah was caught cheating in history class." This is an opportunity to talk about honesty, integrity, and the value of feeling prepared. The opportunity will be lost if a mother responds, "I told you he was trouble. I want your desks separated." More importantly, if this mother's parent alarm blares, she won't see her son clarify his own values and reflect on the fact that while cheating seems like an easy out, it is one he'd rather not take.

It's a Disaster!

Parents sometimes turn something into a catastrophe that needn't be. "Mom, Dad, I might get a C- in history class this quarter," is met with, "You'll never get into college." These parents won't hear about grades in the future because their teens want to avoid the drama. They also may miss the opportunity to learn that dropping grades are often driven by anxiety, self-doubt, or fear of failure, and they'll miss the chance to gain insight into how to help their child perform better in school.

Deep Empathy Feels Like Drama

When you over-empathize or take your child's pain on as your own, they may shut down communication with you out of fear that they're hurting you. As we discussed in Chapter 12, teens try to spare us pain or disappointment, especially if they know we've led difficult or challenging lives. Also, if they vent their frustration about a friend or teacher, strike the balance between listening in a supportive way and rallying to your teen's defense. "I had a huge fight with Jamila. I hate her. I've blocked her from social media, and I refuse to *ever* see her again!" In an effort to align fully with your teen, you might want to say, "I don't blame you! I never liked her. She never treated you well! And honestly, I can't stand her mother." There are 2 problems with this approach. The next day, Jamila may be back in your teen's life. However, you may never know because your teen may be too embarrassed to tell you that she changed her mind. The bigger point is that your teen heard you being judgmental (even if it was taking their side) and saw you were willing to write someone off. They will remember that and may hold back in the future from sharing something they fear will anger or disappoint you, lest they be rejected. For them to come to you in their most desperate moments, they must see that you always consider all sides, won't act rashly, and would never reject them.

Observed Judgments

Remember, teens are brilliant at reading social cues and hypervigilant to spoken and unspoken signals. In fact, they can react too strongly to these signals and, therefore, experience them more deeply than anything we ever intended. Their fear of disappointing us, or of being judged by us, may limit further communication. Even when we are not interacting directly with our teens, they remain hyperalert to our views and attitudes, especially our critical opinions, and they pick up on every clue about how we feel. They observe your reactions to others in their world (eg, teachers, neighbors, their friends, your spouse or ex-spouse, siblings) and may be wondering how they can avoid similar reactions from you. The following example illustrates how a parent's response may be interpreted, or overinterpreted, by an adolescent:

> Fifteen-year-old Miriam comes home from school clearly showing signs that she's been crying. Her mother asks, "You seem upset; what's going on?" At first, Miriam says nothing, but then she begins to unload. Her teacher has said she's improving but should not enter the advanced math group. Miriam is certain she'll never be accepted into college and will become a failure. If her mother responds with, "What does she know? You'll work harder and you'll do it!" then Miriam will believe her parent is deeply disappointed in her and that she is lazy. If her mother responds, "Sweetheart, you are the smartest student in the class," Miriam may feel more pressure to perform well and conclude that her real fears are not taken seriously. If her mother suggests, "Fine, quit math altogether if that's what you want," the situation has turned into a catastrophe that doesn't exist. If her mother replies with, "This shouldn't upset you. It's not that bad," then her mother has minimized Miriam's feelings. Miriam also won't have the opportunity to talk about her real concerns—fear of disappointing her family and discomfort with needing to make friends in a new class. If her mother says, "Your teacher is cruel and had no right to make these decisions for you!" then she has undermined the teacher and may make Miriam wonder what it would take for her mother to judge her as well.

Praise Is Also Judgment

When we praise, we are still passing judgment. To the highly sensitive teenager, praise can sometimes be interpreted as, "This is what I need to do to please my parent, and if I don't do this, I will disappoint them." Praise never backfires when we focus on how pleased we are that they're telling us what is going on. In other words, we focus on the fact that they are sharing their lives with us. We can also note the effort it took for them to meet an achievement, such as, "You worked so hard to get that grade.

Congratulations." On the other hand, when we communicate, "You please me when _____," the unspoken message is, "You wouldn't please me if you didn't _____."

Be a Sounding Board

Parents tell me they often don't know what to say to their teens when their children struggle over a big decision or are deeply troubled. They worry they'll give the wrong advice. My response has always been, "Don't worry about having all of the answers. Being a sounding board helps them figure things out. Sometimes only time will fix the problem or heal the wound. Even in these cases, your listening presence offers the unconditional love and security your child needs now."

The concept of being a sounding board is tightly linked with our belief that teens are the experts in their own lives and that the solutions reside within them. But we also know that people of any age who are stressed operate more on an emotional or survival mode than on a reflective or problem-solving mode. When we act as a sounding board, we create the safe and calm space and respectful tone our kids need to de-stress for a moment. This allows them to access their own internal wisdom and benefit from life's lessons.

You are a sounding board when you create a space for listening—free from interruption, interrogation, or reaction. You offer guidance only when asked and enable your teen to bounce ideas off of you. This helps them clarify their thoughts and consider how things might play out as they talk through the actions they are considering. When we quickly judge (positively or negatively!) or make accusations, teens may stop talking. *"Non-reaction" is the name of the hardest game we play as parents.* Our steady nonjudgmental presence allows teens to express whatever is on their minds. This means that it can't seem as if we are listening only to wait for pauses so we can add our own opinions. But you can check in and reflect on what is being said. Choice words position you as a thought facilitator. Examples are offered at the end of this chapter.

Pass the Test

I suspect that if you follow most of the advice included in this chapter, you will eventually find your previously silent teenager more apt to talk. When we act as a sounding board, we are much less likely to miss the hints conveying that they need us. For example, it is very typical adolescent behavior to float a piece of the story as a trial balloon to see how we'll react. Or, sometimes, they may drop news like a bombshell. In either case, if we jump in, criticize, or judge, we've failed the test and won't learn more.

Rage is a plea for attention. And the rage is sometimes directed at you. Why you? Because you will receive their anger and still love them regardless. Pass their test. Breathe. Respond with something such as, "You needed to let that out. I'm here to listen and to support you." This is a hard test to pass; we will cover how to do this in Chapter 20.

If you are alert to the clues your teen offers, you'll be primed to be an effective listener. But the timing of teens' needs often doesn't match our own schedules, so you'll need to be flexible. When reality gets in the way of your availability, let your teen know that you recognize their need for your time and attention and tell them precisely when you are available to listen.

Availability is an ongoing issue, especially for those kids who don't do as well with those eye-to-eye, "I'm listening; now tell me your feelings" conversations. Don't believe that these teens care less or are inscrutable or unreachable. Sometimes these are the teens who care so deeply that they need to muster more internal courage before being able to share their feelings. They may float more trial balloons and watch your reactions before you'll know what they really need you to hear. Patience pays off.

Words That Say, "I'm Listening"

I want you to benefit from being able to replicate the approach a therapist uses to encourage people to share their thoughts and feelings. First, they thoughtfully use silence. Saying nothing, while fully listening, sends a clear message that you are accepting of the person speaking. It doesn't mean you agree with everything being said, only that you are glad they're sharing. Second, therapists offer brief statements that encourage further sharing by letting people know that they're pleased they are talking and remain receptive to hearing more.

My goal is not for you to sound like a therapist. That's not your role. In fact, practice using the following phrases with another adult before you try them out with your teen. Some of these phrases may feel awkward at first; practice will enable you to use them in a way that feels and sounds more natural and conversational. As you read the following examples, note that they focus on communication itself—that sharing is happening—and that they never praise or condemn (no judgment!) the specific content the adolescent is sharing. Hopefully, they show that you're listening to the words being spoken while trying to understand the emotions beneath them.

- "Tell me more."
- "I'm so glad that I'm in your life and that I can be here for you now."
- "You have an important story to share. I'd like to hear it."
- "Please keep talking. I'm really interested."

- "It sounds like you have a lot on your mind, so I'm glad you're talking."
- "I respect that you're so open and honest with your feelings."
- "It means a lot to me that you feel comfortable talking to me."
- "You're doing a great job of describing what happened."

You'll know when your teen has unloaded all that's on their mind. The pace of their words may slow. They may breathe a sigh of relief, or their body language may soften; they may sit down after pacing, or lean back in their chair. Unexpectedly they may ask, "What do you think?"

Take listening to an even higher level before you share your guidance. First, be certain you have understood the conversation. You might say, "This is what I heard. Did I understand correctly what you wanted to get across?" Then, you might ask, "Is there anything else you'd like to add to help me to better understand?" Check in on their emotions by saying, "It seems that you are feeling _____. Is that right?" If your child is a tween or earlier teen who hasn't yet developed insight, you can facilitate that insight by saying, "When something like that happened to me, I felt like _____. Do you feel a little like that?" Teens appreciate when we want to understand them correctly. They'll know how hard we are working to be there for them when, after we've listened carefully, we check in to recount to them what we've heard and invite them to correct us if we've misunderstood anything. People also appreciate our active listening when we ask for clarification while they are talking, such as, "Could you repeat that? I want to be sure I understand what you're going through," or "I was following you up until _____. Could you explain what you meant after that?"

Sometimes there will be nothing else you should do but be fully present as a sounding board. At other times, though, your teen will need your guidance. To figure this out, ask transparently, "How can I be most helpful to you? Do you want to bounce ideas off of me or hear my thoughts?" Even if they invite your advice, first learn what actions they are considering by asking, "How are you thinking of handling this?" This approach frees you from the unrealistic pressure to always have a ready-made solution to offer. Remember, see your teen as the expert in their own life and see your role as harnessing their expert wisdom. Sometimes that wisdom is not on the surface, but it is there, ready to be tapped into and then shaped by *you*. In Chapter 18, we'll discuss how your words can best guide your adolescent.

Talk Wisely, Learn More

Meaningful communication contains 2 core elements.

1. The ability to listen in a way that makes someone feel heard

2. The ability to speak in a way that someone is able to hear

Adults tend to speak *at* youth, sharing their wisdom and espousing their values. They offer warnings and highlight dangers. They advise how best to reach a narrow definition of success. Adolescents respond when they are spoken with, *not* talked *at*.

Teens want to be engaged as the experts on their own lives and to be heard fully, but they *also* want to benefit from our wisdom. They care deeply about what we think and how we feel. They want to learn from our experiences and apply it to their lives. They want us to guide them to be safe. When we communicate openly with our teens while respecting their increasing wisdom and experiences, they are eager to hear what we have to say.

Effective communication positively shapes our relationships with our teens and positions us to guide them through the adolescent years. It also has sticking power. It will shape our future relationships with our adult children into the kind of *inter*dependent connections through which people thrive. If you communicate well in these years, you'll more likely grow together, learn from each other, and support and protect one another throughout your lives.

Skilled Communicators Understand Development

In Part 2, we covered the importance of honoring development to understand your adolescent's growth and evolving needs. Equipped with an understanding of development, you can be a strategic, if not gifted, communicator with your adolescent. The following key elements of adolescent development directly inform how best to engage with your teen:

- **Brain development.** The thinking centers of the brain can become overpowered when emotions are operating at full throttle. Avoid communication traps that trigger emotional centers to react (see Check the Temperature: Hot Versus Cold Communication section later in this chapter). Instead, use your calming presence to engage emotionally with your teen in a way that generates a sense of comfort and safety. This will allow the thinking centers to operate to their potential. Then, you'll use your knowledge of cognitive development to get those thinking centers working!

- **Emotional development.** Because adolescents are learning to expand their social networks beyond their families, they are highly sensitized to social cues. While this is an enviable strength, it can also go into overdrive, causing them to misinterpret or overinterpret our words or actions. Calm and clear communication increases the odds that we can take full advantage of their evolving emotional brilliance without triggering emotional overreactions.

- **Cognitive development.** Adolescence is a time where cognitive skills— how we think, reason, and plan—quickly develop. Early adolescents still see things concretely, exactly as they are. If you talk too much about the future or pontificate about how one behavior likely will lead to the next, they just won't understand it. Older adolescents can think abstractly; they can visualize the future and make connections between their actions today and consequences tomorrow. Our communication goal is to facilitate their evolving ability to figure things out and help them make the vital connections between their actions and potential outcomes.

- **Moral development.** One of the greatest things to celebrate about adolescents is their growth into caring and moral beings. They refuse to avert their eyes to solvable problems and don't accept things as truth when they know there could be a higher truth. They are our hope for a better world and we must honor the intensity of their passion and idealism. We do so when we listen to their hopes and dreams and ask them to educate us. When a choice or action they take conflicts with the values they espouse, we encourage them to stay rooted in their values. This is covered more in Part 5 but merits mention here because meaningful communication honors their idealism and draws distinctions when behaviors are inconsistent with their values.

Setting the Tone for Productive Communication

Listen: Be That Sounding Board

Listening is the best way to set the tone for productive communication, and that is why we covered it first in Chapter 17. The words you hear and the emotions they reveal to you enable you to share your wisdom and target your supportive guidance more effectively.

Seem Calm (Even if You're Not!)

If you can't be calm, you can't expect your teen to be calm either. If you yell or overreact, your teen may shut down the conversation completely. Even if they let the conversation proceed, they won't be able to think because their emotional centers will overpower their thinking centers. And your teen may feel that they need to take care of you! To spare you, they might withhold sharing what is really going on in their lives.

Staying calm is critical to parent-teen communication because your teen's emotional sensors are so well-developed that they'll borrow your mood—for better or worse. You do not want to push them into panic mode because then they'll be incapable of planning or solution building. We must lend them our calm. This will be thoroughly discussed in Chapter 20, where you'll learn that it is about doing the hard work of calming yourself first (not faking it) and helping our teens learn what skills and strategies we employ to stay calm—even when we're anything but relaxed.

Check the Temperature: Hot Versus Cold Communication

Our children have to know how much we care about them. It is their trust that we care so deeply that makes them feel safe while we offer them our thoughts. If they feel insecure, their emotional brain dominates, their fight-flight-freeze biology takes over, and they won't be able to think. We communicate safety through what is known as "cold communication," which ironically is about showing our warmth. When we are calm, caring, and supportive, our children access their thinking powers better. We must avoid the "hot communication" that triggers the brain's panic button. Remember, one of the greatest strengths of adolescents is how strongly they feel. But it is also their Achilles heel, because when they feel intensely, it is difficult for them to think clearly. Avoid anger or raising your voice, and avoid threats such as, "You can't live in this house if...." Avoid a conde-scending or belittling tone such as, "Why can't you pull yourself together?" or "Why can't you do this right?" When teens feel judged, their rational selves can't take hold. Finally, avoid the dreaded lecture because it is often delivered in anger and makes teens feel belittled and incapable. Lectures are as "hot" as communication gets (more on this soon!).

Avoid the Scalding "D" Word and "G" Feeling

Remember Truth No. 1? Here's a recap: "Adults are the most important people in the lives of young people, and teens like adults. In fact, adolescents care more about what their parents think than they care about anybody else's opinion." Our teens care so much about what we think about them that their fear of disappointing us can be overwhelming. They feel badly when they anger or frustrate us or take more time or resources than they think we can comfortably give. Many parents use the "D" word (as in, "I'm not angry, I'm just **d**isappointed.") liberally without consideration for how devastating it can be to teens. Others believe a dose of **g**uilt will generate the remorse that will get teens thinking (as in, "Do you know what you're doing to this family?"). In fact, the feelings teens have about our **d**isappointment in them and the **g**uilt they have about harming us are highly activating to their emotional centers, limiting their ability to process or problem-solve.

Know Your Own Biases and Assumptions

The guidance you offer should be based on what you hear, not what you *expect* to hear. There likely are topics that push your buttons or topics you feel so strongly about that you can barely listen when they are raised. When these subjects come up, you might jump to your assumptions instead of hearing the details or nuanced explanations that enable you to guide your teen effectively. For example, your tween asking you how you would feel if they became "sexually active" might launch you into a hastily prepared tirade. You'll miss that your tween might think "sexually active" means they have a crush and wanted to hear your thoughts on the right time to start holding hands. Unbiased listening helps you learn what is *really* going on.

Do a Technology Check

Set a standard that certain family times remain sacred and are technology free. You might consider dinner as this sacred time, or it could be a nature hike. Insist that when you are having important conversations, the phones are off and computers are closed. You also must live by the same rules you're asking your teen to follow. Even when the phone is turned over or just in the room, it's common to only half listen. If you're thinking about emails or who is texting, you're not fully connecting. Teens need time where they gain our undivided attention.

Speak the Language of Potential and Possibility

What is our end goal as a parent? Is it to have our child avoid problems during adolescence? To not engage in risk behaviors? No! That is the very base of our expectations. Our goal is to have them be prepared to thrive and to be capable of leading us all into a positive shared future. We mustn't let our conversations be about what they should not do. If we speak the language of don'ts, they'll stop hearing us. We must speak the language of potential and possibility. Even when we have to say, "Don't do this," it must be in the context of guiding them to understand all that they *can* do to live up to their potential. As we will discuss in Chapter 26, we must guide our children and give very clear boundaries but always rooted in the knowledge that we do so because we care about and have high expectations for them.

Time, Spaces, and Places

There is no perfect time to have important conversations with our teens. But a *great* time is whenever they ask for them! More often than not, they don't come to us, so if they ask for guidance, consider yourself blessed. The following are tips for starting conversations when your teen isn't asking for one but you know it is needed:

- Feed them! Hungry teens can become irritated if they haven't eaten. Remember, the emotional brain doesn't dominate when it senses safety. One of the best ways humans feel safe is with a filled belly.

- It's important to not start a conversation when we know they already have a lot on their mind. If a teen is already emotional, too busy (or too relaxed), it's likely not the best time to talk. Ask them for a time to connect. But give them times to choose between both so they can prepare themself and because if you leave it too open-ended, you might find their choice time becomes never.

- Teens can hear things easier when they are not confronted about their behavior or made to "confess" what they have done or forced to explain why they did what they did. A direct approach is best when a teen comes to you with a problem. But for general lessons that you want to teach, look for opportunities that arise. Notice things you're driving past. Watch various media together and talk about the lessons learned from the characters' choices. Listen to music and discuss the subtle and not-so-subtle messages. These offer conversation starters where values can be clarified and developed in a neutral setting.

- Many teens find talking face-to-face uncomfortable. You might start with conversations that don't involve direct eye contact. How about in the car while it's easy to keep eyes forward on the road? Some teens open up best in the dark. Head into their room before they go to bed or suggest some stargazing. Darkness may make it easier for them to tell you what's going on or to hear your thoughts.

- Adolescence is filled with plenty of self-conscious moments. So, it's natural that most teens want privacy when tackling tough topics. Public conversations can lead to public outbursts or shutting down completely. Private conversations allow for feelings to be honestly expressed and sensitive stories to be shared. When we offer privacy, teens know we are sensitive to their feelings.

- Teens often feel more comfortable when they aren't talking directly about themselves or their friends. Use movies or social media posts from people you don't know to start conversations about relationships, love, sex, drugs, or other issues your teens may be questioning.

- Some of the harder chats you'll have may be best broken into segments over time. Consider a text message to keep the conversation going. "It meant a lot that you shared _____ with me. I'm here whenever you want to talk."

Conversation Starters

Ask Open-ended Questions

"How was your day?" *Fine.* Do you like your new teacher? *Yes.*

If you want to keep conversations going, learn to avoid questions that can be answered with one word. Try, "Tell me about your day at school," or "How did you like...?" or "Why do you think...?" to begin a conversation. When we shift our conversation starters to open-ended questions that require more than just a yes or no answer, we signal to our teens that we genuinely want to hear their experiences or views. This will, in turn, make them more likely to share.

Ask Subtle Questions

Let's imagine your teen has just come home from a party. Asking, "Were kids drinking at the party?" is not going to encourage your teen to open up. They may feel attacked or that you are accusing them of something. They may feel the need to lie. Reconsider your approach. Start with less direct questions. "I know the Smiths have a small apartment. How'd they handle all the kids that showed up?" Asking about things that seemingly matter less will help start the conversation. When you respond without judgment to the story that unfolds, you'll pass the test and learn more.

Use Your Math Skills: No More Lectures

It's hard to watch our children make mistakes. We know how complicated life can be and how complex relationships can be. Sometimes we're so concerned about their well-being that our tempers flare and we lecture in a desperate attempt to get through to them. When we lecture—essentially, talking *at* our teens—they hear our condescension, fear, and anger (hot communication!) but miss our intended message. We may push them toward the very decisions we fear, because they'll feel challenged to prove us wrong—"What do my parents know? I have this under control!"

Consider the following sample lecture:

> Parent: "Don't you know that what you are doing (Behavior A) is going to lead to (Consequence B)? I never imagined you being involved with (Consequence B). It makes me wonder what's going on in that head of yours! If (Consequence B happens), it is only a matter of time before (Consequence C) happens to you and possibly even (Consequence D). You never would have even known what (Consequence B) was, let alone (Consequence D), if you didn't begin hanging out with those friends of yours. If (Consequence D) happens, it's a slippery slope to (Consequences E, F, and G). Look at me! I'm not saying this for my own good! The truth is, I'm most worried that you and your friends could begin doing (Consequence H). That can lead to (Consequence I). Do you know what happens to people who have that happen to them? A lot of them die."

What does the young person hear? "Whaa whaa whaa...a lot of them die." Cue a *Peanuts* cartoon strip, but with a gloomy ending. They hear the condescension of our message and the fear in our voices but not a word we are saying. Why do our teens not hear our well-intentioned, heartfelt messages? First, "hot communication" stresses them out, and stressed people can't access their thinking powers. Second, a lecture is abstract, and nobody can think abstractly when they're running from tigers. Further, our tweens and younger teens haven't yet reached the point of cognitive maturity where they can process abstract thoughts.

Don't believe me yet? Consider the lecture in shorthand: "Your behavior now could lead to a terrible outcome depending on whether a series of mysterious variables occur or not." That's algebra! It is abstract by its nature, and an adolescent who is not yet developmentally able to think in that way, or anybody in panic mode, will not be able to grasp an algebra problem.

We can reach our teens, convey the lessons, and help them arrive at and therefore "own" the solutions. Only they can fully imagine their own lives, but we guide them how to get there by adjusting the delivery of our messages to match their stage of development. Instead of a lecture, we support them to understand our thoughts point by point so that they get it...get it...get it...almost there...got it! We accomplish this by changing the mathematical structure of our sentences from algebra to simple math.

Even a panicked person can think in concrete mathematical terms. Even a concrete-thinking early adolescent can follow ideas presented calmly and concretely. They can grasp that 1 plus 2 equals 3. They can easily add another to get to 4. Instead of a string of abstract possibilities (A to B to C to D), break your thoughts into separate steps: "Do you see how A might go to B? Do you have any experience with something like B? Tell me about that experience. Do you see how B could then lead to C? Has that ever happened to anyone you know?"

We need to speak in ways young people understand—short, concrete phrases—and then listen to their responses before moving on to the next step. They'll consider possible consequences step-by-step with their *own* ideas rather than those we dictate. They own the lessons because *they* have figured them out. They learn through our coaching to break down future problems into multiple steps. They can better access their cognitive powers to consider possibilities instead of relying on learning only through experience. They are better prepared to listen to their inner wisdom.

This is a key concept in harnessing the wisdom of earlier adolescents who are not yet far enough along in their cognitive development to grasp an algebraic flow of communication. But this approach also works with our older adolescents because they need us most in stressful moments when their ability to access abstract thinking is limited. We will walk through examples of how to apply this approach for different ages in Chapter 27 when we discuss steering teens toward wise behaviors.

Sharing Lessons Learned

Vulnerability is OK. Your teen wants to know that you are human too. Sharing that you've made mistakes can build trust and reduce shame and may allow them to feel more comfortable being honest about their own situations. You can also underscore that precisely because you've had your share of challenges, you want them to benefit from your experiences. Tell them that although you can't shield them from all of life's curveballs, you want to prepare them as best you can. Be careful, however, with how much you reveal. Anything you discuss (or imply) could be brought up later. If it does, be prepared to share the lesson you learned and state that, while all people make mistakes, you work hard to make safe and moral choices.

CHAPTER 19

Mind Your Body

W e work diligently to be good listeners and spend a lot of energy thinking about our words but rarely consider our body language. This is a major communication trap because our body language reveals our feelings and can undermine effective communication. You'll more effectively guide your child when your body language matches your words. Words convey only about 20% of what we communicate, and the remainder comes through our body language and facial expressions. When our words don't match the signals our bodies send or the expressions our faces reveal, our words are often viewed as insincere or inauthentic. This means that parents can master listening skills and still blow it if a frown, rigid posture, or furrowed brow indicates judgment, displeasure, or even scorn. Off-putting body language can stop a conversation in its tracks just as easily as judgmental words.

People tend to trust others' words least and their facial expressions most. Body language, including facial expressions, is not under conscious control, unless you choose to bring it within your power. You'll never get complete control over your reactions, but you'll learn to manage and consider them as a first step to helping your teen control theirs. In doing so, you will bring your communication skills to an entirely new level, especially with teens.

Teens Are Expert Readers of Body Signals

If anybody knows how to read meaning beyond words, it is teenagers. As social beings, their brains are wired to notice subtle social cues, foster connections, and build empathy. They are also learning how to quickly assess danger and determine whether they are safe.

How does one know how someone else feels? We read a person's body position and facial expression and assess their words. We notice the speed of their speech, the depth of their breathing, and maybe even the size of their pupils. Our ability to quickly determine whether another person is calm, agitated, or even aggressive can be lifesaving. Because this is potentially critical to survival, it may partly explain why emotional development in adolescents proceeds quickly ahead of their reasoning abilities.

Many scientists propose that a set of "mirror" neurons help us conclude what another person may be feeling. These are a parallel set of neurons placed alongside the part of the brain that controls movement, including facial expressions. When we see something, our "mirror" neurons mimic what we see without actually needing for us to move a limb or furrow a brow. Other parts of our brain then determine what we would feel if we held our body in the same manner or had that facial expression. For example, if you see a person with folded arms, shaking legs, a tightened jaw, and sternly arched brows, your mirror neurons associated with those same positions, movements, and expressions would "fire." However, rather than sending signals to those nerves and muscles that would make you actually copy what you see, they'd transmit messages to your emotional centers, helping you make the connection regarding what the other person may be feeling, as in, "If I looked like that person does now, I would be feeling angry and restless. I'll bet that person is agitated and might lose their patience soon."

Adolescence is a time of astoundingly rapid emotional development. Teens are suddenly recognizing the clues that other people are sending about their thoughts and feelings in ways they never had. This explains their remarkable empathy and sensitivity. However, it also explains why parents *sometimes* experience quite the opposite from them. Rather than benefiting from their sensitivity, parents sometimes receive strong reactions from their teens to every parental gesture, movement, and look. "Why do you hate me? I can tell by the way you are looking at me and by how you're breathing!" Let's put this in perspective: they may literally be mirroring your posture and expressions within themselves to better understand what you are feeling. This mirroring phenomenon may partially explain why adolescents can be highly self-conscious. They are so in touch with others' signals that they might imagine being under equal scrutiny.

Teens feel most intensely what they think you might feel and are particularly gifted in reading (and sometimes misreading) you. Why? Because you trained them to pay attention to your subtle signals. Remember how you looked at them as toddlers and used the expression in your eyes, or pursed your lips to say, "No, no, **no**!" without even happening to open your mouth? Your tilted head and serious look shouted, "Don't you dare!" Your child also learned to look back for your approving nod as they ventured to the outer limits of their comfort zone. They also picked up on your mixed emotions when you told them how big they were getting when you took them to the school bus stop for the first time but grasped their hand tightly as it drove up.

Your teen is an expert on themself *and* you. They know the meaning behind your every gesture and expression. The sensitivity they gained as a child heightens to new levels during the tweens. By the early teen years, they might know what you feel before you do. Or they might feel so intensely that they misread your signals, making it that much more critical that you double down on your efforts to send the signals you hope to be communicating.

Mind *Your* Mind First

Although people can shift their body language, it is more challenging than carefully controlling your verbal language. I want to emphasize that you won't have to think about controlling your body language if you get your-self to a calm place before you communicate with your teen. This is rela-tively easy if you can plan when to talk about something. It is much more challenging when you are dealing with a crisis. I'm not telling you to take a vacation to get yourself to a calm place, but I do suggest steps you can take quickly to prepare yourself to deal with any situation in real time. Although this chapter is focused on body language, trust that the same pro-cess of becoming calm can even make a difference in a phone conversation. Anxiety and worry come through in the cadence of our voice and the tone in which we speak.

When You Can Plan

Do the "work" prior to a conversation to get to the point of sincerely believ-ing what you plan to say. When you genuinely hold the beliefs you state, the sincerity of your convictions ensures that the messages your body and words convey will match. If you know what you *should* say but are doubtful or conflicted, delay the conversation. Otherwise, your ambivalence will show through your body signals and undermine your words. Let's consider the following typical examples:

- When you say to your teen, "It'll be OK; you are going to get past this," you have to believe this or you might heighten their fears. They'll wonder whether you are covering up something.

- Don't say, "I am so happy you are seeking counseling. You deserve to feel better. It will build on the strengths you already have and help prepare you for a happier, healthier future," if you haven't yet worked through your own feelings of inadequacy for not being able to solve your child's problems. Furthermore, you should address any issues you might have that mental health care is stigmatizing lest you inadvertently transmit your conflicted thoughts.

- Don't say "I am proud of any grade you get as long as you put in an effort," if you are really satisfied only with the A.

In each of these cases, I am not suggesting that you avoid the topics. These examples are things you *should* say in effective parenting. But I am suggesting you do the hard work *before* these conversations so you can present these critical points while also authentically believing them. *When your teens learn to trust that you mean what you say, it will forever shape your relationships.*

When You Have No Time for Planning

You won't always have the luxury of doing "the work" before you communicate. Life will hand you crises that you need to deal with urgently. And you may still want to say the right thing before you've been able to work through your own conflicting feelings. In that case, let biology come to your rescue. When you are highly stressed or worried, you are in fight-flight-freeze mode and your body will show it. Your body doesn't have a hormone for, "I'm worried about my teen's future," or, "I'm sad my child is suffering from bullying." Concerns that generate sadness, fear, or anxiety in you will activate varying levels of adrenaline—the "tiger is chasing me" hormone. Go for a run (or any vigorous movements) if you can, or run in place for a moment. Because stress hormones respond to the feeling that you're being attacked, sometimes you just can't think until your body believes you've outrun the danger. Another strategy is to fool your body into thinking that you are relaxed. The body has an almost magical switch that transforms the nervous system into a more relaxed state. Deep, slow, soothing breaths are the opposite of the rapid and heavy breathing you do in times of maximum stress. Because this breathing style is the polar opposite of stressed breathing, it flips the switch, making the whole nervous system relax, including restoring your ability to think more productively. This also will prevent your stress from visibly showing through your body movements and facial expressions.

Mind Your Body

When you sincerely believe your words and can deliver them in a relaxed state, nature will do its work on your body language. Nevertheless, let me offer some brief specific pointers on body language for your consideration.

Do This

- If you tell your teen that you have time to listen, show it. Sit down. Be at their eye level instead of hovering. Eliminate distractions. Just be there.

- Consider communicating that you are receptive to being "filled up" by their knowledge. Placing your hands out with your palms up signals that you are open to your teen's input and ready to be filled and that you have a desire to listen and learn rather than impose your views. Try saying, "I'm listening," while gesturing briefly with your hands to underscore your words.

- A warm smile communicates caring. A broad smile, while laughing, says you really enjoy being with your teen and hearing what they're saying.

- Be an attentive listener by working hard to not react with either words or facial expressions that give away your opinion.

- Many people receive hugs as the ultimate sign they are safe and protected. But when a person is in crisis or releasing their emotions fully, they may not want the hug even if they want your presence. Ask.

Don't Do This (If You Can Help It)

- Facial grimaces that signal disgust, or eyebrow creases that reveal worry, will likely stop the conversation.

- Folded arms convey, "I'm not open to listening. I've decided my views and I'll defend them."

- Teens do not like being evaluated or judged. Stroking of the chin or other part of the face signals that you are judging or evaluating. Similarly, hands clasped together, as if in prayer while leaning into your hands and touching your lips, is a strong body signal that can convey, "I am judging you."

- Adolescents may reject suggestions if they feel that they are being told what they must do. The body language associated with this kind of demanding advice includes finger-pointing and other signals of dominance, such as standing over someone.

- A forced smile increases tension. It can suggest you are belittling the other person's feelings or missing the seriousness of the moment. It can communicate discomfort with the power of the emotions present. It can even be interpreted as hostile. Remember, we are primates. Primates bare their teeth as a signal of aggression. If it is a serious matter, have a serious expression.

- Watch the defensive postures that display that you're uncomfortable. Avoid folded arms, finger tapping on the table, or leg shaking, which conveys anxiety or annoyance.

Like a Duck on the Water?

If you're anything like me when reading books, you've already turned the page to see the next chapter's title is "Like a Duck on the Water." Intriguing title for a chapter, huh? It is about how our calming presence helps our teens make the kind of decisions that can only be made when thinking skills are integrated with a steady emotional state.

The first step of being able to lend this calming state was learning how to be an effective listener, as covered in Chapter 17. The second step was learning how to talk to a young person in a way that would foster their thinking rather than trigger their reactions, as covered in Chapter 18. This chapter on body language is critical to lending that calm. Choice words can't paper over a look of terror on our faces. Statements that we're here to listen can't hide the fact that our legs are shaking under the table. Reaching that calm place first is the name of the game. Showing our teens the hard work it takes for us to reach a calm place makes us good players. Now that you've thought this through, you're ready to learn how to look like that duck gliding on the water (even when the water is turbulent).

CHAPTER 20

Like a Duck on the Water

Adolescents bring exuberance, joy, and idealism to our homes and communities. However, so many changes are occurring in their lives that they *also* may experience a great deal of stress. How does one learn to be emotionally stable when it seems that there are so many pushes and pulls from all directions? Young people borrow the mood of others around them, for better or worse.

You'll lend your calm to your tween or teen and then be the one that helps them develop the skills and strategies of self-regulation, so that they become increasingly less reliant on you for co-regulation. These are skills we all need, not just to navigate adolescence safely and successfully but to thrive in every stage of life. When your child experiences your loving and calming presence as their home base—the place where they developed the skills and drew the strength to learn to manage life's inevitable complexities—it will shape your relationship for decades to come. In later years, you'll draw strength and comfort from each other.

Important Vocabulary to Know

Let's define some terms rooted in the science of human connection and stress responses.

- **Self-control** is the ability to pause before thinking or acting while controlling our impulses.
- **Self-regulation** is the layer beneath self-control. It is about the emotional state that underlies whether we can move beyond our initial reaction, especially in stressful or upsetting circumstances. It's about being able to offer attention to a problem, maintain the focus to address it, and then thoughtfully handle the task at hand.
- **Dysregulation** is when we are unsettled. We are so aroused, anxious, vigilant, or worried that we find it difficult or impossible to handle the

task at hand. In a dysregulated state, we are more likely to be reactive, impulsive, hostile, or fully out of control.

- **Co-regulation** is the calming presence of another person. It is an emotional feedback loop where one person lends another person their calming energy, which contributes to the stressed person being able to self-regulate. However, people also can be a disruptive presence, adding to stress load and increasing dysregulation.

Explaining Co-regulation

Emotions are contagious. We want our tweens and teens to "catch" our calm emotions so they can continue to productively think and feel even through challenging moments. In truth, however, all our feelings are catchy. We send spoken and unspoken signals to each other that are read instinctively and affect whether we feel comfortable or unsettled, confident or doubtful, or safe or fearful. In the language of brain science, co-regulation is amygdala to amygdala communication—emotional center to emotional center syncing.

Imagine yourself on an airplane with intense turbulence. Your stomach sinks. You look at the guy next to you and his knuckles are white from grasping the armrests so tightly. Your heart increases and you have hot flashes as you borrow his terror. Within a second or 2, you look at the flight attendants and notice that they're preparing to serve the snack mix. Borrowing their calm state, you return to the book you were reading. Both the guy next to you and the flight attendants lent you their emotions. You want to be more like the flight attendants with your teen, so stock up on snack mix.

Our sensitivity to others' feelings plays out most vividly in our closest relationships. My emotions are tightly linked to my wife's feelings. I feel content when she's happy. When she's upset, I try to find my calm place to restore her state of equilibrium. Sometimes this means putting aside my own reactions and consciously reminding myself I can lose it later. She does the same for me, lending me her calming presence precisely when I need it. We've learned to take turns drawing strength from versus lending strength to each other.

I know it's especially hard to remain calm when your teen is most stressed— or dysregulated. In the moments you're feeling panicky yourself, how can you set that aside? You'll need to draw from well-practiced skills precisely when your own emotions are swirling. Co-regulation is an intentional practice; we learn these skills during our calm moments so they become second nature.

Our Children Look to Us for Co-regulation

Your teen will look to you for a sense of stability; they'll determine how to react by sensing how you feel. There's nothing new here; our children have always looked to us to see how far they could stretch and to ensure they stayed safe. Think of the toddler rambling down the sidewalk who stumbles on her not yet well-practiced chubby little legs. She falls on her bottom and sends her mother that shocked, wide-eyed, pouty-lipped, "Should I cry now?" look. If her mother runs toward her, scoops her up, squeezes her tightly, and checks every limb, her toddler cries hysterically. If her mother remains calm, quickly determines there is no real injury, and says, "Oops! Bump! Keep going!" her toddler giggles, gets up, and toddles away. On the other hand, if your toddler was about to wander into the street, you wisely screamed as loud as you could. Never stop being loud when you have to prevent danger! Worry about regaining your composure later.

Occasionally Be a Duck Gliding on Water

Small children require our unshakable calmness. Our presence, as well as our spoken and unspoken signals, communicate the felt-safety that signal that they are secure. For your small child, you want to create a state of tranquility. Be like that duck gliding effortlessly along the stream. How do they do it? Your small child doesn't care. They just look at the duck and know the world is safe and predictable. Sometimes your teen will also need to see nothing but some-one who doesn't seem affected by the turbulence. When there is a high level of stress in their lives, they need to feel something predictable and that they needn't worry about upsetting you. They need to (falsely, but temporarily) believe you can handle anything and remain unfazed by the situation. Unflappable. Occasionally be like that duck, but only until you can be real.

Be the Duck With Its Paddling Feet

If you make life look too easy, like the duck effortlessly gliding on water, you'll lose an opportunity to guide your adolescent on how to manage stress. And they probably won't believe you anyway because they are highly sensitive to what you are really feeling. To be clear: you'll probably be faking some of it, and they'll know! I don't want you to fake calm. I want you to learn to be calm or even calmer than usual and to pass along what you've learned. Parenting is not about knowing all the answers. Nor is it about being able to handle life with ease. It's about trying to get through complexity as best we can and preparing our children to do the same.

I'll bet that you often feel like the duck who *appears* to be gliding effortlessly on the water, but only because your little legs are paddling like crazy beneath the surface. So, during moments of real crisis, try (as best you can!) to look like the elegant gliding duck. But to effectively parent adolescents, help them understand how much work it takes beneath the surface to stay the course. Offer them the gift of learning self-regulation skills through your example as you transparently discuss all you do to become calm.

Being Real

Be truthful. If you say you've got it all figured out but your lip quivers, your teen won't believe your words. Remember, words are only trusted when they match the signals our body language and facial expressions convey. Use the uncertainty you feel as a starting point of becoming an effective teacher and role model. Say, "I haven't figured this one out. I'm working on it." Knowing you're human makes your teen embark more comfortably on their own journey of learning. It's true! Nobody needs a role model who's perfect because it just makes us feel awful about ourselves. We choose human role models so that we can imagine how to come closer to being our better selves.

It's OK to say, "Right now I'm so upset that I can't make any decisions or even give you good advice. I want to think this through instead of just react. I love you. I know you're going to get through this and I'm going to stand by your side. For both of us, I'm going to calm down first. We'll talk when I'm ready." Go do what it takes to restore your calm as a first step to processing your thoughts and feelings. The real learning will come from you when you share what you did to get yourself to the point that you feel prepared to handle the situation.

Tell them exactly what you'll do on the way to doing it—"I am going to take some deep breaths to relax/go for a run/read a book/call a friend/take a shower/organize my thoughts on paper." Whatever works for you, speak it out loud to make it real. When you come back calmer, underscore what you did. "I'm ready to take this on with you. ＿＿＿＿＿ really works for me." (Fill in the blank with the strategy that worked for you.)

Doing the Work

Stress-management strategies are covered briefly in Chapter 24 on resilience in this book and in greater detail in the book, *Building Resilience in Children and Teens: Giving Kids Roots and Wings.*

The following strategies transform your body into a relaxed state. You'll notice that we covered some of them when we discussed the importance of controlling your body language. That is because dysregulation shows through the signals we send through our body, including our facial expressions.

- **Take a time-out.** They work for 3-year-olds when they need to settle and think about how they've reacted, and they work for you too! Say to your teen, "I'm not at my best right now, so I need a time-out to get there." It's during your time-out that you'll try out all of the other strategies and collect your thoughts and integrate them with your feelings.

- **Outrun the threat.** Exercise works. It uses up the stress hormones that activate our emergency systems when you are feeling most unsettled. It tells your body you've escaped (outrun!) the danger.

- **Activate your calm nervous system.** The calm and emergency systems run in parallel; one is active while the other stands in waiting. When our calm system is activated, the emergency system dials down, allowing our thoughtful, reflective selves to operate. Deep, slow breathing is the magic switch that turns on your calm nervous system. Yoga, meditation, and mindfulness all operate through the power of breathing. Watch an online video on how to take slow, deep, calming breaths.

- **Control your thinking.** You can learn to "catch your thoughts" to interrupt panic-driven catastrophic thinking (see Chapter 25). This is easier after you've burned off your stress hormones with exercise or restored your ability to think through deep breathing.

- **Express yourself creatively.** As long as our feelings stay inside of us, they can disrupt our state of calm and interrupt our ability to think clearly. Learn to access, process, *and release* emotions. Words can organize our thoughts and feelings. Writing or talking can let them out. (That's what works for me!). For you, drawing, sculpting, dancing, or playing music might be the way to restore your calm.

- **Join with others.** In Chapter 10, we talked about the strength of human connection and the power of reaching out to others in our times of need. Sometimes just not being alone is all it takes for us to gain strength and restore calm, knowing that even if we have not yet figured things out, we will ultimately get there.

Be Compassionate With Yourself (It Will Pay Off for You and Your Teen)

Forgive yourself when it feels like you have so much going on that you can't possibly be there for somebody else. There isn't a person who walks on this earth who isn't occasionally dysregulated. (Or if there is, I haven't met them.) Forgive yourself for your imperfections, as it'll be good for you and your teen. The most thoughtful, reflective, and capable teens will have days where they, too, will be dysregulated. On those days, they may push you away precisely when they need you the most. When you learn to be compassionate with yourself on your bad days, it'll enable you to be more forgiving of your teens on their bad days.

Self-regulation Has to Be Learned

Too many adults believe a teen's inability to self-regulate or follow rules is a character flaw. If you believe this, you'll react to their dysregulation with frustration or even anger. (And since your co-regulation is critical to your teen developing self-regulation, these are exactly the emotions you don't want to feel!). Susan Phelps, the director of neuroeducation at the Evansville Vanderburgh School Corporation, points out that *knowing* a rule and *following* a rule are 2 entirely different things. Knowing a car should signal its intention to turn does not make you a good driver. You learn to become a good driver with a lot of practice alongside supportive adults who *calmly* guide you to build your skills. Similarly, knowing you should not be hurt by someone who was never your friend is light-years away from being able to quell the feeling of rejection from a social group that didn't include you. Remember: the messages teens interpret as rejection or judgment can be particularly painful and disruptive to their developing sense of identity. Your calming, unwavering presence conveying that they are fine just the way they are is exactly what this doctor is ordering.

Our Presence Balances Stress Load

The amount of stress we carry is called *stress load*. Stress load affects whether our higher (thinking) or lower (emotional and reactive) brain functions dominate. For people to function they need stress to be within a "window of tolerance" where they can remain regulated. How much stress we have determines whether that stress paralyzes our ability to think clearly (because we are functioning in panic mode) or enhances our focus because it tells us a task is deserving of our attention. Nobody can determine the extent or validity of another person's stress load. It is a subjective experience about what one feels is a threat.

Bruce McEwen, PhD, was a neuroendocrinologist at Rockefeller University who described 3 distinct levels of stress. (Neuroendocrinology is the interplay between the nervous system and our hormones. Among other issues, it studies our relaxation and stress responses). *Toxic stress* is more than we can handle in a healthy way and is disruptive to our well-being. We must protect people of all ages from toxic stress. *Tolerable stress* is uncomfortable but within our window of tolerance because we can cope with it. *Good stress* helps us handle challenges and allows us to stretch just far enough that we are likely to grow from the experience. We should support young people with the skill sets that draw the greatest developmental growth from good stress.

We can make the greatest difference in the window of tolerable stress. What is tolerable is determined by how much someone can handle depending on what else is on their plate and what stress-management skills and strategies they possess. Caring and loving adults can help young people tolerate levels of stress that they may not be able to handle without us. In doing so, we build their lifelong resilience and enable them to solve those situations that create tolerable stress. The power of co-regulation is that your presence changes the equation by making more challenges fit within the tolerable window.

Neurologic science and the spiritual imperative of human connection join as we grasp the power of our calming presence. That calm quiets the emotional reactive parts of the brain by ensuring that there is no danger present. This allows the thoughtful parts of the brain to function optimally. But it also allows the emotional parts of the brain to focus on positive emotions, such as altruism, compassion, and kindness. Our loving presence truly brings out tweens' and teens' very best selves.

Becoming Comfortable With Discomfort

Self-regulation is about getting to calm. It is not about being sublimely happy or even just fine. Well-regulated people can sit with reality and look at it without escalating into undue catastrophic thinking. Self-regulation is about becoming comfortable with your own discomfort. We can dial down our stress responses without denying stress exists.

Your safe presence gives your teen the security that helps them increase their tolerance window to stressful situations. Some actions you'll take to help your teen build their self-regulation skills may run counter to your instinctual need to shield them from discomfort. The following strategy is admittedly challenging to implement because it involves being present while running little interference:

1. Check your own temperature. If what is going on feels catastrophic to you, then take the steps to move yourself to calm. First, state clearly that you are also upset with the situation and need some time to sort out your own feelings. Talk through the steps you'll take to collect your thoughts. Before you take a break, assure your teen that they will not be alone in dealing with the problem. State clearly that you stand by their side and are confident they'll get through it. If your teen is so upset that taking a time-out feels unwise, then remain present but refrain from turning on your fix-it mode. Model that you'll regroup and put your heads together after you've both had a chance to be thoughtful.

2. Consider the challenge your teen is experiencing from *their* point of view. If it feels as if it is a big deal to them but doesn't feel particularly important to you, set aside your own feelings. Otherwise, you run the risk of minimizing your teen's experience and feelings. Similarly, if it feels as if it is a bigger deal to you than it does to your teen, put your own catastrophic thinking in check to avoid heightening their anxiety.

3. Make a statement that acknowledges that you know they are going through something tough. This will decrease your teen's dysregulation, because just being heard and acknowledged sends the clear message that someone is on their team.

4. After you acknowledge what they're going through, sit quietly with them. Remember that your calming presence offers biological feedback to your teen that there is no danger present. If there really was danger, you would both be trying to escape. It can take a few moments for their calm nervous system to take over.

5. Here's the most difficult point: don't try to fix anything or offer solutions. It is in these moments of discomfort that teens learn to tolerate stress, precisely through your co-regulation. This becomes an opportunity for them to problem-solve and consider the complexity of the situation. They will gain confidence just from knowing that you trust in their capacity to figure things out for themselves.

Learning to manage uncomfortable feelings is a developmental opportunity. We have to be careful not to rush in and deprive our teens of the chance to gather their thoughts, develop solutions, and build resilience for future challenges. In each situation, reflect anew whether your teen needs an emergency response to avert danger or if such a response is really about alleviating your own discomfort.

When you try to "fix" a problem, you unintentionally communicate that you don't trust your teen to learn to manage it on their own. In sharp contrast, when you acknowledge a problem and remain quiet and present, you signal that you trust their ability to figure things out. The following dialogues are examples of what you might say to acknowledge discomfort while still leaving your teen room to do their own work. This kind of dialogue stands in contrast to the "I'll solve this problem" dialogue that makes parents feel better in the moment.

Say This (to recognize a current challenge)	Not This (as a way to provide a "quick fix")
That looks like a tough assignment.	No problem; you're smart, you can do it.
I know you're bummed that your friends sat at a separate table from you today.	It's not a big deal; you have a lot of friends. I'll bet they were just working on a project together.
I know you think it's unfair that your brother went out. But he finished his chores and homework. Those are the house rules.	Just begin your work and I'll let you go out.

Say This (to recognize a current challenge)	Not This (as a way to provide a "quick fix")
I know that you're upset because your father wasn't able to do what he promised you. Your father works hard. I'm sure he'll try to make it up to you if you share your disappointment.	How about if I take you out for your favorite meal and dessert?
I see how upset you are. I don't have an easy answer. But I'm here. I'm not going anywhere.	It's not so bad. You can handle this.

We Are Stronger Than the Sum of Our Parts

When we look at each other for calm and seek emotional safety by relying on one another, we learn a central lesson of resilience. Together we are more powerful than the sum of our individual parts. Share your strength and lend your calm to your adolescent. If you are the source of security that enables your teen to develop their self-regulation skills, you'll likely find that the special bond between both of you will continue to strengthen. You and your adult child will mutually draw strength and comfort from each other for years to come.

CHAPTER 21

Staying Close in This New Virtual World

We were once comfortably and predictably dependent on immediate family and close neighbors for our social connections. Some worried when the telephone changed our reliance on nearby family and neighbors, but it also allowed us to stay connected with relatives and friends far away. The challenge has long been to reap the benefit from expanding technologies while minimizing their potential harm.

In this era of expanded communication, the relationship with the individual standing next to you can feel less important. Knowing this, **we must reinforce within our families the value of person-to-person communication.** However, we also know that evolving digital technologies broaden the potential of human connection across the globe and increase our likelihood of staying close when we are not together. It's important that we use the teen years to develop the kind of relationships with our children (digital or not) that will enable us to grow closer wherever their paths lead them.

This chapter does not cover the incredibly complex and nuanced issues that surround social media and digital technology. However, many of these issues raise justified concerns for parents. In this chapter, I briefly acknowledge those concerns while pointing you to credible resources that can help you learn how to support your teen to navigate the ever-evolving world of cyber communications productively and safely.

What the Virtual World Means to Teens

If you view the device in your teen's hand as just an evolution of the phones we used, you are missing the reality of young lives today. That device is a portal to a different world. Whereas previous generations used phones to figure out how to get together in person, many relationships today live largely or entirely online. It is more than just texting; they share their lives through social media. It's their way to connect and find other like-minded peers. Further, communication is no longer between 2 people but involves many people interacting simultaneously through a main thread, multiple side conversations, and shared content, such as posts, videos, and reels on social media. These communications are occurring 24-7 and teens may worry they'll be left behind if they don't keep up with the pace. This can affect sleep and lead to social jet lag.

For some teens, the virtual world is their main source of escape, to have fun, to meet friends, and even to ignite romantic interests. It has become the go-to cure for boredom. The phone has become the portable brain. It is a place that allows you to find instant answers to any question. The digital world, accessed by phone or computer, is also an endless source of entertainment. There are apps for games you can play solo and there are gaming sites that allow you to play with people from across town or across the globe. If you want to experience an emotion—any feeling ranging from inspiration to elation to melancholy—you can find an online video matched with music to fit the mood you seek.

Trying on Virtual Hats

Chapter 7 described identity development as a central task of adolescence. There isn't a more difficult question to answer than, "Who am I?" In the past, teens had very little room for error or experimentation because they existed within a small community or circle of friends. In very sharp contrast, social media and the virtual world provide teens today with a wealth of opportunities to create, test, and re-create various versions of themselves. Teens can use social media or gaming sites to tap into their creativity and imagine new, virtual identities. Some may go online to connect with peers who share similar interests in music, fashion, or other hobbies. For young people who do not have enough local peers who accept them, social media enables them to find others who share their interests, struggles, or developing identities.

What's important to remember if you see a different version of your teen online is that you are not the intended audience for those posts. As teens use online platforms to project themselves to virtual audiences, they may do so in a way that seems inconsistent or out of character with how you see them. The feedback teens receive online is part of the process of identity development. Jumping to conclusions or interpreting their posts out of context may push teens to find ways to hide their online personas from you. If you're concerned, ask them about why they choose to present themselves in a particular way online.

An Opportunity to Never Feel Isolated

Perhaps the greatest advantage to young people in this digital age is that nobody has to feel alone. Remember, there are 2 other key questions of identity development: "Am I normal? and "Do I fit in?" Young people who are different from their peers often feel isolated when they cannot reach beyond their community. As if they are not normal. As if they will never fit in. In today's virtual world, there is a peer group for every young person. People who have endured similar struggles can find strength in each other's company and offer mutual support and advocacy. Young people who experience bullying in school can develop meaningful accepting friendships in the digital world. Our LGBTQIA+ youth with digital access have the opportunity to realize they are far from alone and can develop close friendships in affirming spaces. The virtual world has offered profound benefits for young people with chronic diseases who have been able to connect with others who can empathize fully with their challenges.

Concerns About the Virtual World

In this section, I address dangers to the adolescent well-being in the digital world. The goal is not to stoke your fears but to empower you to consider how to prepare your teen to navigate this world more safely. It is about teaching children to be smart consumers of information and ensuring that they can discern reality from carefully packaged images. Credible resources are listed at the end of the chapter to increase your awareness in these areas and build your skill sets to support your teen.

A False Reality

Very few people are their authentic selves online. They tend to "glamorize" the life they have or to be eternally joyful. They post the perfect pose and may even alter their picture. This can hurt adolescents in 2 ways. First, posting themselves in this way may be internalizing a message that they would not be accepted in their truest version. Second, teens might fail to notice that the online lives they envy are not real. This makes them vulnerable to believing they would be happier *if only* they looked a certain way or possessed certain items.

Influencers

Social media has a multitude of "influencers" who suggest to your teen ways to behave based on the influencer's likes and dislikes. Your teens may be swayed by these social media stars' opinions. They may not know that many of these influencers are being paid by sponsors to have those specific likes and dislikes. It is a new type of advertising to which your child may be particularly susceptible as they search for an identity that fits them.

Fear of Missing Out

Online communication never goes to bed. And online "reality" makes it look as if almost everybody is leading perfect lives except for us. Young people today live with *fear of missing out* (*FOMO*), which can create anxiety, prevent them from sleeping well and make them feel less satisfied with their own lives.

Online Popularity

In the real world, we become popular by being supportive to other people, being a loyal friend, and being somebody others enjoy being around. Online popularity is measured by likes, retweets or reposts, favorites, and the number of times a post is viewed. This quantification of popularity is frightening. First, people can too easily measure their value by these tallies. I reject doing this with tests such as the SATs and reject it as forcefully when based on social media "scores." I deeply worry that earning more likes is something one can do through outlandish behaviors. In fact, many online social influencers earn their clicks through preposterous behaviors and outrageous viewpoints.

Dangerous Supports

One of the greatest dangers of the digital world is that people can find groups that reinforce undermining beliefs about themselves or help them double down on unhealthy behaviors. For example, online groups exist that promote substance use disorder or teach people to starve themselves.

Radicalization

A danger with digital media is that people can become radicalized in the digital space. In fact, some groups prey on teenagers looking for social support and eagerly welcome them into their countercultural groups. Part of the problem is the algorithms that social media uses to deliver content. When someone explores an idea, they continue to be offered similar viewpoints. Once they click on a view that takes the issue to a deeper extreme, they can become drawn into a descending spiral of extremism. For example, a person could be exploring ways to build their own self-esteem. Initial links might talk about the importance of celebrating your own culture. Cultural pride is indeed affirming, and every young person should be proud of their background. If, however, one of the sites they explore writes of perceived advantages their culture offers over others, the process of radicalization can begin. A teen might enter that site as a matter of personal ethnic pride but, once they click on a site with that view, the next set of offerings may present views that suggest their culture is superior to others.

Misinformation and Hatred

It is urgently important that you help your teen discern accurate information from misinformation. It used to be clear which media sources were credible and where in the library trusted encyclopedias were shelved. Now some media sources intentionally spread misinformation. In the digital space, falsehoods can look very much like the truth. Some of the most dangerous content contains enough accurate information to draw in viewers and then exposes them to biased, racist, anti-Semitic, or Islamophobic tropes. The story of biases and hatred is very old; what is new is how quickly it can spread through the internet and social media.

Cybercriminals Using False Personas to Endanger Youth

We must prepare teens to recognize the type of flattery that online predators use to engage vulnerable youth. They must know that many people online lie about their age and identity. This is a "putting your hand on the stove moment" for teens. We cannot allow any room for error. They must know that they should never meet someone in person who they have only met online unless they have an adult present and never share any personal information such as their address or phone number.

Cyberbullying

Prior to the digital world, adults were usually aware when a young person was being bullied. Now, it can happen entirely in digital spaces where adults are not present. Cyberbullying leaves no bruises and creates no visible crowds. But, make no mistake about it, cyberbullying is profoundly dangerous. Young people are living online, and reputations can be destroyed quickly. As a doctor, I remain vigilant that cyberbullying might be the underlying cause of a change in personality or behavior. We must protect our teens by helping them understand that pictures or intimate thoughts posted online or through texts can quickly be shared. Once something is on the internet, it is there forever, even if it's taken down. Talking about cyberbullying with your child is not just about preparing them to not be victims; it is also about reinforcing values. Help them to understand that harming someone's reputation or even embarrassing them is one of the worst things we can do to one another.

The Digital and Real World Can Coexist

As we see our teens become lost in their phones or watch as their fingers furiously tap away, we worry they'll forget the basics of person-to-person communication. You couldn't turn back the clock if you wanted to. Despite having listed dangers of the digital world, it also comes with many benefits.

Forbidding your child from participating in this world is no longer an option. But you can ensure your child never forgets how to participate in the real world.

The following are some tactics you can use to make sure that these 2 worlds can coexist:

- Give your teen the opportunity to continue to have face-to-face conversations. Visit neighbors. Stay longer after community or religious events to visit with people with shared interests. At family events, make sure your teen can tell their relatives about what they're doing in their life.

- Within your own home, create sacred spaces and times when no digital devices are allowed. This includes your own—put them away! Dinner is a great idea. So are movie nights. Picnics. Hikes. Schedule moments where family members are together and need to draw all their needs from one another's presence.

- Encourage participation in real-world activities—theater outings, sporting events, outdoor ventures. Be sure to join your teen in some of these activities. Despite the false notion that teenagers don't want to be around their parents, your presence is exactly why they'll want to participate.

- Make sure your teen understands relationships in the real world are tougher to manage than those online. You can't just power down. You can't hide behind relative anonymity. Real people have real feelings. Real people get hurt when not treated respectfully. Real people are deserving of our full empathy. A beautiful thing about families is that even when we disagree with each other—even become furious with one another—we never stop loving each other. The biggest protection you can offer your child against the dangers of the digital world is to help them understand why families, in all their complexity, remain our greatest source of security. Our homes are where teens can develop safely and be fully accepted.

Benefits to Lifelong Communication

We can use the teen years to shape the kind of relationship with our children that will enable us to remain close long after they leave our homes. This new digital world makes it easier!

The challenge of parenting adolescents has always been about striking that balance between hovering and appropriate monitoring. Later, the challenge of having adult children will be figuring out how to stay close even though you're no longer actively raising them. Turn back the clock a few generations—families that were fortunate enough to have multiple generations living in the same area were able to maintain close relationships. Otherwise, once children left home, there often was not an opportunity to stay in close communication. The telephone enabled us to stay connected. But remember when you were away from home for the first time entering the job world, military, or college? How often did you call home? I called once a week. I stood in line for the phone and the calls were relatively brief.

A lot has changed in the last few decades and many parents are much more involved in their children's lives. Dare I say that some hover? Today's communication gives us an easy answer. Honestly, I communicated with my daughters every day when they were in college. I was able to remind them of my presence without being intrusive. Today, they're 25 years old and now *they* remind *me* of their presence. I've even received 2 text messages from them each while writing this section. That thrills me!

The digital age allows us to check in without hovering, interrupting, or delving into each other's lives. Text messages are easy. They can be quick and funny. You can add GIFs and emojis that convey your emotions. I have a set of emojis that look like me and come linked with preset messages. These easy check-ins allow us to entertain each other, share that we love each other, and communicate that we're thinking about one another. The emojis and GIFs I get in return tell me about their moods without being overbearing. We can take pictures of our surroundings and send them instantaneously, easily sharing our lives. This is how I know what my grand puppies are up to. We can use text messaging to check in to schedule the real conversations we crave and the visits we cherish. Assuming I'm having a good hair day, I can arrange a FaceTime call.

Text messages cannot replace in-person conversations, though. "I'm going to text some sense into that child!" is not a thought that should ever cross your mind. Heartfelt conversations, family wisdom, and discipline should happen in person. But for check-ins, mood checks, and sharing interesting facts or new experiences in real time, text messages are perfect! They also allow you to confirm that quick expectations are received, such as, "I need you home by 8:00 pm today, understood?"

This is a bright, new world for family communication. The digital world can create that unique balance of developing independence and enduring connection. Start this digital relationship with your child as soon as they receive a phone, and it'll pay off during the adolescent years and for years to come.

Recommended Resources

Online Resources

Digital Wellness Lab. This site offers parents the latest science-based resources to learn what you need to know about a specific type of technology or how media can affect children and adolescents' health and well-being (https://digitalwellnesslab.org).

Common Sense Media. Common Sense offers entertainment and technology recommendations for families and schools (https://www.commonsensemedia.org).

Cyberbullying Research Center. This center is dedicated to providing up-to-date information about the nature, extent, causes, and consequences of cyberbullying among adolescents (https://cyberbullying.org).

Internetmatters.org. This organization, based in the United Kingdom, supports parents and caregivers to navigate the ever-changing digital landscape. It offers guidance to help parents engage in their child's online life and manage the risks (https://www.internetmatters.org).

Books

Heitner D. *Screenwise: Helping Kids Thrive (and Survive) in Their Digital World.* Bibliomotion, Inc; 2016

Strasburger VC, ed. *Masters of Media: Controversies and Solutions.* Rowman & Littlefield; 2021

Uhls YT. *Media Moms & Digital Dads: A Fact-Not-Fear Approach to Parenting in the Digital Age.* Bibliomotion, Inc; 2015

PART 4

Guiding

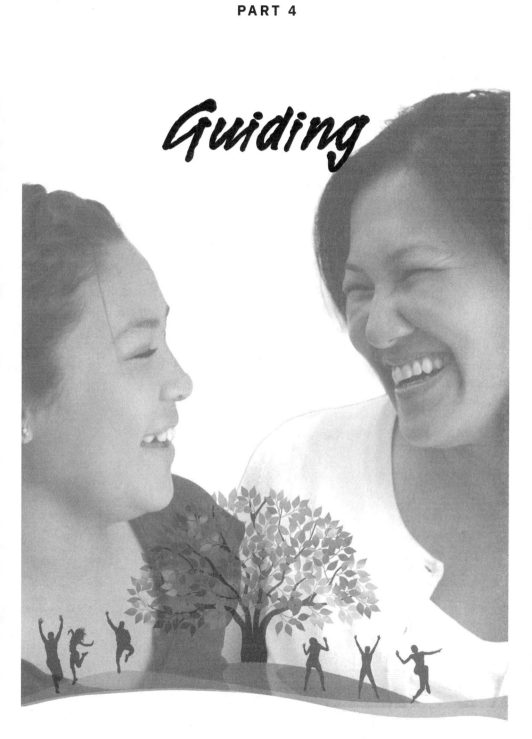

157

The road to adulthood is not a straight line. We want our children to grow to become authentically successful adults. But the journey toward adulthood often involves navigating through challenges. We want to be able to protect our children. And the best way to protect your child is to prepare them to deal with life's uncertainties while also being able to savor life's joys. Resilience. Sometimes you'll get out of the way. Sometimes you'll watch closely. Sometimes you'll set and monitor rules. Sometimes you'll need to enforce a course correction. But do it all with your teen knowing that you guide them because you care.

CHAPTER 22

Guiding Our Teens to Be Authentically Successful

W e hope to instill in our teens the foundations of enduring success—commitment to hard work, tenacity, a sense of wonder, a love of learning, and a collaborative spirit. However, some parents focus on a narrow definition of success, one measured by grades or scores and rewarded with trophies and college acceptances. These parents worry their children have to be résumé perfect to succeed and knowingly or unknowingly transmit this pressure to their teens. While this pressure may fuel effort in some adolescents, others will feel defeated by it and choose to leave the playing field altogether, feigning indifference. Believing they won't be able to be successful later in life, they shut down their efforts in the present. They are left feeling they have failed their parents. For the sake of your child rising to their personal best, I want you to solidify your views on what success *really* means.

Seeing the 35-Year-Old Within Your Teen Takes the Pressure Off

Remembering that you're raising a future adult takes pressure off both of you. Reduced pressure frees them of the anxiety that comes from thinking they're performing for you. They'll be given the privilege to imagine who they could be, allowing them to figure out what they care about. This will increase their success because caring is the basis of motivation and the grist for tenacity and hard work. You will be freed to understand that what disappoints you today may strengthen them for tomorrow. When you feel fully responsible for their success, you'll sometimes feel as if you are the one being graded. When you instead imagine the adult forming in front of you, your role as a guide is highlighted. Your teen has innate talents and interests that may or may not be similar to yours. You are shaping them to be their very best self, not to fulfill the vision you may hold.

What Does "Success" Mean?

When I travel to communities, I often ask parents and teens seated together in an auditorium, "What is success?" Teens initially respond, "Having money"; "Getting into the right college"; "Driving a nice car." A few speak about making the world a better place. Many parents look forlorn as they realize their teens likely absorbed these messages from them, even though these were not the values they'd hoped to instill. When parents take their turn to share what they think success means, they speak of the importance of happiness, service, and relationships, while acknowledging the need for resources to support their family. The gratifying news is that when I speak to teens separately, they speak of repairing the world, having good relationships, and working at a job they enjoy. I interpret the disconnect between what teens say on their own versus in front of their parents as reflecting their desire to please their parents with the "right answer." This hands us the solution. We have to be clearer with our children about how we think about success and to infuse our thoughts with the values we hope our teens will hold.

Merriam-Webster defines success as a "favorable or desired outcome, *also*: the attainment of wealth, favor, or eminence." What if it said instead, "To reach one's goals and to live a satisfying life filled with meaningful relationships, *also*: to have self-worth and self-acceptance and to feel as though one is being their best self; to have a sense of meaning and purpose; to care about others." Imagine if we lived by that definition of success! Those auditoriums would be filled with content people.

Chapter 2 offered thoughts on the strengths we hope our teens would foster to be successful (by the definition I just proposed); the following is a recap. Discuss these ideas with your teen. Try these ideas on for size and add your own. Make sure they understand these are aspirations—what we commit to working toward, *not* a list of items to easily check off. Be certain they know you believe no human being *is* all of these things; perfection is not an option. We struggle to be our better selves, and that is what defines our time on earth.

- To be happy; to be able to experience joy
- To build and maintain meaningful relationships; to have someone you can lean on
- To find meaning in what you do; to act with a sense of purpose
- To maintain a sense of wonder and foster a love of lifelong learning
- To be willing to work hard work to accomplish a goal; to have that stick-to-it spirit

- To be flexible and creative, committed to innovation and open to new ideas
- To be able to experience failure as a correctable misstep and seek guidance on how to do better
- To have tenacity and be able to delay gratification so you can better focus on a long-term goal
- To see constructive criticism as something needed for growth rather than viewing it as a personal attack
- To be self-reflective in a way that allows growth and recognizes we all can work toward being our better selves
- To have self-compassion; to forgive ourselves of our imperfections, thereby maintaining the energy to care for others
- To be generous of spirit; to be willing to share your blessings with others
- To be compassionate; to recognize distress in others and want to alleviate it
- To be driven by a desire to contribute to building a better world
- To care for and about others
- To have an inner compass that guides you to always consider how your actions affect others
- To be a respectful collaborator; to be able to listen, observe, and then share your own thoughts and experiences; to never dominate or belittle others
- To commit to a world in which you don't "tolerate" differences; you *honor* diverse thought
- To never accept inequities and to refuse to avert your eyes to human suffering
- To be resilient; to be able to thrive through good and challenging times

We cannot force these strengths on our teens. Instead, we discuss these with them as developing people who care about forming their own values and want to live satisfying lives. We recognize and reinforce their existing strengths and help fortify the ones they need to build. We model how we live each day with the goal of learning something. We model how we forgive ourselves when we falter in achieving our own aspirational goals. We reflect... and recognize tomorrow is another day.

Fostering Self-acceptance

We have an opportunity during adolescence to help our children gain self-acceptance; from there, they will develop the self-worth that enables them to grow in so many other ways. The aspirations previously listed are not attainable to someone who doubts themself and focuses on their own imperfections. Your teen's self-acceptance will be fostered when they see first that you accept yourself as you are. Next, always see the goodness in your teen, even when they're not hitting it out of the ballpark. They must learn they remain worthy of our love even when they're misbehaving and even when another student in their class received more recognition. They must see that we love them in all of their unevenness, because we see who they *really* are. This will help them relish their accomplishments and conserve energy because they'll lack that inner voice in their head that says they are only deserving of attention and love if....

Failure Is an Opportunity

We mustn't allow our teens to believe that if they experience failure, they *are* a failure. We should reframe failures as mistakes, missteps, misadventures, or misfortunes; all of these words suggest a *temporary* state. Failure can be a wake-up call, and it can feel awful, but it is *always* an opportunity for growth. This idea is richly developed in my book, *Raising Kids to Thrive: Balancing Love With Expectations and Protection With Trust.*

Teens need to experience some failures while still under our protective gaze; otherwise, they'll experience failures later with far greater consequences. Adolescence is the time to learn our limitations and develop the "work-arounds" for them we'll need throughout life. These work-arounds enable us to focus on what our strengths can produce because we'll have fewer stumbles to consume our energy later.

The need for failures and recoveries is about more than preparing us to compensate for our limitations. It is necessary for us to succeed. The best ideas come into focus after multiple failed attempts because each misstep generated new knowledge. "Failures" while stretching occur because we are trying new things and venturing out of our safe zones. In fact, some businesses track a "failure index," hoping to reveal a reasonable proportion of failures. When they have enough failure alongside their successes, they know their innovators considered and tested out-of-the-box possibilities and learned from each miscalculation. Further, many cutting-edge innovators use rapid-process techniques to optimize learning. Test out ideas. Fail quickly. Obtain feedback. Retool the ideas with lessons learned from previous efforts. The goal is to achieve successes that never could be reached without an innovative spirit comfortable with failure.

You may not think of your teen in the same way as you would a leading innovative company, but the lessons are the same. Reach. Stumble and right oneself. Make mistakes and find the solutions. *Do this repeatedly*. When this cycle repeats your teen will face their fear of failure and allow it to be set aside. When they see that missteps do not lead to catastrophes, they'll forgive themself of their imperfections and allow themself to stretch. That willingness to work outside of one's comfort zone is a core strength of successful people.

The Mindset for Success

Our children need to be self-reflective, willing to see their strengths and limitations, and know they are not destined to be "stuck" in one set of circumstances. They must believe in their potential for growth and know the actions they take make a difference.

We begin this discussion by speaking about recognizing and even celebrating our teen's unevenness as a leaping-off point for them to think about their futures and then transition to a discussion about supporting our children to have a growth versus fixed (stuck!) mindset. This discussion is informed by the work of Carol Dweck, PhD, a Stanford University psychologist whose robust research explores the effect praise, and conversely criticism, has on student performance. Her work guides us to consider how to hold young people to high expectations in a way that promotes, rather than undermines, both their performance and emotional well-being. In a book that may shift how you parent, *Mindset: The New Psychology of Success,* she explores what creates a *growth mindset* compared to a *fixed mindset*. She explains how these mindsets influence performance and well-being throughout life.

We Celebrate Unevenness and See It as a Road Map

To reach their potential, people must learn to lead with their strengths while not letting their limitations hold them back. They need to look at their unevenness with curiosity instead of judgment. They'll see they don't always excel and sometimes will fail miserably. Critically, they'll pay attention to how they feel during the process.

Nobody is good at everything. Successful people excel at something. Interesting people also do other things because they are intrigued by them. Our goal is to allow our children to reveal their "spikes"—areas of excellence in which they enjoy working hard and from which they savor making unique contributions. To help uncover their spikes, we should guide teens to discover areas that motivate them to keep learning, dive deeper, and explore the not-yet-answered—even unasked—questions.

To support this process, encourage downtime and suggest "pruning." Downtime creates space for reflection and for life's lessons to reveal themselves. Pruning is about getting rid of those things that may be masking our spikes. It is light-years away from quitting; it is about gaining focus. If your adolescent wants to quit everything, consider whether depression, substance use, or the influence of new peers are driving their

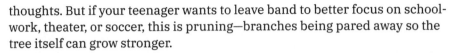

thoughts. But if your teenager wants to leave band to better focus on school-work, theater, or soccer, this is pruning—branches being pared away so the tree itself can grow stronger.

Offer guidance beyond saying, "Just try your best." This well-intentioned phrase is often misinterpreted as, "If you work harder, you'll get straight As." This can generate anxiety, especially in areas that are not their spikes. Guide them to put in their greatest effort and to pay attention to the varied results. Explain that we never trust results—good or bad—without applying ourselves to our potential. Say to them,

- Even if you receive top grades with little effort, ask yourself if you find the work interesting. If not, learn that this is not the career for you. You might think it is the right fit because it comes easily, but you'll get bored doing it over time.

- If you are good at something, love doing it, and want to learn more about it, you may have found your career! Careers are about caring about what you do and working hard to improve your skills.

- If you are not so good at something but find it intriguing and fun, you may have found your hobby. You can enjoy it throughout life and continually strive to get better at it.

- If you are not good at something and don't find it interesting, take the necessary steps to learn it, including seeking extra support from teachers and friends. Learning it will make you well-rounded and allow you to participate in conversations with people who do this work. But don't get down on yourself for an inability to excel in this area, as it will only lead to undue anxiety.

Every teen should launch into adulthood feeling good about who they are and how they might best contribute. That's success.

Set the Bar to Encourage Effort and Recognize Unevenness

What one teen interprets as helpful encouragement might be viewed by another as far too much pressure. Their experience will be influenced by their baseline anxiety or levels of self-doubt. It also may be influenced by whether they interpret your words as being more focused on the results (grades, scores) or their well-being (finding contentment and satisfaction.) Hint: focus on the well-being.

Encourage your teen to "stretch" so they can learn to assess their own reach. But you can guide them to estimate how far their reach is likely to go based on past performance, aptitude, and teachers' guidance. Then set the bar—your expectations—within reach but at a point where a bit of stretching is required to find new talents and reach capabilities. If you place the bar beyond their abilities, they may decide it's not possible to please you and lessen their efforts. If you place it far below what they can do, they'll feel belittled or undervalued. Admittedly, this is a fine needle to thread.

Set an uneven bar. Their potential reach will vary in different areas, and this is precisely what they must learn. Ideally, parents would know when our encouragement and high expectations crossed into pressure. In a perfect world, we'd have an instruction manual where we could learn precisely where and how to set our expectations. In the real world, we get closer when we check in with our teen's teachers and coaches for guidance. We get even closer to the sweet spot when we check in with the real expert. Tell your teen that your goal is to be supportive of them learning about their capabilities and that your expectation is only that they strive to have a satisfying life. Ask for their assessment of their capabilities and how you can be most supportive to them.

A Growth Versus Fixed Mindset

Intelligence is (incorrectly) measured in a way that assumes it is fixed— something that will not change. Dr Dweck, and many others, argue that while intelligence is influenced by genetic potential, it can be built through exposure and experience.

Young people with a growth mindset are willing to put in the sustained work to develop their intelligence. When they aren't met with success, they don't see themselves as failures but as learners. They seek performance feedback from trusted sources so they can learn how to improve. Dr Dweck summarizes, "The passion for stretching yourself and sticking to it, even (or especially) when it's not going well, is the hallmark of the growth mindset."

People with a fixed mindset view things more simply. You're smart or you're not. They experience failure as the proof that they are not. And their interpretation of failure can be alarmingly narrow, such as believing that a B+ is disastrous. They view intelligence as inborn and, therefore, see the need to perform hard work as a sign that they must lack intelligence. Therefore, to avoid discomfort, they may shun tasks that require hard work. They also may not think outside the box because they assume that they should easily find the answers. They may avoid even small stumbles because they seek experiences that confirm they're smart. They may resent feedback because they interpret it as criticism.

Dr Dweck explains that a person with a fixed mindset worries about whether they will win or lose or look intelligent or stupid. Can you imagine how this stifles the love of learning? Can you imagine the stress a teen would experience in school if the stakes felt that high? The mindset of resilience overcomes these voices from within that suggest we are unacceptable *unless* or worthwhile *only if....*

People with a growth mindset feel intelligent when they expand their horizons; and those with fixed mindsets feel smart when they avoid mistakes. The fear that resides within people with a fixed mindset limits their success because they avoid challenging goals. Instead, they find comfort in their achievements from meeting safer goals. We want teens to feel pride in stretching, rather than be satisfied with predictable results. Let me underscore here that we hope for our teens to have a growth mindset not only so they can gain new book knowledge but also so they'll gain self-knowledge and develop new interpersonal skills.

The Research That Helped Us Understand Growth Potential

One of the most important strengths we can nurture is *tenacity*—the "I'll stick with it" approach to challenges. In a remarkably simple experiment that highlighted the dramatic differences in children's performance based on the type of praise they received, Dr Dweck demonstrated how well-intentioned praise can go awry. Fifth graders were divided into 2 groups with no real difference between the groups. Each group was given a series of puzzles that most children would perform well. After the first set of tests, they were told their scores alongside a single line of praise. One group was told, "You must be smart at this"; the other group was praised for their effort: "You must have worked really hard."

The students were then offered a choice of which tests to take for the second round. Students could choose a test that would be harder, but from which they'd learn a lot, or an easy test similar to the first where they'd likely perform well. Ninety percent of children who were praised for their *effort* chose the harder set of puzzles, whereas the majority of those praised for being smart selected the easy test. Next, in round 3, all students were given a test 2 years above their grade level. As expected, it was difficult, and most were not able to complete the tasks. The students praised for their effort on the first test assumed they simply hadn't worked hard enough. Those who were praised for their intelligence took their failure as evidence that they were no longer smart or as proof that maybe they never were. They were visibly anxious and uncomfortable. A final round of tests, as easy as the initial test, was given after the "failure round." The children initially praised for their intelligence performed worse than their first attempt, and those who were praised for their hard work showed improvement. Perhaps this could be largely explained by how the young people interpreted their experience in round 2. The students praised for their intelligence experienced "failure," which naturally hurt their confidence and undercut their focus in round 3. The students praised for their effort instead experienced *practice*, which built their confidence for the final round. They approached round 3 expecting continued improvement.

Consider this: if just one line of praise made a difference in performance in these young students, can you imagine what a difference the style of praise might make in your teen's life when consistently given in the home?

How to Praise to Support a Growth Mindset

It is through noticing, praising, and criticizing that we convey our expectations to our teens. Let's take a step back to think through just how much this work shifted our thinking about praise. We thought that confidence produced effort and that confidence came from self-esteem. To close the loop, we thought self-esteem was bestowed on someone through praise. A generation was raised to feel "special as a butterfly" and "unique as a snowflake." Children's art projects were raved about as if they were budding Leonardo da Vincis, and every hit was celebrated as if the kid batted in the winning run at the World Series. We extolled their bravery as they slid down the sliding board and acted as though the accomplishment was theirs alone, never offering due credit to gravity.

We *should* celebrate their accomplishments, but *over*praising backfired by making 3 mistakes. First, it praised so effusively that it missed the opportunity to offer targeted praise that could have reinforced noteworthy accomplishments. Second, it hoped to make children feel good all the time and neglected to prepare them for the times they wouldn't. A generation was ill-prepared for not feeling "as special as a butterfly." Third, it told children what they were—brilliant, artistic, talented, brave—but missed the opportunity to focus on what they did to get there. Dr Dweck's research gives us pause, allowing us to reconsider the self-esteem movement.

She raised another worry about youth who are overly praised. They might worry so much about losing that praise that they would do whatever it takes to maintain their position, even if it hurt others. How we offer feedback to our own children can affect not only their own success but might affect their integrity—and how they interact with others.

Dr Dweck teaches that every interaction can send a message about how teens should think about themselves. Are we concluding that they have a fixed trait, such as intelligence, talent, or athletic aptitude? (You are so handsome. So brilliant. Such a great player/dancer/artist.) When we do, they feel judged and are more likely to think that their current state is, or should be, or *must* be, permanent. This can generate anxiety that a mishap could have them lose it all. Instead, we want to communicate that we see them as developing people, capable of growth, and equipped to learn from each new experience.

Make the shift in your feedback from, "You are _____," to, "You did _____ and, therefore, _____ happened." For example, rather than saying, "You are so good at science," say, "You studied hard and planned thoughtfully, and it paid off in a fantastic science project." When a young person knows that they have mastered a task through effort, they believe in their abilities, build confidence in their capacity to continue to improve, and earn authentic self-esteem.

Guidance on How to Criticize to Support a Growth Mindset

We must not be afraid to point out how our teens could do better. Two basic points: (1) criticism, like praise, must be specific, and (2) we want to support our teens to get past a shortcoming; it's more effective when our constructive criticism recognizes their strengths as good starting points to overcome their challenges.

This is a good place to remind you of your adolescent's remarkable ability to read (or overread) social cues. Most criticism is not verbalized. Your actions can be unintentionally critical without saying a word. Knowing that you are sending nonverbal signals that are likely to be taken to heart or even exaggerated, it is better to directly verbalize your thoughts.

Criticism should be well-targeted and specific. It should never be generalized. In other words, it has to be about the deed, not the person. It should be about something that occurred, not imply a permanent character flaw. When we generalize criticism, it sounds like "You *are* XXXX." That criticism communicates this is a fixed trait, generating the teen's internal conversation, "Well, if I am XXXX, there is not much of a possibility of change." If, on the other hand, you said, "You *did* YYYY," the teen knows their *behavior* led to YYYY. Therefore, if they direct their effort elsewhere, they might accomplish that as well. Now, infuse some strength-based guidance. "You did YYYY and this is not the kind of behavior I like to see. I know you can do better because I have also seen you do ZZZZ."

Now let's use inaction as an example. "You are lazy!" is a demeaning label that implies a permanent state. More productive and effective feedback would be, "You haven't helped around the house, and all the work is landing on me. I need you to step up." It is accurate and clearly demonstrates that the parent is frustrated by a particular action. It can be followed with the strength-based solution. "I know you aren't lazy. I saw what you did in your group project. I need you to think of me as a member of your group now."

Plan your criticism when you are not angry. While angry, we think inaccurately, and our words are fueled by rage or disappointment. During these moments, we tend to see our teens as thoughtless, selfish, or lazy. In calmer moments, we understand that our teen's behavior does not reflect who they are. See how helpful being rooted in a strength-based approach can be! ☺

When our criticism remains targeted, it is constructive, and our teen's growth mindset is reinforced. When we generalize our rage, our teens (rightfully) feel they are being attacked. The real tragedy would be if they believed our words given in frustration or anger and allowed them to flavor their developing identity.

So, What Do I Say?

To develop their independence, teens have to feel increasingly in control of their lives. When we help them attribute their effort and behaviors to the outcomes they experience, they gain that vital sense of control. When we notice the commitment and work they put into something that generated a result, we support them as a developing human being.

So, what does this look like as we communicate with our adolescents? We must not pass positive or negative judgment, lest we make current circumstances feel permanent or "fixed." For these reasons, avoid saying, "You are _____" (emphasis on the word *are*), or, "Your performance was _____," because both thoughts, even if said with loving intentions, imply full acceptance or rejection/judgment. If I had to write a script, it would look something like, "I'm noticing that you _____ (fill in with some deed or action the teen controlled [eg, focused on studying, put your heart into it your art, practiced your sport until you had muscle memory] and, as a result, you _____ (fill in with desired or undesired outcome)." With this approach, a teen will understand the outcome was the result of their behaviors.

See the following table for examples of what to say and what not to say. Each example

- Praises effort, not results
- Notices process (what was done to get there) rather than product (what the result looked like)
- Is specific and targeted with either praise or criticism and does not overgeneralize

Praise	
Say This	**Not That**
What did you learn in class today?	Did you learn enough to get a good grade?
Do you feel like your grade reflected your understanding of the subject? Did it match the studying you put in?	Did you get back your test? How'd you do?
What are you learning to improve your soccer skills?	How many goals did you score?
Were you proud of your sculpture in the art exhibition?	Did you win the top prize?
I appreciate watching your thinking process. You wrestle to figure things out. That is a skill you'll use forever.	You're so smart.
Tell me about your drawing. It captures so much energy.	You're such a great artist.
I think you did well on your test because you reviewed the problems twice, and you didn't give up on the one that you felt you had never seen before. It paid off.	Math comes naturally to you.
I really respect how you keep turning over the stones to search for the answers. More importantly, you're not afraid to get help until you feel confident.	I'm so proud of your report card.

Criticism	
Say This	**Not That**
I think that you didn't put in as much time studying as you needed. You spent all last evening gaming on the computer.	You got a C– because you don't care.
You need to get your head in the game. You are distracted. Take some breaths and step away to regain your focus.	The way you let that goal past you while you were staring into space makes me feel like you just don't care about the team.
Why do you think you did better on the last exam?	Your grades are slipping. Sometimes I wonder if you're just lazy.
You really let your sister down. She needed your help with homework tonight. She looks up to you and was so appreciative when you helped her with her math tables last week.	You can be so selfish and thoughtless!
The dogs had an accident on the floor. I count on you to walk them when you get home.	You are always thinking about fun. Maybe once, you could realize how busy I am.

Recommended Resources

Challenge Success partners with schools, families, and communities to embrace a broad definition of success and to implement research-based strategies that promote student well-being and engagement with learning. It is a leader in this space and offers valuable resources on its website (https://challengesuccess.org).

Making Caring Common Project. This project's vision is a world in which children learn to care about others and the common good, treat people well day to day, come to understand and seek fairness and justice, and do what is right even at times at a cost to themselves. Read their reports on "Turning the Tide" to learn how your children can navigate the college admissions process while maintaining important values (https://mcc.gse.harvard.edu).

CHAPTER 23

Preparation Is Protection

Our children are born vulnerable and defenseless, making it our duty and privilege to protect them. As they grow into adolescents, they don't depend on us for basic survival needs anymore but benefit from our guidance to learn how to live satisfying, meaningful, and productive lives. But we never stop worrying about their safety.

Protection. The word makes us think of cuddling our babies in soft blankets to ensure they are warm, safe, and secure. As our children grow, it can be a struggle to dial down our protective instincts. But when our efforts to shield them from harm crosses into *overprotection*, we unintentionally communicate, "I don't trust you." For teens especially, if they think their parents lack confidence in them, it undermines their growing independence.

The challenge we face as parents is offering a balance of protection and active guidance, all while trusting your teen's capacity to draw wisdom from their own experiences. One of the hardest questions of parenting is, "How do we protect our children while also letting them learn from life's lessons?" When you genuinely know that the best way of protecting your adolescent is to prepare them for an unpredictable world, you will more comfortably know when to actively guide them and when to observe from a safe distance.

There are times when you should follow your mama bear or papa bear protective instincts. If your child's safety is at immediate risk, jump in with full force. If your teen is doing something where morality is in question, be clear about what you consider acceptable and unacceptable. If your teen is doing something illegal, dive in and make it so your teen clearly understands the consequences and knows where you stand on following the law.

With these critical exceptions noted, you best protect your teen by preparing them to navigate the world. Teens flourish when they've gained the confidence to venture forth in the real world because we have prepared them to make their own decisions and choose their own safe and moral paths. We can then confidently let them approach new experiences, knowing they are equipped with skill sets ready to be sharpened and values ready to be honed.

Be a Lighthouse Parent

So how do you protect your children while also letting them learn from life's lessons?

> Be a stable force on the shoreline from which your children can measure themselves against. Look down at the rocks. Make certain your children know the rocks are present, so they do not crash against them. Look into the waves and trust in their ability to learn to ride them. But prepare them to do so.

The concept of being a *lighthouse parent,* first introduced in my book, *Raising Kids to Thrive: Balancing Love With Expectations and Protection With Trust,* will be addressed in greater detail in Chapter 26. For now, know that unlike fad parenting styles with catchy names, this concept is rooted in decades of research about *balanced parenting,* which is proven to produce the best academic, behavioral, social, and emotional outcomes for children and teens. And, critically, it produces the strongest family relationships.

You've balanced between enforcing safety and allowing safe experimentation from the moment your baby began crawling. You learned early on that children learn best when they test and manipulate their environment and "stretch" into new territory. But you also learned that they felt safest stretching when they entered territory you had assured was safe for them. Even as they ventured forth into new territory, they kept checking back to read your unspoken signals to be sure you didn't seem worried. You acted as a lighthouse—a stable, secure presence that allowed them to assess their own security. You looked down at the rocks, imagined what might go wrong, and warned of any dangers. You looked into the waves and kept a mental note of what you needed to do to prepare them to manage them on their own, knowing you would not always be in their direct view. Perhaps, above all, you've learned that your children often copy what you do to imagine what it feels like to be an adult. Your role modeling is the defining feature of what it means to be the lighthouse "from which your children can measure themselves against."

Teens Knowing Who They *Really* Are

Adolescence is a time of trying on many hats. Teens sometimes do what they think it takes to fit someone else's expectations. This can put them in danger. It is for this reason that being grounded in their *own* values is highly protective. Remember, adolescence is a time of growing independence and, therefore, teens can *temporarily* reject their parents' values; this means your opinions and values may not be as protective as helping them clarify what *they* value. Your role as a lighthouse is to remind them of who they are capable of being. In other words, the most important thing you can do to prepare your child to make wise choices is to help them truly know themself.

Performance Character Strengths

Grit

Angela Duckworth, PhD, professor at the University of Pennsylvania and founder and CEO of Character Lab, has demonstrated through extensive research that perseverance, tenacity, diligence, and a commitment to hard work, consistent effort, and practice can predict real-world success. Dr Duckworth calls this *grit.* Recognizing that intelligence and talent contribute to our potential, she states in her book, *Grit: The Power of Passion and Perseverance,* "Our potential is one thing. What we do with it is quite another." Perhaps the critical point here is that people will exhibit tenacity and commit to the hard work when they really care about something.

Dr Duckworth describes gritty young people as those who see life as a marathon rather than a sprint. They have a passionate desire to reach a goal and have that "I'll stick to it" attitude. They are willing to work hard and even plan ahead to reach a goal, even if it means delaying or forgoing immediate gratification. Sprinters can see the finish line from the moment they take off. The end point is clear. Marathon runners have to imagine the finish line as they round the curves and struggle to make it up the hills. They run knowing that perseverance itself is an accomplishment; self-improvement is the reward. A goal that may not be immediately visible drives the effort.

Let's take this one step further. Successful people are those who can recover when they stumble. When a sprinter falls, the race is over. A marathoner can trip, dust themself off, and make a full recovery. A marathoner may even plan a better route.

I highly recommend Dr Duckworth's book, *Grit: The Power of Passion and Perseverance,* for guidance on how to support your teen's development of grit. The following are key thoughts I draw from her book:

- **Set goals.** Support your teen to be genuinely goal oriented, to care about something so much that they will pursue it with passion. It is critical to note here that we cannot define the goal or interest, as it has to reside within them. But we can support them fully to reach *their* goals.

- **Find their passion.** Help your teen to understand that finding a passion is a process, not an event. Inspirational speakers focus on "finding your passion," as if it is hidden somewhere in a drawer. It takes time, effort, and open-mindedness to find it.

- **Focus on the present.** Don't overfocus on the future with your teen because it's...just...too...much...pressure. Instead, focus on what they care about, notice their strengths and interests, and provide the opportunities and exposures to see what people in the real world do with those interests.

- **One step at a time.** Dr Duckworth advises young people to take the steps to "foster their passion." This includes listening to their inner voices and paying attention to the questions they choose to explore and problems they want to solve. Which adults do they see who they'd like to model themselves after? From whom do they crave guidance and mentorship? What are they successful at already but still want to improve their skills? What makes their hearts sing, and just as importantly, what do they dread? What are their strengths and what are their challenges? When do they most appreciate guidance and constructive feedback? Avidly seek mentorship?

- **A world of possibility.** Help your teen experience life. There is time in the future for specialization. If you want your teen to prepare themself for a satisfying life, help them understand the teen years are for sampling life. It is from seeing the possibilities now that they will find their dreams later.

Perseverance and Delayed Gratification

What may feel good in the moment can get in the way of success. Your teen is more likely to invest in the choices that will lead them to a successful future and to avoid dangerous diversions or impulsive actions if they can delay immediate gratification.

However, if putting off something pleasurable feels like sacrificing, your teen will not be eager to delay gratification. Eran Magen, PhD, scientific director at the Center for Supportive Relationships, and James Gross, PhD, professor of psychology at Stanford University, suggest that teens who enjoy the challenge of testing their willpower or who gain satisfaction in sticking to their values will take pleasure and experience pride in the strength it took to overcome their impulses. Your teen likely offers you lots of opportunities to recognize and reinforce their willpower. For example, every time they choose to complete their homework instead of going out to have fun with friends, they demonstrate internal strength.

You can guide your teen to make it easier on themself to resist temptations by changing their environments. Dr Gross teamed up with Dr Duckworth and Tamar Szabó Gendler, PhD, professor of psychology and cognitive science at Yale University, on research that looked at situational self-control.

Because we struggle less with our impulses when we are not triggered by reminders of what we want, we can better avoid temptation by changing the situations we find ourselves in. For example, if a person doesn't want to be tempted to drink, they shouldn't attend an unsupervised party. If they want to avoid homework distractions, they can leave the cell phone in the other room or switch on the Do Not Disturb function. Out of sight, out of earshot, out of mind. This strategy may not make controlling our impulses easy—just easier.

None of us should delay gratification all of the time. You don't want your teen to feel guilty for having pleasure. Hold the discussions about persevering, but also talk about the importance of fun and the necessity of relishing life. Even better, model this balance!

Thinking Skills That Build Resilience

In Chapter 11, we discussed how adolescence is a time of remarkable cognitive (thinking) growth. In Chapter 26, we discuss how to help teens consider the natural conclusion of their actions all through thinking—*without* having to learn from real-life errors. In this chapter, I focus on 2 very specific thinking skills that will prepare your children to remain emotionally healthy even when things are not going smoothly.

Avoiding Catastrophic Thinking

People who view issues realistically can access their internal wisdom to better resolve them. We don't have to remain stuck in negative thoughts when we become frustrated, worried, anxious, or sad. As we discuss in Chapter 25, when we are not certain of an outcome, we sometimes have catastrophic thoughts. Our fears spiral to the worst possible outcomes, and we begin to imagine that as reality. We can learn to use our cognitive abilities to reframe the situation, "decatastrophize" our thoughts, and find workable solutions.

I suggest you read the classic books, *The Optimistic Child: A Proven Program to Safeguard Children Against Depression and Build Lifelong Resilience* (Martin Seligman, PhD, with Karen Reivich, PhD; Lisa Jaycox, PhD; and Jane Gillham, PhD) and *The Resilience Factor* (Karen Reivich, PhD, and Andrew Shatté, PhD). These works offer deeper dives into how to support adolescents to have healthier thinking patterns. Some key points from these books are summarized in the following text:

It is important for teens to have an accurate, rather than catastrophic, interpretation of a situation. This helps them distinguish when they have control in a situation versus when they do not. In turn, this enables them to harness their resources when they have control and to conserve their energy when they do not.

Automatic thoughts fly through our minds and influence how we feel about ourselves and how we interact with the world. Four steps can help us take control of our thoughts.

1. Learn to recognize negative thoughts when they begin to race through our heads. They often begin with key phrases such as, "I better," "If I don't," or "I should." This is called *thought catching.*

2. Stop. Pause. Evaluate whether these thoughts are accurate.

3. Brainstorm more accurate explanations when difficult things happen. Take away self-blame.

4. Decatastrophize. Let go of those harmful thoughts that suggest that a mistake or failure will lead to inevitable disaster.

How we talk to our teens will help them become aware of their thinking patterns. Developing their insight into their thinking patterns is a first step toward preparing them to develop healthier thoughts. It also helps them identify inaccurate beliefs that drive much of their distress. Dr Reivich points out that, in adult conversations with children, we often focus on the A ("What happened?") and C ("How do you feel now?" or "What are you going to do?"). Because of our teens rapidly evolving cognitive abilities, we can help them better understand the B connectors. They can learn to pay attention to the silent self-talk that drives their beliefs, determines how they interpret situations, and, therefore, shapes what will happen next.

The following is an example of being an effective teacher by modeling the process of bringing your thoughts under control. If you lose your focus while preparing for a work presentation, you might say, "I was working on this presentation, and I suddenly began to panic. I began thinking, 'What if I mess up?' Then I began imagining them laughing...or even criticizing me. I actually imagined getting fired because I messed up so badly. None of that happened! It was all my imagination. I stepped away, took a deep breath, and put those self-defeating thoughts away! And I got back to work."

If your teen experiences negative thought patterns in a way that interferes with their well-being, speak to your pediatrician or school counselor about a referral to a cognitive behavioral therapist. Preparing your teen to embrace healthier thinking patterns will pay off throughout their lifetime.

A Word That Shows Change Is Always Possible

Self-defeating thoughts often begin with words such as, "I never," or "I can't." This undermines hope. Help your teen add the transformative word "yet" to their thoughts. "I can't solve this problem" becomes, "I can't solve this problem *yet*." Hope. Now your teen can free their mind to create an action plan. Successful people see the fact that they haven't accomplished a task or learned a skill as an issue of not having had the practice as opposed to being tied to an innate inability. Throughout their lives, we want our children to see their limitations as challenges they have not *yet* learned to overcome or work around.

Interaction Skills That Prepare Teens to Follow Their Own Wisdom

I think a parent's greatest fear is tied to the effects of peer pressure on their teen. In reflection, Chapter 12 offers 2 reassuring points. First, peer influence can be a positive force as easily as it can be a negative one. We should ensure that our teens are surrounded by positive peers. Second, most peer influence is internally driven by a teen's desire to fit in. Occasionally, however, it looks more like coercion as portrayed in made-for-TV movies, where one child forces the other to do something. Please refer back to Chapter 12 to review the skill sets that your teen needs to follow their own wisdom.

··

Recommended Resource

Character Lab turns scientific discoveries about the mindsets and skills that develop character into actionable advice for parents and teachers. On this website, you'll find Playbooks, organized by character strength, with information and activities based on rigorous research studies. This site has a playbook on Grit as well as other character strengths (https://characterlab.org).

CHAPTER 24

Build Your Teen's Resilience

We couldn't protect our children from every skinned knee when they were in grade school, and we can't prevent them from being emotionally hurt now or in the future. We can, however, help them to build resilience—the capacity to bounce back from life's challenges. But having children who can recover from difficulties is not our end goal. We want them to grow stronger from each challenge so they are less likely to be scathed from the next round life may throw at them. Even that, however, must not be our end goal. People who possess the skills and strategies to recover from difficult times also have the capacity to make the most out of good times. To thrive. That is our goal, to raise our children to thrive.

When we think of building resilience, we don't deny difficulty or tell others to set aside their frustrations. We mustn't imply they should "just get past it." The language of resilience does not sugarcoat realities. It guides others to create hope and generates a sense of control by encouraging them to take actions that will change their experience. It helps others express their emotions in healthy ways and learn that buried emotions only lead to a loss of the ability to feel. Above all, it highlights that when circumstances are tough, we do better when joined with others.

Roots of Resilience

Our teens aren't fragile. They possess strengths and can learn to cope with challenges, grow from their mistakes, and mature into adults who are capable of thriving. But to activate their inner resources, they must be exposed to challenges in which they can develop and practice coping skills. Remember, preparation is protection. We can't solve all their dilemmas or overprotect them, lest we send a damaging message—"I don't believe you're capable." Instead, we must support them to strengthen their resilience muscles by pushing them just a bit further than what they are used to.

Ann Masten, PhD, one of the leading thinkers on resilience, calls it "ordinary magic." It doesn't need a rocket scientist to craft a brilliant formula; resilience exists and can be fortified through human connections. Briefly,

- **Unconditional love** offers the deep-seated security that allows young people to weather their own uncomfortable thoughts and feelings and to withstand external pressures or undermining messages. It allows them to comfortably stretch into new territory as they need to adapt to evolving circumstances. Your love is the safety net; other things in their life might falter, but they know they will never lose you. Unconditional love doesn't mean you accept all behaviors. But the security offered to your teenager from knowing that they are worthy of being loved and that your love will never be withdrawn or threatened enables them to launch into adulthood ready to face what comes.

- Young people live up or down to the **expectations** adults set for them. We are not demanding things easily measured, like grades, scores, or trophies. This is about being a good human being—the character strengths you hope your teens have. It is about recognizing and reinforcing all that is good and right about your child and holding them to the standards of being their best self. As they grow, it is also about standing alongside them as they strengthen and solidify their values.

- We do our best teaching when we **model** responding to stress with resilience. When we are transparent about the steps we take to calm ourselves, manage life's complexities, and move forward, they learn how to adapt from us.

Resilience Is a Theme Throughout This Book

Although only 2 chapter titles contain the word *resilience*, resilience-building strategies are interwoven throughout this book. You're reading this book because you want to be an adult who can bring out the "ordinary magic" in your teen. You want to be able to offer that solid foundation from which they can launch into adulthood. That's what resilience building is about, and that is the underpinning of this entire book. Dialogues rooted in the language of resilience about how to handle various situations are woven throughout this book. If you want to frame all parental interactions in the context of building resilience or study the "teachers guide" on stress management, read *Building Resilience in Children and Teens: Giving Kids Roots and Wings.*

Seven Crucial Cs of Resilience

There are 7 Crucial Cs—competence, confidence, connection, character, contribution, coping, and control—that contribute to building resilience. Many of these Cs are borrowed from thinkers on positive youth development and resilience whose paths inspired mine. The original 4 Cs—competence, confidence, connection, and character—were coined by Rick Little, who founded the International Youth Foundation. I have been most influenced by Richard Lerner, PhD, a personal hero of mine, whose research demonstrates that adolescents who possess these Cs are better prepared to thrive.

Competence

Competence is the ability to handle situations effectively. It is acquired through the development of skill sets that position people to trust their own judgments, make responsible choices, face difficult situations, and navigate the personal and professional world.

Confidence

Confidence is rooted in competence. When young people possess the skill sets that make them competent, they earn a deep-seated confidence. Confidence is not something we can bestow on a person; it is something they need to find themself. We can, however, notice their existing strengths, helping them to understand they are deserving of confidence.

Connection

People with close ties to others are more likely to have a solid sense of security that produces strong values and prevents them from seeking harmful or unhealthy relationships. Family is the central force in any young person's life, but connections to people they meet in civic, educational, religious, and athletic settings also increase their sense of belonging. Adolescents thrive when peer relationships are healthy and supportive.

Character

People need a fundamental sense of right and wrong to ensure they are prepared to make wise choices and contribute positively to the world. Young people with solid character strengths enjoy a strong sense of self-worth and confidence. They are more likely to adhere to their own values and demonstrate caring toward others. Adolescents who are future-oriented may find it easier to work harder and make wiser decisions.

Contribution

Adolescents who learn that they can make a difference in others' lives or in the well-being of their communities gain a motivating sense of purpose. They receive reinforcing thank-yous instead of the low expectations too many teens endure. As they experience how good it feels to give, they'll have less shame when they need to receive, because they'll have learned that the giver does so not out of pity but out of purpose.

Coping

People who learn to cope with stress in a healthy way will be better prepared to overcome life's challenges. The best protection against turning to unsafe, worrisome behaviors when stressed may be possessing a repertoire of positive, adaptive coping strategies.

Control

Adolescence is about gaining increasing independence—control over their own lives. When teens gain insight that their decisions lead to real-life consequences, they learn to wisely consider their actions and, over time, gain self-control over their impulses. If parents make all the decisions, teens are denied opportunities to learn control. Parents should create safe spaces within which adolescents can safely learn self-control.

Managing Life's Inevitable Stressors

Many of the behaviors we worry about most in adolescence are misguided attempts to diminish their stress. When we are stressed, our first impulse is to relieve our discomfort with any quickly accessible coping strategy. There are positive and negative coping strategies. Most negative coping strategies are highly effective—in the short-term—at relieving discomfort associated with stress. However, negative strategies perpetuate and intensify the cycle of stress because they have harmful consequences to our teens, to our families, and to society. Anything that solves a problem "quickly" and easily has the potential to be addictive. It is our job to raise teens with a variety of positive coping strategies that will *also* minimize their discomfort but in ways consistent with their values.

We have to stop simply telling teens what not to do. It doesn't work. First, it denies them the opportunity to explain the whys behind the behaviors— why they are feeling the need to manage stress, why they are feeling overwhelmed, what they feel they need to escape. This is our chance to engage and to co-regulate with them to increase their windows of tolerable stress. Teens need to learn effective and satisfying ways of coping that are consistent with their values, will keep them healthy, and bring families together rather than tearing them apart.

I can't guarantee that your teen won't try a worrisome behavior even if they possess good coping strategies, because some of these negative coping strategies *also* are fun or feel good. An adolescent may try drugs to test limits or to have fun with friends. We hope they will move beyond this phase quickly. But a young person who seeks comfort through drugs, or who is using them to mask their feelings, may be destined for long-term problems. People with safer, healthier means of coping with stress don't need to avoid their problems; they can confront them with confidence, thereby better controlling their destiny.

If your teen is engaged in worrisome coping strategies, lovingly invite them to learn healthy ways to manage their feelings. If you're reading this when your child is a toddler, 7 years old, or 17 years old, in crisis or without a worry in the world, you're reading this at the right time. *Now* is the time to build positive stress-management skills. It is about more than preventing problems; it is an essential strategy to building resilience and preparing young people to thrive.

Stress Management and Coping: Powerful Strategies to Take Control Over One's Life

Assess the Stress

There are crises that demand every drop of our energy and others that only feel like a crisis. Core to resilience is being able to focus our concentration and resources on real problems rather than those that have been unnecessarily heightened by our catastrophic thinking.

Three questions can control your teen's thinking (and ours as well) to enable a more realistic assessment of our situation.

1. Is this a real tiger or paper tiger?
2. Is this problem temporary?
3. Is this good situation permanent?

Real Tiger or Paper Tiger

We are designed to run from tigers. But the thinking, rationale part of our brain shuts down because we are ready to escape, not negotiate. And our empathy can be dampened because this is not the time to ask the tiger to explain his perspective. We must ask ourselves, "Is this a real tiger or a paper tiger?" If the situation can't cause real harm, the answer is paper tiger. Once we realize that, we can regain our thinking capacities.

Is This Problem Temporary?

Some people imagine that each problem may lead to far-reaching and long-lasting consequences. Ask yourself, "How will I feel in a week or even a month?" If the answer is, "I won't be upset about this," then reassurance is warranted: "This too shall pass."

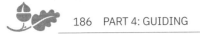

Is This Good Thing Permanent?

Sometimes people feel anxiety about losing their good fortune. This expectation of impending loss or failure reinforces a lack of control. Instead, we want people to remind themselves that good things *can* be permanent. The challenge is to continue creating the circumstances where good things will come to them.

A Comprehensive Coping Plan for Adolescents

A comprehensive stress-reduction plan should include strategies that would prepare youth to

- Accurately assess the stressor (as previously described).
- Effectively problem-solve to address the stress-inducing issue.
- Maintain a state of health optimal for managing stress. Strong bodies are needed to have resilient minds, and those bodies are built through exercise, good nutrition, proper sleep, and routine relaxation.
- Manage emotions in a healthy way. This includes strategies that offer healthy ways to avoid feeling and others that enable full emotional expression.
- Give people a sense of meaning and purpose. This enables them to maintain perspective and reinforces that their well-being matters to others.

The plan has 10 points that include ways of doing all of the previously mentioned strategies. It is not a 10-step plan meant to go in any particular order. Rather, it offers a repertoire to draw from at appropriate times. *Building Resilience in Children and Teens* offers a variety of activities and actions in each category.

Category 1: Tackling the Problem

Point 1: Identify and then address the problem. Actions that address the problem diminish the source of stress. An effective strategy is to name the problem and then divide it into smaller pieces, committing to work on only one piece at a time. Strategies include making lists and timelines followed by a plan to address each component of the problem. Metaphorically, this is about revisualizing problems from being mountains too high to be scaled into small hills situated on top of each other. As we stand atop each hill, the summit appears more attainable.

Point 2: Avoid stress when possible. Sometimes triggers to stress can be avoided entirely. If, for example, there is a person who bullies in a classroom—a place that cannot be avoided—a young person should find an adult authority. If a person who bullies is in the neighborhood and only acts up when you walk past their corner, plan a new route.

Point 3: Let some things go. People who waste energy worrying about things they can't change don't have enough energy conserved to address problems they can fix. People who focus on the things they can change gain a sense of control versus the powerlessness, frustration, and anger that comes from trying to fix things they cannot affect. The serenity prayer summarizes this point.

> *"Grant me the serenity to accept the things I cannot change; the courage to change the things I can; and the wisdom to know the difference."*

Category 2: Taking Care of My Body

Point 4: The power of exercise. Exercise is the starting point for someone whose stress hormones prevent their thinking powers from resolving an issue. When a stressed person does not exercise, their body is left feeling as if they haven't run from the "tiger." Therefore, their body senses the tiger is still lurking and they remain nervous. It is not surprising, therefore, that exercise is so tightly linked to emotional well-being and positively affects stress, anxiety, depression, and attention-deficit/hyperactivity disorder.

Point 5: Active relaxation. Deep breathing is the portal to relaxation. Managing stress is sometimes about quieting the mind. This is a mainstay of yoga, meditation, and the martial arts, where it is used to gain focus. Young people can be taught: *"You can flip the switch from being stressed to relaxed if you know how to turn on the relaxed system."* There are many digital apps or programs that can guide people to learn effective breathing techniques.

Point 6: Eat well. Proper nutrition is essential to a healthy body and clear mind. Guide your teen to understand that good nutrition keeps you alert throughout the day and keeps your mood steady. People who eat mostly junk food have highs and lows in their energy level, which harms their ability to reduce stress. Eating more fruits, vegetables, lean proteins, and whole grains can keep you focused for a longer time.

Point 7: Sleep well. Proper sleep is key to stress management. Some people do not sleep well from having too much stimulation in their bedrooms and keeping irregular hours. Another source of lost sleep is stress itself; people sleep better when they resolve their problems before bedtime in a place other than the bed or by setting them aside before going to sleep (see Point 9).

Category 3: Dealing With Emotions

Point 8: Take instant vacations. Sometimes the best way to de-stress is to take your mind away to a more relaxing place. Young people can be taught to take advantage of their imagination and ability to focus on other interests. Books are proven ways to escape current thoughts and feelings. This healthy disengagement strategy is key to drug prevention because it offers a healthy escape.

Point 9: Release emotional tension. A person needs to be able to express emotions rather than letting them build inside. This includes connecting to others and letting go of feelings through verbal, written, nonverbal, and creative expression. We want young people to be able to express their emotions with anything that completes this sentence, "I _____ it out!" Strategies that can fill in this blank include the following: prayed/laughed/talked/cried/drew/sung/danced/rapped/wrote/screamed.

Category 4: Make Your World Better and Help You Feel Better

Point 10: Contribute. *The importance of this point draws directly from the 7 Cs.* Contribution to others pays off in many ways. First, those who experience the personal rewards of service tend to feel better about themselves. Perhaps more importantly, they may be more comfortable asking for help during a time of personal need.

Stress Management in a Crisis

A highly stressed teen is unable to access their best thinking skills. To get there they should

1. Exercise first. If stress hormones are surging, our brains are communicating, "RUN!" and are unable to think. Adrenaline turbocharges the body. Until that fuel is used up, the body cannot feel settled.

2. Breathe. Flip that switch. Breathing done correctly calms the body and activates the mind.

3. Now, think. Now that the turbocharged fuel is used up and the body has been put in a relaxed state, problem-solving can begin. It starts with a self-reminder, even amid panicked thinking, "I am not in danger." Once the brain is calm and self-talk has reinforced safety, you can think through a solution.

4. Express emotions in a healthy way (see Point 9).

The Language of Resilience

Our words express when we see our teens as vulnerable. Broken. Incapable. We also communicate when we see them as strong. Thoughtful. Capable. Deserving. When we say, "Let me help you out," we communicate, "I don't think you can handle this." When we say, "It'll be alright. I'll fix this. Let's hug it out," we may belittle the situation and imply that comfort and solutions rely on us. Instead, we want our teens to know that we see their problems as real but maintain faith they'll be able to handle it with our support.

The language of resilience is offered throughout this book in the suggested dialogues. As you consider each one, imagine how your teen would react differently if you said something similar to the suggestions versus those words not suggested. I don't want you to use the suggestions as scripts; rather to understand the underlying principles that explain the chosen words. You'll notice a few things.

- We check our own temperature to make sure our unspoken signals don't undermine the words we hope to say.
- We reinforce that our presence is reliable.
- We express comfort with emotions.
- We sit comfortably with discomfort.
- We trust that our teen will get through these uncomfortable moments.
- We do not supply answers and sometimes admit we don't have them.
- We recognize teens as experts in their own lives and occasionally ask them to guide us in how we can be most supportive.
- We trust that our teen in time will come to their solution.
- We speak in a way that the young person can understand. We are sensitive to their developmental stage and their ability to understand each of our words. We know even the most intelligent person in crisis needs things to be presented in very simple terms.
- We never catastrophize a problem, and we don't sugarcoat it.
- We disapprove of behaviors while making it clear we approve of the person.
- When we offer corrections or discipline, we are very specific about the problem being addressed so the teen doesn't think we believe that the behavior defines them.

The following table depicts how each of the 7 Cs flavor the language of resilience:

The Critical Element of Resilience	Language That Elevates the Element of Resilience
Competence	When we speak to our teens, we elevate the skill sets they possess by reinforcing how they could be helpful in the current situation. If they do not yet possess a skill set, or the one they are using requires adaptation, then this becomes the focus of our conversation.

(continued)

The Critical Element of Resilience	Language That Elevates the Element of Resilience
Confidence	We build our children's confidence by noticing what they are already doing right, including noting their competencies. We use praise wisely and focus on effort they're putting in rather than the result. We never praise something not worthy of praise but can always find something positive to highlight.
Connection	Even in the most difficult moments, we reinforce that our presence is reliable. In fact, that is all we can guarantee. Whenever possible, we reinforce that all people are stronger when they join together and support each other or wiser when they collaborate to arrive at a solution.
Character	We always hold our children in an aspirational light. We do not judge the current behavior as defining them; rather, we can highlight all that is good and right about them. When necessary, we point out when a current behavior is not consistent with the person we know them to be. When our kids are stuck and trying to find a solution to a problem, we root our proposed solution in their existing strengths.
Contribution	We know young people with a sense of meaning and purpose in their lives are more likely to make wise choices. Therefore, we listen to our children's interests and encourage them to do good for others.

The Critical Element of Resilience	Language That Elevates the Element of Resilience
Coping	When our teen is involved in worrisome behaviors, rather than condemning them we explore the whys behind the behavior. We guide our teen to consider positive things they can do to deal with uncomfortable thoughts and feelings rather than only telling them what they must not do.
Control	We approach our discussions by recognizing that our teens are the experts in their own lives. We guide them to arrive at solutions and offer opinions only when asked. However, we insist on and monitor clear limits beyond which they cannot stray. We do this with the understanding that they will have more control over their lives within safe boundaries.

Recommended Resources

The Center for Parent and Teen Communication through parentandteen .com offers practical strategies rooted in what is known to work to strengthen family connections and build youth prepared to thrive. It offers materials to help adults guide youth to build their stress management skills (https://parentandteen.com/category/health-prevention/helping -teens-cope).

It also offers an interactive stress management plan that guides young people to build their own repertoire of stress management strategies. Their personal plan is sent back to them in PDF format. It does not substitute for the protective power of human relationships nor replace professional guidance (https://parentandteen.com/teen-stress-management-plan).

CHAPTER 25

Building Resilience in Difficult and Uncertain Times

O ur desire to protect our children is embedded in our parental bone marrow. Unfortunately, we cannot control the circumstances they will face. The best way to protect them, therefore, is to shape the lessons they gain during difficult times and build the resilience skills they benefit from throughout their lives.

Uncertainty creates deeply uncomfortable feelings. We are designed to confront imminent danger—the real tigers in our lives. With our fight-or-flight responses, including increased heart rates and widening pupils, our bodies quickly transform to deal with discrete emergencies. We are not designed, however, to know precisely what to do with the tiger who *might* be lurking in the grass. We must remain ready to jump in an instant. The changes in our body required to remain in a state of readiness to escape and the stress on our minds to remain hypervigilant take a toll on both our physical and psychological well-being.

It is how we handle struggles that teaches our children how to manage uncertainty in their own lives. It is how we handle our emotions that creates the opportunity to build resilience. It is how we respond to feelings of confusion and self-doubt, anxiety, and frustration that models for our children how they, too, might manage their own future difficulties. It is how we reach for support and draw nearer to those we love that instills within our teens the values that will enable them to navigate the most difficult challenges. **Every emotion that is not set aside or denied is an opportunity to build resilience.** In this chapter, we'll look at common emotions that arise in difficult and uncertain times, pair them to the potential lesson it offers our children, and underscore how we rise to best model resilience.

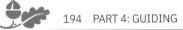

"I feel like I am failing": Learning Self-forgiveness

You've become used to juggling many balls; however, in stressful times, extra balls keep coming. We can't possibly keep them all in the air. **In uncertain times, we have to become satisfied with good enough.** Know that if you forgive yourself and are genuinely intentional about seeing the good in yourself through self-compassion, your adolescent will learn that when times are tough, it is OK to give ourselves a break. They will understand that when we care for ourselves, we are in a better position to care for others. Perhaps the greatest benefit is that they will feel safer including you in the details of their lives because they have seen you forgive yourself of your human frailty, reassuring them that you will offer them the same compassion when they, too, make mistakes.

"My kids are frustrated, and so am I": Learning to Empathize

The best way to gain empathy muscles is to experience empathy firsthand. In other words, you help your child build empathy for others by working to understand your child's thoughts, feelings, and behaviors. Adolescents can suffer in unique ways during difficult times. The way they react can be challenging for adults. If we learn to understand the *whys* behind their behaviors, our empathy for our children can help them build empathy for others, precisely because they have benefitted from ours.

You may find it easier to support younger children through challenging times than you do adolescents. Children know something is worrisome but easily draw comfort from you. They are less likely to ask unsettling questions that have no answers. When there are answers, we can keep our responses simple yet reassuring. Adolescents, however, may remain more on edge because they understand what we adults worry about. During stressful times, we keep our families near. Adolescents may rebel against our protective restrictions because these limits fly in the face of adolescents' needs to be exploring, gaining independence, and building peer relationships. So, we should expect them to push back harder. **Give them as much freedom of choice as is safe and as much independence as the situation allows.**

Your adolescent also wants to understand the "whys" of large unanswerable questions such as, "Why do we allow people to go hungry if there is enough food for everyone?" The most challenging times often pose questions nobody can yet answer. It is understandable that adolescents will struggle with these unknowns. Knowing this, we are reminded that, even as we grow weary, we need to have deep, thoughtful discussions with our tweens and teens. You'll get to know your adolescent better, strengthen your connection, and encourage their inquisitive nature.

"I don't have it as bad as someone else": Understanding Is a 2-way Street

Suggesting that another person does not have the right to experience their own feelings and frustrations just because someone else has it worse minimizes their feelings. Such an approach leads to shame and can cause feelings to be suppressed, which can result in psychological distress.

To thrive, people need to grasp that understanding is a 2-way street. That means that it's important that our teens also understand what we are going through. Just as we provide empathy to them, they need to understand we also deserve their empathy. Everyone should acknowledge we are *all* going through something and deserve to be forgiven for our less-than-stellar performances.

"I don't know how to handle how I feel": Acknowledging, Processing, and Releasing Emotions

A time of uncertainty with heightened emotions is precisely when to demonstrate emotions are not to be ignored. Too many young people receive messages that strong people need to contain their emotions and that genuinely experiencing feelings is a sign of weakness. In truth, bottled up emotions fester and lead to unresolved feelings. **Our children must learn that having emotions is OK, talking about them is necessary, and being honest with them is healing** (see Chapter 10). With our words, we express whether we see youth as vulnerable, fragile, and incapable or as safe, strong, and capable. When we say, "It's not that bad. Let me give you a hug," we minimize the situation and imply that comfort is dependent on us. Rather, we want young people to know that their problem is real and that they'll be able to handle it with our support. When we jump in quickly with solutions, we deny space for teens to arrive at their own solutions. On the other hand, when we act as a sounding board, we give them the opportunity to express and process their thoughts and feelings (see Chapter 17).

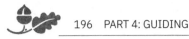

"I want to pull my hair out": Creating a Safe Haven Within Our Homes

Parenting is tough and often is tougher in challenging times. Sometimes precisely because teens feel most comfortable within our homes, they express their frustrations loudest right in our living rooms and their anger right to our faces. When events outside of your home seep through your walls, it is critical to create a safe haven.

Resilience is about taking control of what you can. **We cannot control the outside world, but we can be intentional about creating sanctuaries within our homes.** We have to speak frankly: "The world feels frightening right now. Therefore, we are going to make our home a safe haven. We're going to choose to be kinder and gentler. We're going to gain our strength from each other. We're going to speak openly about how we love and care about each other. There still will be things about each other that get on our nerves. But we will do our best to let them go. **We are going to get through this together because we will create peace in this house."**

A haven is not a place to tuck away or ignore emotions. To the contrary, it must be a place where heightened emotions are processed in healthy ways. You can love everything about your teen or partner and still sometimes want to tear your hair out. It is the fact that we are committed to working through tension and focusing on each other's strengths that adds an even deeper layer of security to our relationships. When we create safe havens in our homes, teens learn you can have conflict and recover. They learn that there is a place where they can temporarily be their worst selves and still be cared about. They learn that love is not only about praise but also about active, even firm, guidance.

Home also has to be a place where people can safely unplug. Check in routinely with credible sources, but do not let bad news consume all the oxygen in your home. Create a place where your family can study, reflect, and enjoy time together.

"I need a time-out": Being a Calming Presence for Others

In moments of uncertainty, when our minds begin racing toward worst-case scenarios, the presence of a reassuring and caring person makes all of the difference. Chapter 20 covered the importance of co-regulation in detail. We can't be co-regulators, however, unless we first become calm ourselves. That isn't easy and often takes a time-out to access our own self-regulation strategies. Our children benefit from seeing which strategies we use to become calm as much as they benefit from our calming presence. As your teen learns to borrow your calm, they will learn the benefits of reaching out to others, and that is an additional resilience tool. In the future, your teen will take the initiative to lend their own calm to loved ones.

"I don't know how to respond": Being Clear and Honest With Yourself and Others

The last thing you want to do in a time of uncertainty is to pretend you are certain. Calm, yes. Thoughtful, yes. Hopeful, always. Certain? Only if you want to lose the trust of those who are relying on your judgment. **Instead, say what you do know. Admit what you don't.** And discuss how you plan to find credible information.

- "You're asking the right questions. I don't know all the answers. But I trust that there are wise people trying to figure out what to do right now. Let's search for answers together and make sure we are looking in places we can trust."

- "You want to know which experts I trust? The ones who have the training to find the answers. But also the ones who are clear about what they know and what they are still working to figure out. It makes me believe what they tell me."

"My mind feels out of control": Maintaining Physical Health Strengthens Emotional Health

We cannot control what happens to us, but we can control how our bodies support our minds to best navigate the circumstances we confront. We optimize our mental dexterity and emotional capacity when we maintain an exercise routine, prioritize sleep, and eat nourishing food. Occasionally say out loud, "I can't sit on the couch all day. Taking naps just makes me more tired. I'm going to get up, get dressed, exercise, and do normal things."

"I keep thinking about the worst-case scenario": Stay Present and Live in Reality

Uncertainty can sometimes make our minds race to the worst possible outcome. Catastrophic thinking then becomes our perceived reality and our stress responses are activated as if the worst circumstances already occurred. This interferes with our ability to think and plan. Catch those thoughts and say, "I am imagining the worst." Take a few deep breaths. Then ask, "What is happening *right now*? What is the worst-case scenario? What is the best-case scenario?" The truth is probably somewhere in between. Notice that what I am calling for is *realistic*, not optimistic, thinking. **Realistic thinking generates hope and empowerment because it enables you to thoughtfully plan out solutions. It doesn't sugarcoat or minimize real problems.**

Resilient people can distinguish when they have control over a situation and when they do not. They gather their resources for situations in which they do have control and conserve their resources when they do not. They can assess when something will pass easily and quickly; they're able to
talk themselves down when they start to magnify events in their minds to catastrophic proportions. All of this can reduce stress levels.

Model how thinking patterns affect your ability to deal with difficulties. Talk out loud to help your children see the connections between inaccurate thoughts and uncomfortable feelings. For example, if you become unnerved while watching the news, you might say, "My imagination just took over. I was listening to the news and began to feel panicky. Then I realized those thoughts were all in my head. I took a deep breath, caught the panicky thoughts, and put them away! Then I focused on what we are doing to stay safe."

Finally, remember young people have not *yet* had the experience to know that crises come and go. Amid a crisis, it is usually hard to see past it. Say what older generations have passed down to us: "This too shall pass," coupled with the line about your unwavering presence, "And I know we'll get through this together."

"I feel helpless": Finding What You *Can* Do

Few things create discomfort more than feeling like there is too much to do...or nothing you can do at all. And few things restore comfort more than tackling what you can. As long as you view a problem as insurmountable, it will always feel like a mountain you can't climb. Each mountain, however, can be broken down and thought of as a few hills on top of each other. The first step is to choose one hill to conquer. Once on top of that hill, the summit of the mountain won't feel so unattainable.

Incorporate the word "yet" into your thinking. It serves as a reminder that the current reality does not prevent us from moving to the next step. "I'll never _____!" transforms into "I haven't _____ yet." **We want our children to possess a mindset that doesn't accept failure or disappointment as permanent but instead views setbacks as opportunities to try *yet* again.**

"I can't do everything": Learning to Let Go

Remember those balls you've dropped on the ground? Look up in the air and see which balls are still there, because this likely reflects what matters most to you. Taking care of those around you who are vulnerable. Letting your family members know they are precious to you. Doing what it takes to keep a roof over your head and food on the table. **Now look down on the ground at the balls you've allowed to drop. Leave some of them there.** You can wait to pick them up or may wisely determine that what may have felt important to you before does not matter much now or never really mattered as much as you thought. Letting go of some things frees you to focus intently on more important matters.

"I am so disappointed": Find Joy, Give Service, and Maintain Purpose

Life is full of disappointments. It is OK to feel them fully. But even in the toughest of times, find space for joy. Sometimes that comes naturally simply by opening our eyes to the loving presence of those around us. Other times it is about making a choice, such as deciding to play a game or cook a favorite recipe. Sometimes it is finding solitude. But be intentional about including joy in each day. We also must fill our lives with reminders that we matter to those around us. Contributing to others' lives is a time-tested way to maintain purpose. It is a sense of meaning and purpose that can bring us joy every day and get us through the toughest times (see Chapter 32).

"I had so many plans that aren't working out": When You Can't Change Things, Adapt

Resilient people know when they have the power to change something by doubling down on their efforts and when they should conserve energy by focusing instead on what *can* become a reality and what *can* be done. Some things are simply beyond our control, leaving how we choose to react as the only thing we can (somewhat) control. Often, the best thing we can do in these situations is move ahead without tearing ourselves apart. It's in these moments that you remind loved ones that when life becomes tough, you rely on each other.

"I miss my family and friends": Relationships Strengthen Us

Uncertainty is frightening, but knowing that we are not alone brings comfort. Any individual can be vulnerable, but, together, we are stronger than the sum of each of our individual strengths. People can take turns between drawing strength from others and being a source of strength. Young people should see that wise adults actively reach out to others during stressful times.

I have high hopes for the generation of teens affected so deeply by the 2020 pandemic. I believe the lesson drawn will be how much relationships matter, precisely because social distancing made them aware of much of what we've taken for granted and previously undervalued. This generation will understand and appreciate the simple joy of being with grandparents, extended family, friends, and community. If they appreciate togetherness just a bit more and cherish relationships more deeply, they will forever reap the benefits. **This could be the generation that leads us into a better shared future—one in which we hold those we love nearer and offer those who are vulnerable the extra support they deserve.**

"Will things ever be the same?": Hope

Resilience is about more than surviving, bouncing back, or recovering. It is about adapting. Growing. Becoming stronger. Being ready for the next challenge, but also being prepared to savor all the good life has to offer. Each challenge holds the potential of generating hopelessness and powerlessness. But we cannot let that be the end result. Imagine if this world views problems previously seen as insurmountable as awakenings and learns that if we join together with resolve—as we must—even the toughest issues can be addressed.

CHAPTER 26

Balance the Expression of Your Love With the Wisdom of Your Monitoring

Truth: Adults are the most important people in the lives of young people, and teens like adults. In fact, adolescents care more about what their parents think than they care about anybody else's opinion.

You are an indispensable guide in your teen's journey toward adulthood and I hope to solidify your confidence in how to fill that role. A challenge is that sometimes the most important ideas in parenting seem to contradict each other. It *is* critical to unconditionally love your teen and expect them to rise to their own standards. The best way to protect your child *is* to prepare them to navigate the world on their own. And your teen knowing you trust them *is* critical to your relationship. But does that mean that love, high expectations, preparation, and trust are all teens need to remain safe and make wise decisions? No. We are *also* obligated to monitor our teens to ensure they stay within safe territory. Parenting is about striking the right balance to meet your teen's needs.

If you wonder how your child will feel about your guidance, remember another **truth** about teens: Young people care deeply about safety and want to avoid danger but need guidance as they learn about risk. This chapter, as well as Chapters 27 and 28, positions you to effectively offer guidance about safety and risk.

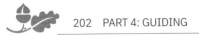

The Secret Is Out: We Know Which Approach to Parenting Works Best

If you watch daytime TV, you might think parenting approaches change with the season. The tiger and helicopter approaches to parenting made some parents double down and say the heck with moderation (there was no moderation in those styles!). Some thought, "I'm going to be a snowplow parent and clear the path for my children." Others adopted the free-range parenting style committed to getting out of the way. While these battling approaches to parenting attract media attention, sell books, and earn online clicks, they are disruptive and disorienting to parents. Not surprisingly, these media-favored approaches are rarely rooted in science or long-term experience.

This book is rooted in a balanced approach to parenting. Decades of research and experience tell us how to balance our love with clear expectations and our need to protect our children with their need to earn our trust. Most critically, we know that parents who get this balancing act right foster open communication within their households and, therefore, strengthen their families. If you prefer a catchy phrase, consider *lighthouse parenting*, a term that metaphorically conveys the best of what is known of balanced parenting—a style backed by what is likely the largest body of parenting research and has consistently shown meaningful benefits across cultures. Tell your friends,

> *I like to think of myself as a "lighthouse parent." A stable force on the shoreline my child can measure themself against. I see it as my job to look down at the rocks and make sure they do not crash against them. I look into the waves and trust they will eventually learn to ride them on their own. But I will prepare them to do so.*

Balanced Parenting Makes a BIG Difference

Balanced parenting leads to children achieving greater academic success, fewer behavioral risks, and a higher level of emotional well-being and reduced emotional distress. Teens raised with a balanced parenting style have the following:

- Better emotional and mental health, including reduced depression and anxiety
- Higher levels of resilience and better self-esteem
- Improved grades and better engagement with teachers
- Increased participation in after school and extracurricular activities
- Less substance use and less exposure to violence

- Later initiation of sexual activity and safer sexual behaviors
- Safer driving behaviors and half as many car crashes
- Less experience being bullied; less experience bullying others
- **The closest, warmest, and most communicative relationship with their parents**

What Is Meant by "Parenting Style"?

Parenting style was first explored in the 1960s by Diana Baumrind, PhD, a renowned developmental psychologist, and, since then, generations of psychologists have studied its impact on raising children and teens. Parenting style is about the balance between expressed love (warmth), responsiveness (flexibility and willingness to respond to changing needs), and demandingness (expectations and how rules are set and monitored).

We know adolescents do best when parents *both* express their caring and monitor their safety and behaviors. Achieving this balance takes real thought. There is often tension between parenting approaches that focus on loving attachment and those that take a step back to foster independence. Similarly, there is a balance to strike between high levels of parental oversight and allowing teens to learn from life's lessons. Your teen's needs coupled with your family's unique circumstances may influence how you strike that balance. Cultural values and safety in your community will also influence your approach to parenting.

You come to parenting with a strength no book could teach—the innate love for your child. My goal is to build on that strength while guiding you to apply the parenting lessons research has shown leads to the best outcomes for teens in a way that works for your family.

The 4 Parenting Styles

Which of the following statements sounds like what you might say to your teen or like the thoughts that best describe your approach to parenting?

- "You'll do what I say. Why? Because I said so!"
- "I really enjoy you. I couldn't always speak openly to my parents. I know that if you think of me as a friend, you'll feel comfortable coming to me. I will spend lots of time with you and we'll have good times together. I trust you to make your own decisions."
- "Kids will be kids. I figured it out and so will they. If they get into serious trouble, I'll get involved then."
- "I love you. I am not your friend, I am your parent, and that's even better. I'm going to let you make your share of mistakes, but for the things that

might affect your safety, you'll do as I say. And if something you do is not consistent with our values or could compromise your morality, we are going to sit down and think it through together. My job is to keep you safe and stand by you as you become your best self."

Starting by recognizing the strengths of each style allows you to make changes more easily in how your teen is parented for the following reasons. First, we all copy (or reject entirely!) how we were parented. However our parents raised us, they acted with the best of intentions. In recognizing the strengths of each style, you can rest knowing your parents did not act with malice...and then you can move on. Next, if you start from the strength of your existing style, you'll know you are partway there and can then build your repertoire. Finally, you'll want to effectively compromise with other adult caregivers. Knowing they are grounded in some strengths will allow you to better work together to move toward a balanced style.

You'll do what I say. Why? Because I said so! This is called *authoritarian parenting*. It is high in rules but low in warmth. These parents hold the authority and don't want to be questioned. Their word stands. Its strength is that young people know that their parents care enough to pay attention to them. They know that they will be watched over.

I really enjoy you. I couldn't always speak openly to my parents. I know that if you think of me as a friend, you'll feel comfortable coming to me. I will spend lots of time with you and we'll have good times together. I trust you to make your own decisions. This is called *permissive parenting*. It is very high in warmth, and love is palpable, but permissive parents set few rules. These parents worry that enforcing limits will create conflicts that may harm their relationships. So, they allow their teens to be responsible for their own decision-making. The strength of this parenting style is that parents and teens care about each another and tend to have warm relationships.

Kids will be kids. I figured it out and so will they. If they get into serious trouble, I'll get involved then. This is called *disengaged parenting*. Disengaged parents neither express their love nor watch closely over their teens. They often have other stressors and find it difficult to closely monitor their teens. This parent may think, "They'll do what they want to do, regardless of what I say." (This is part of the reason all parents must understand how much they do matter!) They remain hands off until their teen is in serious trouble and lay down the law in crisis situations. The strength of this parenting style is that it allows youth independence and enables them to learn from the natural consequences of their actions. (Note: Young people learn better when an adult helps them think through a situation.)

I love you. I am not your friend, I am your parent, and that's even better. I'm going to let you make your share of mistakes, but for the things that might affect your safety, you'll do as I say. And if something you do is not consistent with our values or could compromise your morality, we are going to sit down and think it through together. My job is to keep you safe and stand by you as you become your best self. This is called *balanced parenting* or *lighthouse parenting*. This parenting style is warm, loving, and responsive to an adolescent's needs and is proven through a robust body of research. It includes clear rules and monitoring to protect the teen. Its strengths are that teens raised in this way have the best relationships with their parents and communicate most openly with them.

Why Do the Other Parenting Styles Underperform Compared to Balanced Parenting?

There are likely many reasons that adolescents raised with a balanced parenting style do so well. Teens raised by *authoritarian* parents tend to be well-behaved...*until* they rebel. They delay a lot of concerning behaviors in the early teen years but then, to assert their independence, may participate in negative behaviors in the mid to later teen years. Others do not rebel but feel powerless to make their own choices and decisions and, in worst cases, seek others who will control them later in life.

Teens raised in *permissive* households feel loved but long for boundaries. They may be anxious about letting their parents down by making mistakes. They may engage in risky behaviors, mistakenly assuming they have permission to do so. Most concerning is that, despite parents using this style precisely to foster open communication, repeated studies reveal that teens do not turn to their permissive parents for advice on the most serious subjects. They worry about letting down their parents and, therefore, skip the conversations altogether.

Adolescents raised by *disengaged* parents often have the worst outcomes of all. They may not be aware of the stressors in their parents' lives or the competing demands on their parents' attention. They are unlikely to view their parents' hands-off approach as a nod toward their growing independence. Instead, they may feel ignored or even neglected. They may misbehave and engage in the riskiest behaviors to get their parent's attention.

Remember: love counts most when young people know without question that they are cared for. Monitoring is most effective when adolescents know that the rules exist not to control them but to keep them safe.

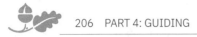

Responsiveness: A Fancy but POWERFUL Word

One of the reasons a balanced parenting style strengthens families is that teens appreciate parents who are responsive to their needs. "Responsive" is a fancy term for flexible. In contrast, controlling or rigid parents can push their children away. Teens appreciate flexible rules that meet their unique needs and recognize and reward their growing displays of responsibility. Perhaps most critically, responsive parents foster open communication within the family. Teens share more fully with their parents when they know it may make a difference. For example, if they make a reasonable case for increased privileges, backed by their proven displays of responsibility and agreement to being appropriately monitored, they may be given increased privileges.

Part 2 of this book offered a foundation in adolescent development. I hope it increased your comfort level with being responsive. Once you can recognize your teen's new capabilities, inflexibility doesn't make a lot of sense. Rigid rules don't allow for growth. Understanding development allows you to better gauge how to link your flexibility to your teen's capabilities. For example, if your tween cannot yet make the connection between their behaviors and consequences, you cannot yet safely loosen your reins.

Prepare Your Teen to Navigate Today's World

You know best the world your child needs to navigate. If your teen is engaged in worrisome behaviors or lives within a dangerous environment, your boundaries *need* to be tighter and your monitoring *needs* to be stricter. If your teen experiences systemic and structural racism, microaggressions, or overt hatred, then raise them to maintain a strong sense of self despite these undermining forces, helping them to stay safe within a world that is not. In these cases, your guidance takes on a justified level of urgency. There is less room for your teen to learn lessons through experience and you may need to be firm about what they can and cannot do. In other words, there are more potential "hand-on-the-stove" moments when you have to jump in quickly or offer explicitly clear warnings.

Being strict or speaking with urgency *does not* make you an authoritarian parent. As you express your passionate thoughts and clear boundaries, make sure your teen knows they come from a place of caring. "I love you, and for that reason, _____," or "You will not _____ because I care about you and cannot allow you to put yourself in danger," or "The world is too dangerous and unpredictable, and you need to know _____ to deal with that reality. You have too much to give to the world and are too precious to me to lose." Key word: balanced. As long as they know your vigilance comes from a place of caring and not a desire to control them, your teen and your relationship will benefit from your approach as a lighthouse parent.

Build on Your Existing Parenting Strengths

I hope you are ready to move toward parenting with a more balanced style. First, reflect on what's been working well and what hasn't. Next, ask yourself from where you've adapted your parenting approach. Most of us parent very much like our parents—or commit to being completely different. Ideally, we'd imitate those aspects of our parents' style that felt right to us and adjust those that didn't. Let's consider your strengths.

- If you currently lean authoritarian, you have a firm commitment to knowing what's going on in your teen's life and to ensuring that they behave appropriately.

- If you currently lean permissive, you care about having a close relationship with your teen.

- If you are less engaged than you'd like, you understand that young people sometimes need to learn from life experiences and gain confidence in knowing how to pick themselves up.

- No matter how you currently approach parenting, you know your cultural values, your community, and the resources available to your family.

Building from these strengths, you can add new communication skills and parenting approaches that will help you achieve that balance of warmth, rules, and responsiveness known to benefit your adolescent and strengthen your family connection.

Adding Balance to an Authoritarian Style

Your strength is that you care about protecting your teen and are committed to guiding them firmly. You will better meet your parenting goals if your teen knows why you feel so strongly about this. When they know it is rooted in your love for them and your concern that their environment or behavior might put them in danger, they will more likely invite your guidance and better understand, perhaps even appreciate, your rules. Keep much of what you are currently doing, and openly share how much you care about your teen by connecting it to why you so fiercely protect them. Remember: balanced parents have the most authority over their adolescent's behaviors.

Adding Balance to a Permissive Style

Many parents today who were raised in strict authoritarian homes opted to have more laid-back relationships with their own teens. In many ways, it paid off. You may have a close relationship, and that is irreplaceable. But many teens raised in this way can become anxious because they learn to self-monitor through guilt and deeply worry about disappointing their parents.

When parents don't set boundaries, teens must set their own but lack the wisdom to know where those boundaries should be placed. By setting appropriate limits, not only do we keep them safer but we remove pressure from them. With a balanced approach, we can be warm and extremely loving while still setting, explaining, and monitoring the rules. When you feel conflicted about being firmer than you'd like, remember 2 things. First, clear boundaries allow adolescents to more safely experiment within limits we've set for them. Viewed from this angle, it offers them freedom and a clearer path toward independence. Second, saying "no" can be a loving act when spoken in the name of protection.

Adding Balance to a Disengaged Style

Your strength is that you know teens need to learn some lessons on their own to develop their increasing independence. And you may have learned some of life's most important lessons on your own. Know, however, that involved parents don't take away independence or diminish lessons; they ensure that life lessons take hold. They hear their teens' thoughts about the choices they are making and then discuss the consequences they experience. Further, balanced parents allow their children to make mistakes and learn how to self-recover. But the clear boundaries they set ensure their children will make those mistakes within safe territory. Finally, when adolescents know they are cared about, they gain the confidence to stretch into new territory in which life's greatest lessons are found.

Bring Other Adults on Board

When I speak at events, I am consistently taken aside by parents who tell me they are personally committed to balanced parenting but struggle with another adult who has a *very* different approach to parenting. I advise them to set aside their frustrations and approach the other adult (spouse, former spouse, grandparent, etc) with the understanding that everyone wants the best for the adolescent. From there, they can both agree that their shared goal is to do what is best for their teen. This strength-based approach leads to the most effective compromises.

If you find yourself in this situation, use the same strategy to nudge that other adult toward a balanced approach that I used with you in the Use Your Existing Strengths and Build New Parenting Strengths section. First, recognize the existing strength of their current approach to parenting. This gives them something to build on and leaves room to add new communication skills to their repertoire. Finally, motivate them by sharing that decades of research and experience has shown balanced parenting leads to the best academic, emotional, and behavioral outcomes for our children and strengthens our families. Invite them to consider how they could balance out what they are currently doing. Perhaps they only need to tell your teen that they watch closely and make rules because they are committed to protect what they love.

A Lighthouse Parent Knows...

You could microchip your teen, put a GPS tracker on the car, and track their phone. You could follow their texting, social media, and computer usage. But a savvy 13-year-old can run circles around most adults with technology. Also, you may make your teen feel like you don't trust them or are trying to control them.

Effective monitoring is about being the kind of parent with whom a teen chooses to share what's going on. We want them to see us as a safety check—so that they can stretch without straying too far. We want being honest to make sense to them. The way we listen tells teens they are free to talk. Controlling our reactions tells them they can talk without fear of being judged.

Your ability to protect your child is not about what you ask; it is about what you know. You can ask questions, but your teen can choose silence or even lie. You want your teen to *choose* to come to you. Lighthouse parents are the most effective monitors *because* they practice the kind of open communication that makes their adolescents include them in their lives. To understand why, you need to remind yourself of 2 key points: (1) teens care about your opinion and (2) they want to be safe. (Remember: we have discarded the myth that teens believe they are invincible!) But they don't want you to intrude on their personal lives, as we discuss in Chapter 27. They want your guidance when it is about keeping them safe. They want you to support their need to venture forth but be ready to pull in the reins when needed.

Imagine, if you were a teen, that you want to "check in" with a parent to get that safety stamp of approval and are open to guidance but do not want intrusion into your life. Who would you turn to? You wouldn't go to the authoritarian parent for advice or permission because you already know the answer—it's no! You wouldn't turn to the permissive parent for nuanced wisdom or the safety check because you know they'll reflexively say yes and you fear disappointing them. You wouldn't go to the disengaged parent because you (perhaps mistakenly) believe they'll respond with, "I don't care." You will go to the lighthouse parent for advice because you know they care and will be thoughtful about safety or actions that might undermine your values.

A Lighthouse Parent Says...

Teens rely on us to consistently hold them to high expectations and for our firm commitment to keep them safe. Above all, they want to be loved. In those moments when our teens push us away, never doubt for a moment that what they need from us remains the same. In fact, they may need it all even more urgently.

WORDS MATTER. Love is most protective when our teens know they are loved. Don't assume they'll know that your actions and decisions are rooted in you caring; use your words to tell them! Our boundaries are closely followed when our teens know *why* we have put them in place. Teens want to know the whys! Sharing the reasoning that drives your decisions also helps them develop their own decision-making skills. Hearing their words matters too! Express yourself clearly and then engage in healthy give-and-take conversations. You'll be amazed hearing your teens' growing wisdom. You'll likely be relieved to know that they are *also* deeply committed to their safety and appreciate you watching out for them. As you hear them out, you'll also learn what steps you can take to be responsive to their needs. Don't be surprised when your teen tells you that your rules are too restrictive, even if they know you set them because you love them. This pushback is part of their growing independence. Respond with, "I hear you that you think my rules are too strict. I am setting them only because I love you and want to keep you safe. As you demonstrate to me that you can stay safe within these boundaries, my goal is to give you more room to stretch." (That's being responsive!)

A LIGHTHOUSE PARENT IS AN ACTIVE GUIDE. You watch out for your child, are firm when you need to be, and loosen the reins as they are able to handle increasing independence. You are always clear that your monitoring is in place because of how deeply you care.

"I cannot allow you to _____ because it is my job to keep you safe and to raise you to be the very best YOU. I love you and that is why I am insisting on _____. I think you can _____, and when you demonstrate that you can handle _____, I will support you fully."

. . . .

Recommended Resource

The Center for Parent and Teen Communication is committed to strengthening family relationships and building youth with the character strengths that will prepare them for healthy, successful, and meaningful lives. It is rooted in lighthouse parenting (https://parentandteen.com).

CHAPTER 27

Steer Them Toward Wise Behaviors

Adolescents appreciate our efforts at keeping them safe and value our desire to raise them to be good people. They welcome us steering them toward good decisions. However, they reject our actions if they feel restrictive, controlling, or belittling.

Teens must figure most things out on their own, but we hold the conversations and create the spaces for them to build their decision-making capacities. We must craft our conversations to ensure we are talking *with* them rather than *at* them. These conversations must recognize their evolving wisdom and growing expertise in their own lives. We must set boundaries with their safety in mind while offering enough flexibility within those boundaries that they know we have no intention of controlling them or keeping them dependent on us.

Adolescents who feel they are being talked *at* or controlled instinctively push back. Why is this an instinctual rather than well-reasoned response? Because being limited defies their developmental needs. They are wired to have their growing wisdom recognized and to be rewarded with increasingly expanded limits. This chapter focuses on striking that sweet spot where *our* protective instincts (we have instincts too!) are satisfied, our need to teach our adolescents valuable life lessons is met, and *their* need to develop is honored.

Permission to Enter Their Lives

The best way to monitor our teens is to have them choose to tell us what is going on in their lives. The book *Adolescents, Families, and Social Development: How Teens Construct Their Worlds,* by Judith Smetana, PhD, shares her research on what adolescents consider parents' "legitimate authority." Breathe; I know that's hard to hear. This means that there are subjects we are welcome to approach and others where we are not. Equipped with this knowledge, we can learn how to optimize our influence in those welcomed areas and to adjust our strategy in those areas we are not.

Good news: teens believe parents should be involved with their safety and have a responsibility to teach society's rules. Hard but important news: teens do not believe parents have free rein to enter personal territory. If the issue is about their friends or personal choices that don't affect safety, laws, or values, your teen may interpret your involvement as an effort to control them or intrude on their growing independence.

This knowledge informs us how to wisely present rules and boundaries— whenever possible, make them about safety or following the law. While some rules will be *always* or *never* rules, those will be limited to dangerous situations. We explain that most rules are in place until adolescents gain more experience or demonstrate the responsibility that shows they can safely manage expanded limits. "Always wear a seat belt. Never drive with any mind-altering substance in your system. You may not drive in bad weather until you gain more driving experience."

This leaves peer relationships as the toughest area to tackle. Adolescents may not believe you are entitled to influence their friendships or what they do with their free time. When possible, frame conversations, even about these topics, as related to safety. "I worry about your hanging out with Jon because he fights a lot, and I don't want you getting hurt." If, however, there is no safety issue to focus on, your efforts to restrict a particular friendship may backfire. You can work on shaping your teen's values and peer-management skills. But when you condemn a friend, you might make that relationship more enticing to your teen as a way of demonstrating their willfulness. Further, they may choose to not share what they're doing in their free time or make up misleading stories. They justify their actions as, "This is my personal life, and my parent never should have gotten into my business."

Basic Knowledge Is a Good Start

We wish knowledge alone ensured wise behavior. If it did, we'd only have to inform young people of the ravages of drugs, for example. Unfortunately, behavior is affected by many other forces. In the case of drugs, a youth might know their dangers but still turn to them to avoid uncomfortable feelings or to break into a new crowd.

But knowledge *is* a great starting point. Find accurate sources to ensure your teen knows how they can be harmed by risky behaviors (eg, harmful substances, putting information on the internet, sexual behaviors). Sharing how these behaviors can be harmful ensures you have the "legitimacy" to address them as safety concerns.

Discipline Is About Teaching

If you were to stand on the sidelines of a high school sporting event and say, "I think my kid needs some discipline," I'm pretty sure the person you'd be talking to would ask, "What did they do wrong?" *Every* young person needs discipline, and that has nothing to do with them doing anything wrong.

The Latin word disciplina, meaning "to instruct or train," is the root of both the words *discipline* and *disciple.* Knowing this, we understand discipline is primarily about teaching or guiding in a loving way, not punishment. It is our privilege to discipline our children because it is how we guide them to walk down good paths. They are deserving of discipline because they are worthy of our loving guidance.

Honoring Their Expertise and Honing Their Wisdom

Good discipline works best when the goal is for the young person to be their best self. If you think about it this way, you'll see that we've been talking about discipline from the very first pages of this book. Through recognizing all that is good and right within them, you created the standard by which they should live. It was not imposed by you; it was merely recognized by you. Next, by viewing them as the expert in their own lives, you acknowledge that they possess wisdom. Your job is not to install wisdom but to help hone theirs.

An Up-front Investment

Our children want our attention. As they grow older, however, they spend less time with us because more of their day is spent in school and at after-school activities. And we may be busy at work, leaving only a short time to focus on them. Because time is limited, we begin focusing on "high-yield" interactions. We tend to focus on school performance or behaviors. Let me be clear: you *should* spend time and energy addressing their behaviors. But if this is the bulk of time you're spending with your teen, they'll learn to act out, intensifying their behaviors to draw you in.

Everything you needed to know about discipline you learned when your child was in kindergarten; catch them being good and redirect them when they're not. Make your high-yield time a pleasure. Be together. Honor the adult taking shape in front of you. Answer their incessant whys and celebrate their idealism. If you do, I suspect you'll see your teen feeling confident that they already have your attention.

If you suspect that your teen acts out to get your attention or is experiencing emotional distress to seek comfort from you, give it to them. I have seen too many parents ignore distressing signals because they didn't want to reinforce attention seeking. If they need it, give it. Moving forward, offer your attention as an investment in your relationship rather than in reaction to a difficult circumstance.

Parenting Style That Supports the Wisest Behaviors

In Chapter 26, we discussed parenting style and its effect on behavior and emotional health. Children raised with *authoritarian* parents toe the line until adolescence but then may rebel with higher rates of worrisome behaviors. Children raised with *permissive* parents may participate in unsafe behaviors and believe they have their parents' implied permission to do so. Those with *disengaged* parents may push their behavior to the extreme to get the attention they crave. Children raised by *lighthouse* parents have the least emotional distress, engage in fewer negative behaviors, and are most likely to talk to their parents about what is going on in their lives.

Don't Get Caught in a Lot of 3rd, 4th, or 10th Chances

To display flexibility (or be nice!), we may offer teens 3rd, 4th, or 10th chances when they don't follow our expectations. Let's look at what this "flexibility" and kindness does to our family relationships. (But first, remember that your teen wants to maximize your attention, for better or worse.) If you make a demand and your teenager doesn't follow your wishes, you'll calmly repeat yourself. Your teenager learns to recognize the pattern and can anticipate how many times you'll repeat yourself before you escalate to anger and possibly give consequences. Your teen will force you to repeat yourself until right before you would reach that escalation point. This means that your relationship will include a lot of nagging and repeating. If they feel they still have not gotten your full attention, they'll take it to the next level with misbehavior. Now you begin threatening consequence. How many times will you threaten? Your teen already knows. It may be 1, 2, or 3 times before they'll worry about receiving a consequence. That's a lot of wasted communication nagging and fighting when you could have been building and strengthening your relationship.

What does this all mean? It means we should make as few rules as possible with our teens so we can invest instead in high-yield interactions. But our teen must follow those rules we do make or receive immediate consequences. I know this seems inconsistent with the tone that I've been setting in this book. Remember my goal is to strengthen your family.

Therefore, I don't want your family interactions wasted in cycles of nagging or hostility. I believe you can make these clear requests and tie them to immediate consequences when your teen knows both your *expectations* and the *consequences* in advance because they helped you set the family rules.

Set Clear Expectations *Together*

Setting expectations for good behaviors and what it means to be a contributing household member improves communication with your teen for several reasons. First, discussing how to help your family function better positions it as a priority. Second, you'll have the opportunity to hear what your teen believes they can handle and learn how they hope to stretch. Also, you will frame this as your need to know that they're being safe and responsible, granting you the legitimacy to set and monitor rules and expectations. This approach also lets your teen know you're willing to trust them and consider their ideas.

Consider sitting down with your teen to craft a written agreement that addresses both your expectations and their desire for increased privileges. Explain that you want to come up with a plan that ensures that (1) your teen will receive greater privileges as they demonstrate they can handle them; (2) you'll be reassured they will be safe and grow to be increasingly responsible; and (3) the household will function better because everyone will know their role in making it run smoothly (ie, chores!). Use this opportunity to let your teen clarify their goals as well. Expect things like, "I hope you notice I'm growing up and can handle more," or, "I want you to learn to trust me more," or, "I want you to allow me to make more of my own choices."

Together, you'll draw up lists of what you each want to achieve your respective goals. You'll match their "wants" with your "needs" to ensure safety. You'll discuss these, negotiate, and come up with a written agreement. This agreement will ensure expectations and consequences are clearly laid out. The agreement helps the teen understand, "I will earn this privilege by showing responsibility and expand it by proving my responsibility. I know I'll lose it if I behave irresponsibly." This makes corrective actions far easier to take. (We discuss this further in Chapter 29.)

The final agreement has 3 columns. The first is the parents' expectations or wants. The second is the teenager's "wants." And the third is the consequences for the teenager not following the expectations. The more input your teen has, the more likely they'll happily implement the agreement. This is an opportunity for your teen to consider what they are ready to handle and what they cannot. It will help them think through the benefits and disadvantages of certain actions. This is discipline in the truest sense of the word because it catalyzes learning.

The following are some useful tips when creating your own family agreement:

- All adults in the home should speak with a common voice. Adult disagreements should be handled privately beforehand.

- Let your teen know you will listen to their wants, but you will decide what you consider safe and reasonable.

- Clearly state your "absolutes." These are permanent rules that exist for your teen's safety (for example, not being a passenger of an impaired driver).

- Let your teens take the lead in stating the privileges they think they can handle. It is your job is to determine if their request is reasonable or too far of a reach. With each request, you place clear boundaries. They may need guidance into which areas you consider open for discussion. Possibilities include phone/computer privileges, curfew, car privileges, going places independently, and dating.

- After your teen has laid out their wants, fill in your needs. You can also start new points listing your "wants."

- Let your teen run through some what-if scenarios. "What if I come home late and haven't called?" "Well, what if I am going to be late but call to tell you what the problem is and how I'm handling it?" This will help your teen solidify their understanding of the rules and know the limits of your flexibility.

- Encourage your teen to negotiate. You are the ultimate limit setter and certain misbehaviors are nonnegotiable, but they will more likely follow through on understandings they've had a role in reaching. Also, they will have learned useful give-and-take skills for future negotiations with peers, teachers, or bosses.

- Let your teen know that when they demonstrate responsible behavior for 2 to 3 months, you will revisit the agreement to consider expanded privileges. This will make them more motivated to follow through on commitments.

- Try to focus on verifiable items. For example, you'll know when your child arrives home. You won't know if they use unacceptable language outside of the home, so don't put that in an agreement.

The following table is an example of just a few elements of what might be in a much longer agreement.

Jason's Family Agreement		
Mom and Dad's Wants/Needs	**Jason's Wants/Needs**	**Consequences**
We need to know you'll be a safe driver. We insist on the following: No passengers in your car for 6 months No cell phone use while driving Following the graduated driver licensing laws in the state, including curfew laws	Now that I have my license, I want to be able to drive on my own.	Jason understands that having a license is a privilege and if any of these rules are not followed, he will lose driving privileges for at least 30 days.
For the house to run smoothly, we need you to empty and fill the dishwasher every night and do your own laundry. We also need you not to leave your sports equipment in the living room.	I agree to help with the assigned chores. I can't promise my room will always be spotless, but I'll keep the shared spaces clean.	Jason understands he can't leave the house until the dishwasher is filled and his laundry is thrown in the hamper. If he is unable to keep this commitment, he won't be allowed to leave the house the next day.
We agree to these curfew requests if your schoolwork is completed before you go out. We need to know where you are going and who you will be with. We need you to be easily reachable by phone.	I want to be able to stay out until 11:00 pm on weekends and 9:30 pm on weeknights.	If Jason is unable to handle the responsibility of staying out late, his privileges will return to the curfew he proved he could handle—10:00 pm on weekends and 8:30 pm on weeknights.

Teens *Do* Appreciate Our Watchful Presence

You need to know your teen is staying within safe boundaries. Your teen has the developmental need to stretch their limits. This creates a natural tension between our need to keep them safe and their need to grow. Well-thought-out boundaries, however, give them more room to grow! Within safely prescribed boundaries, they can confidently have new experiences and comfortably learn from their mistakes. To get this right, you'll expand your teen's boundaries as they can safely handle more freedoms—more room for growth! They'll likely not tell you, but they'll appreciate your presence in their lives and may use it as a safety check to ensure they have an excuse to do the right thing. You know who *will* know you're a good monitor? Their friends. Your teen may say, "I'm being watched like a hawk. I could never get away with that!"

Steering Them Toward Their OWN Solutions

In Chapter 18, we discussed how lectures were *not* the way to go when guiding our teen's behaviors. Recall that when we talk *at* them with lectures, they hear, "Whaa whaa whaa...and you will get hurt or die." Why? Because the lecture follows an abstract mathematical structure: "Your behavior now could lead to a terrible outcome depending on whether a series of mysterious variables occurs or not." Our goal is to help adolescents "own" their solutions because they have thought things through themselves. We get them there by adjusting the mathematical structure of how we guide them so they understand point by point until they get it...get it...get it... almost there...got it! I call this the *cognitive aha experience*. Our goal is to help them think through real-life consequences of what may seem like casual decisions.

To achieve the cognitive aha, we talk *with* them as we break our thoughts into separate steps and invite them to engage with us. "Do you see how A might go to B? Do you have any experience with something like B? Tell me about it. Do you see how B might lead to C? Has that ever happened to anyone you know? What would that feel like to you?" Pause after each point and give them time to think things through and express their thoughts. The pauses could last seconds, hours, or days. What matters is that the guidance happens at the pace they can absorb. The following scenarios point out some lectures to avoid followed by strategies better suited to help your child understand your concerns, while allowing them space to understand the issue for themselves:

Avoid the Lecture on Drugs

"If you even begin trying drugs, it's a slippery slope toward the rest of your life falling apart. First, you'll fall into the wrong crowd and be influenced by them in ways you can't imagine. Then it's only a matter of time until your grades slip, you'll lose your focus, and many of your future plans won't come true. You're dreaming of becoming an architect. People don't get through college being addicted to drugs. It tears their families apart and many of them end up dead."

Try This Conversation Instead

"I worry so much about drug use because I've seen it devastate people's lives. I care about your safety and your well-being and can't imagine you doing anything to mess that up. What are your thoughts about drug use?" Pause. Listen. "Do any of the kids in your class use drugs?" Pause. Listen. "What have you noticed about how their behaviors changed once they began using drugs?" Pause. Listen. "I want to make sure you know why I worry about drugs. Do you feel like you understand why they can be dangerous?" Pause. Listen. "A lot of young people know they're dangerous, but they also think they can't get hooked. How do you think people first become involved with drugs?" Pause. Listen. "Well, what would you say if your friends asked you to try it once so you'd know what it would be like?" Pause. Listen. From there, you can move into peer negotiation skills.

Avoid the Lecture About School

"There is only one good way to reach your dreams and that's through your education. But you have to stay focused and put your heart into it. All I'm seeing from you, frankly, is laziness. You're not focusing on your homework and I am worried your grades are going to drop terribly. Colleges care about grades—it all counts now. If you don't get into the college of your choice, then there's a good chance you're never going to get to the career you want. Too many people work at something they don't even care about and you're headed there if you don't quickly change your attitude about school."

Try This Conversation Instead

"I've noticed you're spending less time on your homework. Am I right about that?" Pause. Listen. "What do you think explains why you're not focused as much on schoolwork?" Pause. Listen. "School is just a phase of your life. What kind of things interest you that you could imagine being part of your future career?" Pause. Listen. "What kind of an education do you think helps you enter that career?" Pause. Listen. "What will it take for you to get to that next step in your education?" Pause. Listen. "How can I support you now?" Note: if a barrier such as a difficult subject or an overly critical teacher is raised, this is your opportunity to help your teen navigate through that issue.

Avoid the Lecture About Peers

"I know you're having fun with this group of kids, but they're a terrible influence on you. I don't know all of them, but I do know Lisa and I know her family. She is allowed to get away with everything. She talks back to her parents and I'm not going to have that kind of behavior in this house. I even heard she was caught shoplifting and drinks a lot. If you begin hanging out with kids like this, it's only a matter of time before your grades begin dropping and you'll think that our rules don't apply to you."

Try This Conversation Instead

"I know you're hanging out with a new group of friends. What are they like?" Pause. Listen. "I notice you're less focused on your team than you used to be. Am I right about that?" Pause. Listen. "My concern is, and will always be, that you follow your own values. What kind of things are most important to you when you choose a friend?" Pause. Listen. "In life, you will always have relationships with people with different values or who will push you to do things against your better judgment. How do you handle it when that happens with your peers?" Pause. Listen. "Is there anyone in your group who you're worried is pushing the group in the wrong direction? I don't need their name; I just want to know how you plan on still maintaining your own values." Pause. Listen. Advise if asked.

••

Recommended Resource

The Center for Parent and Teen Communication offers a deeper dive into discipline strategies including guidance on holding family meetings (https://parentandteen.com/category/communication-strategies/discipline-monitoring).

CHAPTER 28

When to Jump In (and When to Watch From a Distance)

A dolescence is a time seemingly designed to allow humans to make mistakes so they can learn to recover from them. First, the developing teen brain drives adolescents to stretch into new territories. In parallel, their quest for independence pushes them to challenge boundaries. Above all, teens seem to have an inborne ability to rebound from errors and grow from challenges and in the process become intensely aware of their limitations and begin to see their strengths. However, for adolescents to optimally reap the benefits from their experiences, we adults have to let them gain the knowledge they've *earned*. But it can be difficult to watch from the sidelines. It becomes easier when we remember adolescents are much safer making their mistakes under our watchful eyes than if they made those mistakes in adulthood when the stakes would be much higher.

Your challenge as a parent is to let your child experience the natural consequences from their actions while continually protecting them from circumstances that could cause irreparable harm or threaten their safety. This means you have to create limits beyond which they cannot stray and have a game plan for when you will jump in.

So, When *Do* I Jump In?

I imagine the "Who am I?" question of identity as a 1,000-piece jigsaw puzzle. Your teen finds all the pieces laying haphazard and (mistakenly!) believes that they have a limited time to complete the puzzle. Your first role, therefore, is to offer guidance before they even begin to grapple with the pieces. Offer reassurance that these questions of identity take a lifetime to answer and that each of us are given ample opportunity to reconsider our roles and remake ourselves as we grow. Share that it is sometimes our missteps—even failures—and the reflection that follows that provide us the opportunity to rebound even stronger and come up with wiser solutions. Your point will be taken more to heart if you demonstrate that even you remain committed to continued personal growth because you see yourself as a work in progress. (That's a good thing, not an insult ☺!)

Although these reassurances might give your teen a chance to catch their breath, they are likely still going to get to work to complete that puzzle as quickly as they can. There are just too many pressures to ignore. So, what is your role? Think about where they'd begin putting together what seems like an incredibly complex puzzle.

The Edges: Creating Clear Boundaries

They'd likely get started with the corners and then build the edges. *A parent's job is to create the edges of the puzzle.* You do this by defining clear boundaries and making sure your teen does not stray beyond them. In fact, they must understand there are consequences for attempting to go beyond those boundaries. Flexibility is an important part of being a responsible parent for a teen. So, it is likely you will expand those boundaries later, when it is clear they can handle new limits. But it is vitally important to know when flexibility hurts our adolescents. We need to create firm, consistent, and inviolable boundaries surrounding issues that involve safety and serious challenges to moral behaviors. Your adolescent might complain that your boundaries are rigid, but, if you've correctly placed them around safety and morality issues, they will, in truth, make your teen feel secure. These clear boundaries offer them the security to take healthy risks elsewhere. It offers them the edges they can push against but never stray beyond (see Chapter 29 for advice on what to do if they do stray).

Similar Colors: Show What It Means to Be an Adult

Now that the borders are in place, what's their next step in putting together the puzzle? They'd gather together the pieces of the same color. They'd look at the red pieces and wonder, "Will they be roses, balloons, or fire engines?" Lacking the patience to find out, they might cheat by looking at the picture on the box. *You are the picture on the box.* Remember, you are raising your teen to be a healthy 35-, 40-, or 50-year-old. When you model what it means to be a thoughtful, caring adult, you allow them to understand what it looks like to be an adult. When you model an adult who is reflective and considerate of how your actions affect others and how your choices are made with consideration for future consequences, you paint them a vivid portrait of the kind of adult they might be in the future.

The Middle: Watching and Trusting From Afar

What's next? The borders are in place, and they've grouped those pieces that easily hang together. They've reminded themself of the vision and have a picture in their mind's eye that they can strive toward. They look at all the leftover pieces and become frustrated by their irregular and jagged edges. The matches are no longer easy to find. They try to fit them together and sometimes find the perfect match. Other times, they force some pieces together but realize they'll have to look further to get it right. Placing together those inner puzzle pieces involves imagination, experimentation, trial and error, and mistakes. It often involves starting over.

The middle of the puzzle is your teen's job. It is within the safe boundaries you've set. You can get out of the way as they master the puzzle piece by piece and ultimately accomplish the task. You support your teen's development most when you watch from afar, trusting in their ability to solve the puzzle. But you remain available for guidance when asked and lend your calm and emotional support when their frustration rises to the point of discomfort.

This is yet another balancing act. But now you have language you can ask yourself as challenges arise. In fact, it has become the language of many of the families I have cared for as a pediatrician. Parents ask themselves, "Is this issue on the inside or outside of the puzzle's edge?" If it's inside, breathe…and remind yourself that you have ensured that your child is safe. Many of my teen patients, in fact, have learned to say to their parents, "I've got this. This is within the puzzle edges." If your teen is having an outside-the-edges moment, dive in!

You May Not Like This...

The fact that something is inside the puzzle edges doesn't mean it's easy for your teen. It just means that it is important they try to handle it on their own. Here, I offer 2 examples, and I suspect they will both feel uncomfortable because not fixing your child's discomfort may go against your parental instinct.

- School is on the inside of the puzzle edges. In fact, an effective education will sharpen your teen's talents by helping them learn more about their strengths and limitations. This process will certainly involve your teen experiencing some failure, but there is no real safety issue and little possibility of irreparable harm. Further, your teens are surrounded by youth development professionals—teachers and counselors—who know how to support them.

- The social slights your teen will likely endure will be devastating to them but are also within the puzzle's edges (bullying is not!). Through these unpleasantries, your teen will build skills to manage unpleasant personal interactions that they'll find throughout their lives in workplaces and community settings. They'll learn what matters to them in relationships. They'll also likely be given opportunities to clarify their values.

In both cases, be there with your unwavering support. Offer guidance when asked. Lend your calm, but do not dive in to fix problems. If you become involved with every one of their missteps, your teen will not gain the most out of the opportunities they are given to grow while still under your protective—but not intrusive—gaze.

If it's outside the puzzle edges, follow your protective instinct. Turn the page to learn when and how to react.

CHAPTER 29

Course Corrections and Corrective Actions

O ur goal is to have our teens learn self-control and develop wise behaviors. If something provides a lesson, it is discipline. If it only makes people feel badly, it is a punishment—which is not discipline. Discipline can involve *course corrections* or *corrective actions*. Course corrections steer toward a safer or wiser direction and include conversations or seeking professional help. Corrective actions are the consequences given to solidify a lesson. They are also meant as guidance but are specific actions given in response to a misbehavior or clear demonstration of irresponsibility.

Our message of unconditional love, even in the face of disappointment over a recent behavior, remains critical. If our goal is to teach our teens, we have to draw them nearer precisely in the moments their behavior is most challenging. The core message must be, "Your behavior is unacceptable, but I love you and you remain fully accepted." We approach discipline with firm values and an unshakable commitment to our teen's safety but with a soft touch.

Remember that it is our love that drives our anger when our kids are misbehaving. Reflect on that. We become angry because we love so much and care so deeply. We become angry because we know our kids can do better. Let your anger be a reminder of how much you care. That will move you to the calmer place from which you can think through the best course corrections. If, on the other hand, your decisions are made while angry, you may overshoot with consequences and your teen may feel punished and, if so, will not have learned anything.

Course Corrections

As a lighthouse parent, you are keeping an eye on the horizon. There are times you will watch from a distance and times when you will gently (or quickly!) ensure your teen steers away from a problem.

When *Not* to Offer a Course Correction

There are moments when life is the best teacher. Stand from the sidelines and be available for guidance when asked. Model a learner's mindset from which you try to grow from inevitable error. Talk out loud about this. Your teen will be listening.

Also know that you may see backward movement first from your teen in key developmental moments—acting out, moodiness, or a loss of confidence. To a young person, each major step in development can feel as though they must cross a 10-foot-wide chasm. Knowing they'll need a running start to travel across it, they'll first take a few steps back to pick up enough speed. Then, as they leap, they'll likely cover their eyes. So don't assume a bit of backward movement is a sign of danger. It might be the first sign that real forward movement is *about* to happen. Remain watchful to ensure your teen doesn't slip too far backward, but stay cautiously optimistic that you'll like what you see when they reach the other side.

Another time not to take any action is when you don't *yet* know what to do. Don't act out of anger. Don't guess what to do. It's fine to say, "I/we need to think about this. Right now, I need to ensure that you'll stay safe, so for now you must _____. After we've had time to calm down, we'll sit down with you and together come up with our best thought-out plan." This gives you time to reflect and models a thoughtful and collaborative way to deal with challenges.

Steer Quickly in the Face of Danger

If your child is having a "hand-on-the-stove" moment, there is no room to think, and quick action is needed to guarantee their protection. This will likely be for circumstances unexpected by you, even if you have agreements in place and solid boundaries set. It's OK to act before you've had time to reflect, even if you're boiling hot angry. You can pull out the firmest consequences, including grounding. Typically, grounding is a poor teaching tool because it is too broad and is not clearly associated with "the crime." But it makes sense when your teen needs to be pulled from a dangerous environment or separated from peer interactions. It buys you time to sort things out and figure out what extra support your child needs to stay safe or to lessen their emotional distress. It also gives your teen a peer-management skill where they can say, "Of course I want to meet you, but I'm not allowed out of the house. If I leave, I won't be able to use the car for a year! They're making me check in with them every hour while they're at work to prove I'm home."

The Most Important Course Corrections

When your child is in serious emotional distress or is engaging in dangerous risk behaviors, they are deserving of more support than I can offer through this book. However, I will guide you on how to support your teen to accept professional support in Chapter 39 and address how to strengthen your relationship even through these challenging times in Chapters 36 through 39.

Many parents experience self-blame when their child is not doing well. I plead for you to let that go. **Good parents can't prevent all challenges in their children's lives, but what they can do is stand by their side and provide the support they deserve.** If you see your child's struggles as a personal failure, it will become a barrier for you to do what you need to do. Hear this: it is also likely an inaccurate interpretation of what created the problem. Know this: you *are* a critical part of the solution.

Your role in crisis situations can boil down to the following essential elements:

- Help your teen know they will get through this time with you by their side. Your knowledge of all that is good and right in them will remain their North Star.

- Steer quickly to prevent your child from being in immediate danger. This involves putting firm, inviolable boundaries in place and finding emergency professional evaluation if necessary.

- Be open to exploring the *why* behind their behaviors. Acting out behaviors are often masks for intense feelings. In the middle of a crisis, you are likely better off just remaining present instead of asking questions. But with ongoing issues (such as drug use), learning the *why* positions you to create a better plan for moving forward.

- Engage professional support for long-term treatment or healing.

Corrective Actions

Corrective actions teach lessons through consequences. Wisely selected consequences can be lessons in cause and effect and in personal accountability. On the other hand, if the corrective action does not logically follow what your teen did, it can't teach personal accountability, and it's not a consequence at all. It will be experienced more like a punishment designed to exact a toll rather than teach a lesson. In a teen's mind, parents cede the moral high ground when the corrective actions feel worse than the "crime." They'll become frustrated, resent how random and unfair your behavior is, and may even want to get even ("I'll show them! I'll never...").

Common Corrective Actions

Overly harsh or illogical actions sends the message to your teen, "You aren't in control. We, your parents, control what happens to you. There's no logical connection between your actions and what happens to you." This undermines the point of discipline. Let's consider a couple of common corrective actions to see the difference between their use as punishment versus their appropriate use as a consequence.

Cell Phone Use and Other Electronics

Parents often take away cell phone privileges for relatively minor infractions. To parents, it makes sense because they know this will sting their children a bit but, in the grander scheme of things, feels like a minor consequence. After all, there are many other things to do than text friends. But to a teen, this cuts off their contact with the world and it is a *very* big deal.

Loss of Cell Phone Privilege as Punishment

Bobbi was supposed to help her mother clean the house for a family reunion. She became caught up in decorating for a party at a friend's house and arrived home late. Bobbi lost the use of her cell phone for a week. Debrief: helping around the house is not connected to having contact with friends. Bobbi was engaged in an activity that felt important to her and got distracted. She wasn't thoughtful of her mother's needs but had no ill intent. She broods in her room in anger and refuses to attend the reunion.

Loss of Cell Phone Privileges as a Consequence

Arun has been falling asleep in class. He plays video games until midnight and then does his homework into the wee hours of the morning. His parents restrict his cell phone and computer use until his homework is completed, unless it is being used for schoolwork. All computers and phones are docked in a common space after 11:00 pm. Debrief: Arun understands that his parents care about his schoolwork and his well-being and see the phone and computer as distractions. They don't restrict him from all social connections with his friends, but they set boundaries to protect time for homework and sleep. Arun misses being able to game in the evenings. But he realizes he has been struggling in school because of daytime fatigue. At first, he complains about the restrictions. After a couple of weeks, he realizes he is learning more in class because he is less fatigued. This enables him to breeze through homework, leaving some time for gaming.

Grounding

Parents ground their children for serious infractions. It makes parents feel better because they don't have to worry about where their kid is. But to a young person, it is entirely taking away their ability to be social and to meet their developmental need to stretch their wings.

Use of Grounding as a Punishment

Petra was supposed to be home at 9:00 pm but didn't arrive until 10:30 pm. She hadn't called to say she was running late and wasn't responding to texts, which was unusual for her. Her parents became worried sick. They were on the phone with the police when she walked in. Angry and frightened, they shouted, "Petra, you are grounded for 2 weeks!" Debrief: her parents acted out of anger, and grounding their daughter made a lot of sense because, in their mind, she was in danger and doing anything, such as grounding her, to protect her seems perfectly reasonable. The problem is that Petra knows she was never in danger and, therefore, the punishment doesn't make sense to her. She storms off to her room and pledges to herself that she will sneak out.

Use of Grounding as a Consequence (and Protection)

Jayden was supposed to be home at 9:00 pm but didn't arrive until 10:30 pm. He was drunk and disrespectful to his parents. When they said they wanted to talk to him, he told them they had no right to interfere with his life and that he had friends who really understood him. His parents had noticed his behavior had been changing since he was hanging out with a new friend group. They were worried he was putting himself in danger with these friends and grounded him for 2 weeks, making it clear that if he broke those rules there would be much greater consequences. They expressed concern about his safety and stated they needed time to sort out a plan to ensure his safety. Debrief: Jayden feels like he's being treated like a baby and his parents don't understand what it's like to be a teen nowadays. He'll never say this to them, but he appreciates that they are paying attention. He is angry for a couple of days but he also gains the opportunity to reflect because he is in a safe environment. He thinks that the guys he's been hanging out with are really cool and he's flattered that he's been welcomed into this friend group. But he also notices that they haven't been taking school seriously. He dreams of being a lawyer and doesn't want to mess that up.

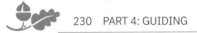

Sticking to Predetermined Consequences

We can create written agreements, as described in Chapter 27, that essentially say, "I will earn this freedom or privilege by showing responsibility and will keep this freedom by continually proving my responsibility. I know I will lose this freedom when I do not show I can be responsible." This makes applying consequences easy for you. If your teen has behaved irresponsibly, you revoke a privilege until they demonstrate responsibility long enough to earn it back. Even better if you don't need to take away a privilege entirely. Pay attention to what your teen can handle so you can return them to their point of demonstrated responsibility. Cause and effect in action. It will make full sense to your teen and, even if they don't like it, they will know it's fair because you're letting them operate at the limits of their demonstrated responsibility.

Revise the contract every 2 to 3 months to create a clear record of past successes— levels of freedoms your child has proven they can handle. When you need to come up with a fair consequence, you can revert to a freedom your child proved able to handle in the past. This works most seamlessly for privileges related to time. For example, "You said that if you stayed out until 8:00 pm, you would have time to finish your homework. You didn't finish your homework. You'll have to begin coming in at 7:30 pm again."

Is It Too Late to Make This Shift?

I am often asked whether it is possible to begin this approach to discipline if a teen is already 16 or 17 years old? Yes. Tell your teen that you've noticed how they have matured and that you want them to safely stretch into new territory. Tell them this approach is what gives you the confidence to increase their privileges as they can handle them, because you'll remain confident that they are safe. Most teens will get on board when they understand these are not new restrictions; these are paths toward their developing independence.

CHAPTER 30

Helping Our Teens Rise Above the Noise and Find Their Own Rhythm

Maria Veronica Svetaz, MD, MPH
Tamera Coyne-Beasley, MD, MPH
Kenneth R. Ginsburg, MD, MS Ed, FAAP

*This chapter is written with Maria Veronica Svetaz, MD, MPH, and Tamera Coyne-Beasley, MD, MPH, who are 2 of the great leaders and visionaries in adolescent medicine. I (Ken Ginsburg) focus in this chapter on bullying. Drs Svetaz and Coyne-Beasley focus on preparing parents of Color to guide their children on how to surmount racism and undermining expectations. Both Drs Svetaz and Coyne-Beasley are parenting children of Color, and both are personal heroes of mine. You can benefit from reading this chapter, whether or not your own child has experienced bullying or racism. We **all** gain from better understanding the strategies to build resilience in the context of unique challenges. We **all** need to learn how to be allies to teens and families enduring challenges.*

We've spoken about recognizing all that is good and right in your teen. We've spoken about the security your unwavering and unconditional love offers your adolescent as they launch into adulthood. We've underscored this point with the message that the reason your love holds so much power is that it enables your teen to know they are worthy of being loved. Knowing that the person who knows them best sees them as they deserve to be seen, as they really are, confers lifelong protection.

Your love exists in the same reality in which your teen may be navigating deeply undermining forces, which we will call "noise." This noise most often is a sound that is noticeably unpleasant, unwanted, disruptive, distracting, and disturbing. Your presence helps them especially when they receive troubling messages or noise from other sources. There are many potential sources of undermining noise, but it can be broken into

2 broad categories, *interpersonal interactions* and *structural and systemic biases,* that convey low expectation or even denigrate individuals or groups. These destructive biases tear people down. Although people who endure them may display resilience, they do so at a significant cost. Young people exposed to these biases can internalize negative messages about their own worth, leading to negative self-talk where they blame themselves for their victimization. We will use bullying in this chapter as the example of destructive interpersonal interactions and racism as the example of destructive structural and systemic biases.

Your love *is* protective, but we also must prepare our teens to navigate these noises. We must build within them the shields that will lessen the likelihood that these noises will touch their sense of inner value. We all need to commit to eliminate these biases from the lives of our teens for good. After all, we belong to each other, and advocacy for all is the way to ensure we all do better as a society.

This chapter cannot do justice to the topics we are about to touch on. We encourage you to pursue further knowledge through some of the suggested resources at the end of this chapter and to join in solidarity with other families navigating the same waters.

Family Connection Is Vital, but Teens Have to Be Prepared for a Complicated World

Although young people equipped with internal motivation and surrounded by adults who believe in them will rise to be their best selves, that doesn't tell the full story. If the complete story is not told, we run the risk of harming our teens. If our internally motivated teenagers believe the only extra ingredient needed for them to succeed is being surrounded by caring adults, how are they to interpret it if low expectations from a teacher or bullying from a peer knocks them off-kilter so that they cannot function? How will they interpret it when barriers make it harder for them to succeed? If they believe all they need is internal determination and external validation from their family, then the only thing they have left to blame when their dreams are not realized is themselves.

We must tell young people the whole truth, because it is liberating from the pain of thinking they are deserving of low expectations and negative perceptions. We must not allow our teens to believe it is their fault that others hold stereotypes and biases about them. There is no doubt young people respond positively to the unconditional love and high expectations they get in caring homes. But that may not be enough to counter the noise of low expectations, distorted reflections of their being (stereotyping), and barriers that exist outside of the home. Teens should recognize these negative biases, name them, and, as best they can, put strategies into place to not succumb to them, while we work to dismantle them.

Responding to Interpersonal Interactions

Bullying

As I (Ken) pointed out in Chapter 12, bullying is *not* a normal rite of passage for young people. It is a toxic stress and is unacceptable. It harms identity development and runs the risk that adolescents internalize their tormentors' views.

The following are key tips to help your teen deal with bullying:

- Do not tell your teen to ignore the bullying. You likely would not know about it if they were able to successfully ignore it. Let them know that you understand how hurtful it can be and offer them your empathy. Check in on their level of distress and help them understand they are deserving of professional support (see Chapter 39).

- Listen to your teen describe what they are experiencing. They may hold too much shame to tell you specifics about what is being said about them or the discomfort they are experiencing. Do not push them to disclose, but let them know you are comfortable hearing anything they want to share.

- Because being a victim may (falsely) make someone feel weak, acknowledge their strength and courage in sharing their story with you.

- Let them know that being a victim of bullying is *not* their fault; bullying is a problem owned by the person who bullies. This person feels as though they have to make others feel powerless. They are missing how important it is to treat every person with respect.

- Tell your teen that you love them fully and accept them completely. (This is urgently important if your teen is being bullied about their sexual orientation or gender identity.)

- If the bullying is happening in school or another adult-supervised activity, insist that the setting adopt a "no-bullying" standard and implement evidence-based interventions as described in Chapter 12. These approaches do more than reduce bullying; they ensure there are more peer champions in these environments. This will prevent your teen from feeling isolated, because the community of peers will stand behind them.

- Do not expect your teen to take the steps to initiate anti-bullying policies; these should be driven through your advocacy and school or program personnel.

- There are circumstances where your teen can take active steps to prevent the person who bullies from having access to them. If the bullying is coming from a virtual platform, the person who bullies can be blocked. If people who bully do not have access to the person they are interested in hurting, they may lose interest. If nothing else, it truly "shuts out the noise," preventing exposure to the hurtful, undermining messages. When cyberbullying occurs and is unresolved, it is important to document and report the behavior so that it can be addressed. Reports can be shared with schools, online service providers, and law enforcement. If there is a person who bullies in a non–adult-supervised space that can be avoided, your teen should take steps to avoid contact. An example is your teen avoiding the corner or part of the neighborhood where a person who bullies prefers to hang out.

- Ensure your teen spends time with positive peers who affirm and accept them. These teens are likely found in the same setting where the bullying might be happening, such as school, but also can be found in different settings, such as sports, clubs, or places of worship. This is another reason why young people should have more than one circle of peers.

- Use your teen's new awareness around bullying to learn to be an ally for those who are being bullied in their presence.

- If your own child or teen is a person who bullies others, they also need a space to heal. Ensure they receive the psychological support and care that addresses why they are behaving in this manner.

Responding to Structural and Systemic Biases

Racism

Racism will create noise and pain for your teen, and it will likely impact you in the same way. Race itself is a social construct. In other words, it is not rooted in biology. There are strikingly few biological differences between races. Rather, "race" is something that has been created to justify the inequitable distribution of power and resources among different communities. These imbalances limit the ability for some to reach their full potential and, in the end, harm everyone in our society, as we are interdependent beings.

As a parent, racism affects you on both a personal level and as a caregiver. Think about the drill we all learn before a flight: when necessary to use, you need to put on your oxygen mask first, so you are best able to help your children. We need to protect ourselves first to buffer our children from the dangers and undermining forces in their lives. Experiencing racism (bias, discrimination, and/or stereotyping around race or ethnicity) can be exhausting and can erode your energy and affect the reserve you need for parenting.

As we feel the toll of holding spaces and bearing witnesses to too many acts of racism, we must invest in our own healing as a key step to restore the energy needed to protect and eventually empower our children. We recommend the book, *Mindful of Race: Transforming Racism from the Inside Out*, by Ruth King, to support our healing. We should also reach out to find or create common spaces where other parents from similar cultural and spiritual backgrounds support each other. We best meet challenges when standing shoulder to shoulder!

Racial-Ethnic Identity

There are many identities our child can choose, and many ways they might want to belong. Our teen's *racial-ethnic identify* refers to how they identify with or feel they belong to an ethnic group. Developing a *positive* racial-ethnic identity is essential to a teen's well-being as their sense of self develops. Parents and caregivers can be critical guides in coaching them to successfully achieve this task.

Ethnic identity is a journey—one that needs reflective, thoughtful consideration about our world and where we feel welcomed or where we feel excluded. One needs to process the meaning of belonging to a group, while exploring the beauty of strengths passed to them from their parents and family. Ultimately, we all need to decide where we fit in. Usually, this is an ongoing process, and, most of the time, it starts to be explored during adolescence. As parents, we need to allow room for our children to explore this, without judging, without despair, but with safe and open hearts.

Racial-Ethnic Socialization

The process of transferring roots and traditions to our children should start early and through all types of conversations and actions, from combing hair to preparing food; from discussing and analyzing how groups are represented, misrepresented, or not represented in media and social media to discussing and analyzing how racism affects our schools, neighborhoods, and families. These conversations should include what we can do about this, as individuals, as families, and as societies. Actions can include participating in a march and voting for leaders committed to building a stronger society. As we support our teens to take positive, meaningful action, it helps them become agents of change. This whole process is called *racial-ethnic socialization.* It serves as a potent antidote to internalized racism. The best way to make sure our young people will be able to reject negative noise and biases is to have a positive, affirming racial-ethnic identity. This will not block the undermining effects of racism entirely, but it will shield our children whether they witness discrimination, experience it directly, or recognize it in negative mass media (mis)representations of people who share their background. Conversations can help young people process past encounters and make sense of future experiences. Most importantly, it positions us to address their questions.

Racial socialization messages can be distinguished in 4 general categories.

- **Cultural socialization:** promoting ethnic pride and transmitting knowledge about cultural history and heritage.
- **Self-worth:** emphasizing positive views of oneself.
- **Preparation for bias:** preparing children and youth to adapt to and operate within a world in which race plays such a large role, including exposure to prejudice and discrimination. This prepares youth for experiences of racial discrimination and provides strategies for coping.
- **Egalitarianism:** emphasizing that all people are equal and deserve equal rights and opportunities.

Research on racial-ethnic socialization has shown that enhancing cultural pride and preparing young people to recognize and deal with bias is associated with better outcomes in teens—better adjustment, including higher self-esteem, improved academic engagement and performance, fewer behavior problems, and reduced depressive symptoms. This means that strategies that provide youth of Color with positive parental modeling and clear messages that emphasize racial-ethnic pride and promote learning about one's heritage offer powerful protection. A well-developed racial-ethnic identity may help youth of Color distinguish between actions directed at them as individuals versus those directed at them as a member of their group. Ultimately, it prepares them to lead an effort to dismantle biases and racism.

Racial-ethnic socialization incorporates *political socialization*—the development of critical thinking that allows youth to recognize and analyze dimensions of power and authority. These socialization processes have been well documented among African American youth and their families, and several authors (particularly Janie Victoria Ward) have described this work as "raising resisters." Ward has extensively researched how to prepare youth to resist and has written work on how to support parents of Color in this process. The word "resist" here is not used to imply that any action should be taken toward any other person or group. Rather, it is about resisting the internalization of undermining messages or evaluations. It is about the "self-creation" of a new positive and valued identity. It is about developing the ability to hear and incorporate elevated messages rooted in accurate assessments of who they really are, rather than incorporating into their sense of selves harmful messages rooted in bias or discrimination. It can involve creating an "oppositional gaze," where one figuratively looks away from destructive noise while looking toward those who will share the truth about who they really are.

Although resisting can be highly protective, it also takes a serious toll on our children and teens. Maria Trent, MD, MPH, a professor of pediatrics, public health, and nursing at Johns Hopkins University and the lead author of the American Academy of Pediatrics policy statement, "The Impact of Racism on Child and Adolescent Health," states, "The concept of 'shutting out the noise' means that youth (and adults) of Color must continually learn how to evaluate other people's behavior toward them or those like them, decide the important outcome to consider, and choose their actions or their battles carefully. Isabel Wilkerson describes this moment when parents of children of Color realize that they must shatter the innocence of childhood so their children can learn to protect themselves at very young ages." She goes on to explain the difficult balancing act youth of Color must achieve as they learn to self-advocate, while limiting how doing so interrupts their own goals. Dr Trent continues, "Shutting out the noise may also mean that a youth navigating adolescence in environments with limited diversity must make careful decisions about the daily acts of conscious and unconscious bias that permeate their school and friendship experiences. They must consider how to create change without moving them off their educational goals or isolating themselves from peers."

Telling Our Children the Truth

While we parents must stress the importance of personal effort and responsibility, we also recognize that this does not necessarily translate to success because of undermining social inequities. By honestly sharing this with our youth, we provide them with insights that decrease the potential of self-rejection and, therefore, foster their self-esteem. It will also promote the development of their *critical consciousness*, which is about achieving an in-depth understanding of the world, including social and political contradictions. Critical consciousness also includes acting against the oppressive elements in one's life that are illuminated by that understanding. Parents must recognize that our children regularly receive messages of a "Color-blind meritocracy" where the ability to succeed is portrayed as linked only to their effort. We must value and promote effort but caution that effort is not always enough in a society marked by inequity. This preparation enables youth to better navigate systems that are often blind to the forces of inequity. We can equip our children and adolescents with the critical consciousness that allows them to identify and analyze dimensions of power and authority and to remain resilient in the face of barriers imposed by society. Parents, as coaches, can do the following:

- Intentionally instill racial-ethnic pride and self-respect.
- Steep children in the knowledge that they are deeply loved. The security gained from having someone's absolute and unconditional love can buffer against biases.

- Create spaces to talk about discrimination and bias in developmentally appropriate ways. Janie Victoria Ward shares that this "liberating truth-telling" approach has a "transformative quality"—it can create stronger individuals at the personal level and foster a sense of belonging with peers, the community, and even in institutions and organizations within society.

- Instill in youth the ability to detect racial stereotypes. This helps them understand and challenge racist ideologies and the harm they inflict. In sharp contrast, keeping expectations high and praising children while providing new challenges adds to their self-esteem. Teens internalize our expectations and turn them into their own aspirations.

- Teach independence. Children who have a sense of control over their environments also feel that they have the ability to influence or improve it.

- Let them know that it is OK to seek help and express their feelings (see Chapter 39).

- Promote the development and application of critical consciousness to their examination of the popular and news media, especially how such outlets create messages that "obscure the truth" and contribute to the creation of "implicit bias." *Implicit biases* are subconscious assumptions made about members of a group solely based on their belonging to that group.

- Engage in your teen's desire to debate you on difficult issues. When we ask questions, our children learn their opinions matter and that we care about their views. Valuing and hearing their perspectives holds meaning in a world where they will experience being marginalized. Above all, listening offers insight into what is important to them and with what issues they struggle.

- Counter the biases that promote the internalization of negative messages by providing positive affirmations and promoting the development of critical consciousness and agency through liberating truth telling.

- Counter negative encounters with alternatives by modeling and describing their own experiences (eg, through storytelling about real-life events) or coaching youth how to channel feelings of rage and hostility into pro-social action, such as voting or advocating for social change.

We can acknowledge the reality of discrimination and bias and prepare our children for negative encounters by offering concrete examples of where and how they may occur and discussing how they can best respond. This allows youth to identify what is happening, recognize their emotional reactions, and deploy appropriate coping responses instead of internalizing the harm (eg, "Ah, I wonder if this is what my dad was talking about with stereotyping!" instead of accepting a negative comment as a real reflection of their actions). These encounters can include role-playing and discussion about how to assess situations. Discussions can cover the importance of how to handle situations that can turn life-threatening, such as encounters with the police.

Shutting Out the Rumblings of Microaggressions

We must prepare our teens to learn what to do with the rumbling noise of microaggressions. What are *microaggressions*? They are common insults and degrading and derogatory messages sent to marginalized groups by individuals external to the group. The noises of microaggressions might be heard throughout the day. They come in the form of a word, a look, and/or an exclusion. They may suggest an "othering" of someone, implying that one does not belong. An example is, "Where *are* you from?" when the tone underscores that the questioner believes they are an outsider. Or they might note an accomplishment and suggest the individual does not deserve what they have earned. "How did *you* get into this class?" The noise is like the drip-drip of a faucet.

Do not interpret the "micro" in the term microaggressions as though these insults have a small effect. Ruth King talks about the cumulative impact of microaggressions: "It's like a repetitive motion injury that occurs daily, weekly, and generationally, impacting the capacity of the body and the mind to function optimally." These repetitive insults keep the body in a state of constant alertness to danger or insult. When a person needs to be always on high alert, their stress hormones remain constantly activated. This largely explains why people of Color have increased health concerns, including hypertension and diabetes, and, in the end, decreased life spans.

The person who is the source of the microaggression may be unaware of the implications of their statements or actions because they are often rooted in unconscious biases. Further, people who are the sources of microaggressions have likely not been victimized by them and, therefore, don't perceive why they are so harmful to others' well-being. As a first step, people can educate themselves about the damage these subtle forms of exclusion create. Then they can begin to engage in critical self-work that explores their racial biases (both unconscious and conscious). This process of deep self-reflection is nicely guided in the book, *The Racial Healing Handbook,* by Anneliese Singh, PhD, which helps the reader engage in work that confronts racism and promotes collective healing. *People can do better, but only when they take the steps to become their better selves.*

Microaggressions are a lifelong reality for people of Color. Therefore, we need to coach our teens on learning to be present and aware of what is going on so they can take the steps to cleanse their bodies from the increased stress hormones that these daily events generate. In parallel, adults who are victims of microaggressions must care for themselves, both because they deserve to be well and whole and because we are role models for our teens. One of the most important actions is to control the reactivity or state of constant alertness awakened by these injuries. This means that healing involves tending to both our minds and our bodies. Once in a less reactive or vigilant state, we can decide whether to tackle that aggression in the moment or choose to let it go to be dealt with at a different time.

In her book, King describes a meaningful strategy, the RAIN exercise, to center our thoughts and calm our body's reactions.

> **R—Recognize** what's happening and name it. Become an observer rather than an actor. Does your body feel heat, a racing heart, heavy breathing, chest tightness? Just notice that. What emotions do you feel? Do thoughts of anger or shame rise within you?

> **A—Allow** the experience to exist without judging what you are experiencing. Allow yourself to have the full experience without being angry at yourself for being affected by others' thoughts. Practice self-compassion.

> **I—Intimately investigate.** Allow yourself to be in touch with what is happening. Notice your perceptions, thoughts, and emotions. Name the feelings you are experiencing: pleasant, painful, and others. Think about which of these sensations you wish to think through and which you want to let go.

> **N—Nurture.** Now is the time to think of yourself. Ask, "How do I care for this distress?" Separate yourself, however, from the experience you are having. Don't own it as you being the cause of the distress; it is not yours. It is suffering or "noise" placed on you. Ask what you can do to nurture yourself and reduce the suffering? Do you need to practice forgiveness of those who have caused you harm to free yourself of anger and hurt? How can you release these painful feelings? Do you need to just take the time to relax and remove yourself from these feelings through imagery or other steps of active relaxation?

Individuals who experience racial microaggressions are often taxed with additional questions that play out in their mind, such as the following:

- "Did this really just happen?"
- "Did they really just say/do that?"
- "Am I being too sensitive?"
- "Should I say something or just let it go?"
- "If I respond, will I be perceived as the angry person of Color?"
- "If I say nothing, am I failing the other people of Color?"
- "If I stay quiet, will they continue this type of behavior?"

- "When and how do I stop the cycle?"
- "Why didn't the people who witnessed this situation (bystanders) speak up or be an ally?"
- "Do I teach the person how and why their look or comment was harmful?"

This is a delicate balance to learn for ourselves and to teach our teens. We need to make sure we are not reinforcing the "tax": communities of Color are (unfairly and wrongly) expected to create the teaching and the changes for a more just society while simultaneously feeling the direct impact of racism. We must prepare bystanders to act as allies to stand against racism—and we must raise our teens with permission to not engage. Teens must know it's OK to save their energy and choose not to react or to respond in the moment. It is always their choice. Caring for themselves is enough!

Your teens can be taught how to react to a microaggression if and when they choose. Roberto Montenegro, MD, PhD, a psychiatrist at the University of Washington and Seattle Children's Hospital, offers a strategy to respond to microaggressions in a way that is structured enough that it can conserve our energy. He emphasizes that a person should first ask themself if it's worth it. Is it the right time? Will the person who delivered the microaggression be receptive to feedback? The choice of walking away can be a good one. When the time feels right, he refers to the DEAR method as a way of remaining organized in our thoughts and simultaneously effective while expending less energy. Although he warns this initially may be experienced as "robotic" or "too structured," it becomes easier and flows more naturally with practice.

> **D** stands for "describe the situation," meaning stick to the facts of what occurred.
>
> > If I heard you correctly, last week during math class you....
>
> **E** stands for "expressing the feelings" that were experienced as a result of the statement or event.
>
> > When I heard that, it made me feel uncomfortable.
> > I felt that your statement made it sound like....
>
> **A** stands for "asking or asserting." This is about addressing the specific microaggression.
>
> > I just wanted to bring this to your attention and ask that you be more mindful about not making these kind of hurtful statements....
>
> **R** stands for "reinforcement," to make sure the listener is open to feedback.
>
> > I believe you care about our relationship/partnership/friendship, so I appreciate you being open to this feedback....

At first, Dr Montenegro recommends that people write their DEAR statements and practice reading them aloud. Eventually, with enough practice, this can become an automatic process in which responses to microaggressions are structured in a manner that is clear and absent of emotions that may hinder difficult conversations. The goal is to communicate a clear ask that empowers the victim of the microaggression, while also potentially helping the individual who is the source of the microaggression.

Take, for example, the seemingly innocent touch or comment on another's hair. Such acts disregard personal space and may lead the recipient to feel like an object of curiosity, unable to freely express their own identity.

> *"Hey John, can we talk in private? Last week during math class, while we were in a big group, you told me you really liked my new hairstyle; you asked me if my hair was 'real' and touched my hair without my permission. Although I know you were probably trying to give me a compliment, I felt uncomfortable with you commenting on my hair like that in public and touching my hair without permission. In the future, I would appreciate you not making comments like this in public or touching my hair without my permission. I'm sharing this with you because we are just getting to know each other and I want to make sure that we can tell each other things that can help our friendship. I know this is probably uncomfortable for both of us, but it's important for me to tell you how I felt. I really appreciate you hearing me out, John."*

In preparing our children (and ourselves) to navigate a world with microaggressions, we should fully believe the words of Shivani Seth in the article, "Am I an Imposter, or Am I Oppressed?," written for restforresistance.com:

> "I was always enough.
>
> I am always enough.
>
> I will continue to be enough."

We Must Stand Together

If you are a White parent reading this chapter, you may be asking yourself: How can I be an ally?

- Expose your children to as many different experiences and cultures as possible. This can include travel to other countries or local communities, purchasing books and movies, and visiting museums that represent other cultures and diverse individuals.

- Examine yourself and your family for your own biases and work to dismantle them.

- Discuss stereotypes with your child and dispel myths when you see or hear these biases. Help your adolescents understand that all people are beautiful and strong and intelligent and worthy of love and respect.

- Develop new relationships and friendships. It should include advocating for or supporting a family or teen who is experiencing discrimination and actively advocating for equity.

- Help your adolescents understand their own family history and the experiences of their ancestors. Youth with pride in their own people and secure sense of selves will more easily celebrate the differences and similarities they have with others.

- Expose your children early on to the reality of our multiracial society. We must not perpetuate the myth that we exist in a color-blind society. That well-intentioned effort teaches that it's best to behave as though racial differences don't exist and, therefore, denies a large piece of others' experiences. All parents should speak to their young people about the realities of the world we live in. Starting these conversations can be difficult. EmbraceRace (www .embracerace.org) offers resources for parents and teachers who want to prepare youth to be brave, informed, and thoughtful about race.

The Uplifting Truth

To raise resilient youth of Color, you need to be prepared to discuss and counter racism and injustice whenever you see it. If your teen sees you do this, they will gain personal empowerment through your modeling. All of our children must hear elevating messages that they will be stronger when they celebrate their own cultures and appreciate the cultures of others. We must see all of our children as they deserve to be seen and build a better world where every one of them can rise to be their very best self.

And when we all get there, we will have moved toward a better, more equitable society, where all its members can contribute fully through the uniqueness of their strengths. Children learn in middle school that, in nature, an ecosystem is more resilient to external challenges because of its diversity. This is the same in our communities—diversity brings different strengths that make our communities stronger. We should rely on those strengths and, in so doing, cultivate a culture of care for all.

Critical Closing Thoughts

One of the most wonderful things about raising adolescents is that we're raising people who can change the world. All adolescents are exposed to undermining forces whether as victims or observers. When observers are encouraged to do good—to become allies—there is power in joining together and becoming change agents.

Our actions, love, and support provide noise-canceling effects for our children and adolescents. Our continued rhythms—the strong, regular, repeated patterns or movement of positive messages and sounds—help our teens build resilience and resistance against racism. It ultimately positions them to rise above the noise to dismantle it and find their own rhythm.

Recommended Resources

The American Psychological Association created the RESilience Initiative: Racial and Ethnic Socialization as a journey that promotes resilience (https://www.apa.org/res/parent-resources/racial-stress).

Comer JP, Poussaint AF. *Raising Black Children: Two Leading Psychiatrists Confront the Educational, Social, and Emotional Problems Facing Black Children.* Plume; 1992

King R. *Mindful of Race: Transforming Racism from the Inside Out.* Sounds True; 2018

Racism and its harmful effects on nondominant racial-ethnic youth and youth-serving providers: a call to action for organizational change: the Society for Adolescent Health and Medicine. *J Adolesc Health.* 2018;63(2):257–261

Stopbullying.gov offers strategies on how to identify bullying and stand up to it safely. The following article offers guidance on identifying and responding to cyberbullying: https://www.stopbullying.gov/cyberbullying/how-to-report.

Trent M, Dooley DG, Dougé J; American Academy of Pediatrics Section on Adolescent Health, Council on Community Pediatrics, and Committee on Adolescence. The impact of racism on child and adolescent health. *Pediatrics.* 2019;144(2):e20191765

Ward JV. Raising resisters: the role of truth telling in the psychological development of African American girls. In: Leadbeater BJR, Way N, eds. *Urban Girls: Resisting Stereotypes, Creating Identities.* New York University Press; 1996:85–99

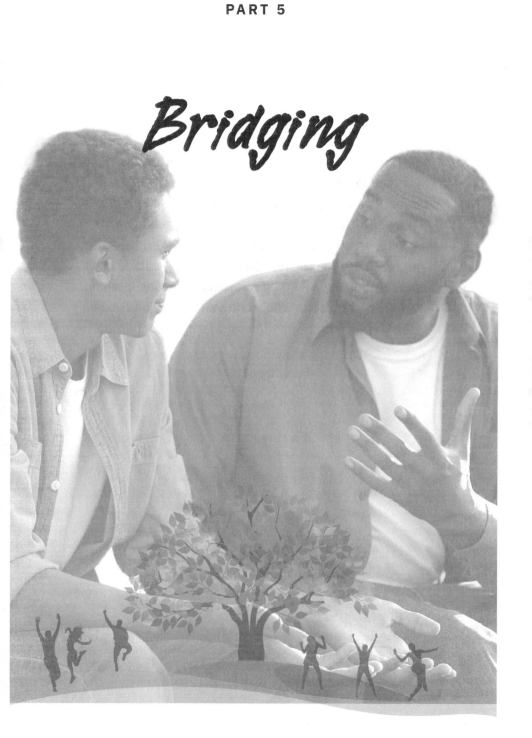

PART 5

Bridging

Adolescents are our path to a better shared future. Allow yourself to see and celebrate your teen's idealism. Be thankful that they refuse to avert their eyes to problems not yet solved. When you trust that your child might have the solutions, you will be building our bridge to the future. Honor your teen's sense of wonder, satisfy their curiosity, and support their passion for lifelong learning. Help them reflect on what matters to them, and you'll raise a child with clear values and a sense of purpose.

CHAPTER 31

A Bridge to the Future
A Generation Prepared to Do Good and Be Good

Parents want their children to be good and do good. You are privileged to witness your adolescent's developing values and sense of purpose. But you don't sit entirely on the sidelines. You play a meaningful role in supporting your teen to shape themself into the person you know they're capable of becoming. It is not about telling them what to believe or what to do; it's about remaining their North Star. You know who they are—and have always been—you see their core goodness. Adolescence allows them to build on that and to develop new capabilities that position them to make a difference.

There are many strengths that help people hone their values, become moral beings, and display character; each enables them to live richer, fuller lives and to be better poised to contribute to the world. As parents, we are lucky to have experience and family and cultural traditions that teach us how to do and be good—traits we can pass along and instill in our children and future generations. Our family stories guide them how to follow in their ancestors' footsteps while lighting a path for their descendants. Earned wisdom from our own lives also guides us.

In this part, I focus on the strengths that will enable your child's generation to be the bridge to our shared future. We need them to care about people and be endowed with a sense of noble purpose. We need to nurture a generation whose curiosity ensures they never stop seeking new knowledge. We need our future 35-year-olds to maintain the humility to consider answers to questions they had not yet known to ask. We need young people who can imagine that the best solutions might *currently* be found outside the box. We need dreamers.

- This chapter offers you a general background on character and moral strengths but focuses on **caring**—one of the foundations on which other strengths rely.

- Chapter 32 addresses ways in which parents can support their teen's developing sense of **meaning and purpose,** which drives people to do good for others.

- Chapter 33 covers those strengths that support **lifelong learning**. It includes the importance of **curiosity** as a driving force to seek solutions as well as the intellectual humility that allows people to remain open to new knowledge.

- Chapter 34 explores how a **sense of wonder** and awe allows people to marvel at possibilities and join with others in thinking on a grand level.

- Chapter 35 reminds us that *all* young people have a role in **building a better world** and that we magnify our effect as caring adults when we support all teens.

A Framework of Character Strengths

The Character Lab, led by Angela Duckworth, PhD, defines character with remarkably simple clarity: character is "everything we do to help other people as well as ourselves." I would also add a phrase I first heard from Richard Lerner, PhD, who leads the Institute for Applied Research in Youth Development: "Character is about doing the right thing even when no one else is looking."

The Character Lab separates character strengths into 3 dimensions: Strengths of Heart, Strengths of Mind, and Strengths of Will.

- **The Strengths of Heart** are described as the "giving" strengths. They are the source of human contentment. They enable us to see others in a positive light and to possess the interpersonal skills to reach, support, and impact others. They include gratitude, kindness, generosity, honesty, and a sense of purpose. The capacity to love fully and to remain caring about, and empathetic toward, others are also strengths of the heart.

- **The Strengths of Mind** are the "thinking" strengths that position us to reason and to create. These strengths include judgment and decision-making. They also include strengths, such as curiosity and creativity, that enable us to think outside the box and consider ideas beyond our comfort zone. Perhaps most intriguing is the critical importance of intellectual humility, which is about recognizing our own limitations—knowing what we know and what we don't know is the first step to being open to others' ideas.

- **The Strengths of Will** are the strengths within yourself that make it more likely to achieve your goals. Character Lab describes these as the "doing" strengths. They include grit (discussed in Chapter 23), growth mindset (discussed in Chapter 22), and self-control (discussed in Chapters 20 and 23).

Although we don't know the precise recipe to build these strengths, science helps us better understand how these character strengths can be supported. Bear in mind that, like all things human, we are uneven in our character strengths. But if we possess a growth mindset, we trust that we can at least improve in each of these areas.

It Matters What We Say. Kids Are Listening.

Research suggests that nearly all parents are deeply invested in raising caring children, and most parents view moral qualities as more important than achievement. But do our teens know this is what their parents most value? The alarming—and actionable!—answer may be no. The Harvard Graduate School of Education Making Caring Common Project, led by Rick Weissbourd, EdD, surveyed 10,000 middle and high school students from 33 schools representing diverse youth from across the nation and observed scores of youth, parents, and teachers over a decade. The majority of youth reported that they valued aspects of personal success—achievement and happiness—over caring for others. A majority of young people also believed their parents were more concerned about achievement than caring, even though their parents reported valuing the development of their teens' caring more than their achievement.

The Making Caring Common Project, which conducted the study, stated that "any healthy civil society depends on adults who are committed to their communities and who, at pivotal times, will put the common good before their own. We don't seem to be preparing large numbers of youth to create this society." The good news is that adults hope their children prioritize caring as a core value. The challenge is that there is a wide gap between what parents and other adults say are their top priorities and what young people are hearing. The Making Caring Common Project states, "The power and frequency of parents' daily messages about achievement and happiness are drowning out their messages about concern for others." They go on to conclude: "The challenge is for adults to 'walk the talk,' inspiring, motivating, and expecting caring and fairness in young people day to day, even at times when these values collide with children's moment-to-moment happiness or achievement."

Why does it matter that we walk the talk and are clear about what we value? Because young people respond to our expectations and what we model. To be clear: it is OK to want your child to achieve in traditional ways (academic, economic), and certainly you want your teen to be happy. Them caring for and about others doesn't preclude achievement or happiness; rather, it puts it in perspective. When young people are too preoccupied with their own happiness, they may be less likely to do what's right, generous, and fair because they may feel entitled to place their own needs first. This can have consequences, such as exhibiting signs of selfishness or being less likely to stand up for a person being bullied. Stanford researcher Denise Pope, PhD, one of the founders of Challenge Success and coauthor of *Overloaded and Underprepared: Strategies for Stronger Schools and Healthy, Successful Kids,* found that high numbers of achievement-focused high schoolers trivialized certain types of academic cheating. They may have seen cheating as acceptable because it was on the path to the higher scores they viewed as critical to achievement.

As much as we want our children to achieve, we also care that they have integrity. As much as we want our teens to be happy, we also want them to consider others' needs.

A Strategy to Develop Character Strengths

Marvin Berkowitz, PhD, director of the Center for Character and Citizenship at the University of Missouri-St Louis, has spent decades exploring how to develop moral character strengths in young people. He states, "No society, community, or family can thrive, perhaps even survive, if its members don't have basic moral qualities necessary for effective and nurturing interaction." In an interview with the Center for Parent and Teen Communication, he described the model he advises parents to follow to build character strengths in their children. You will find it consistent with strategies offered throughout this book.

He suggests following the acronym DENIM, which stands for *demandingness, empowerment, nurturance, induction,* and *modeling.* Taken together, it describes a set of behaviors, all well supported by research on parenting, that serve as the scaffolding for your teen to develop character strengths. Ask yourself, "What should I be doing in each of these categories to offer my teen what they need to develop into moral beings?" In response to the call for action from the Making Caring Common Project, we will later apply it to nurturing teens to be caring.

Demandingness

Morality cannot be dictated, but we can have high expectations for our teens. And we need to be sure our teens understand our clear expectations. In fairness, we should set the bar with expectations we know they can reach with the appropriate resources and guidance. This is another reason why it is helpful to root your expectations in what you know is good and right in your child. You are expecting them to be their best self.

Dr Berkowitz emphasizes that "we must provide resources to help them have a chance—not a guarantee, just a chance—of meeting our high expectations. This isn't a 'throw-them-in-the-pool-and-they'll-learn-to-swim-or-drown' strategy. While we want them to know it's important to meet our expectations, they also need to feel safe to fail. They need to know that you won't hate them if they make a mistake or push them away if they misstep."

Empowerment

Adolescence is about developing independence and a sense of control over one's life. Part of that is knowing that your opinions matter enough to be heard and honored. As we discuss morality, teens have to be invited to be part of the discussion. Moral development relies on people thinking through their values and often doing so in discussion with others. We have an opportunity to listen; people who are heard experience empowerment. We have to create the safe spaces where emotions can be expressed and thinking can be developed. We can't just set expectations; we have to support their ability to meet them. This may involve helping them develop new skill sets or exposing them to resources that enable them to follow through on their decisions. Then, we have to create room for them to make their own decisions.

Nurturance

It is our unconditional and unwavering love that gives our teens the security to develop their own values. Your child needs to know that you love them and that no behavior will cause them to lose your love. In fact, it is because you love them so much that you pay attention to their behaviors and care so much about them developing into a good person. Remember, you can disapprove of a behavior while never rejecting your teen. It is often not enough to just tell them that you love them; they need to believe it from how you treat them.

Induction

Dr Berkowitz describes *induction* as "a technical term for something really basic at the core of good parenting. It is about how we let kids know how we feel about their behavior, good or bad." According to Merriam-Webster, the word itself is defined as "the act of causing or bringing on or about." Tying this together, one key way to "bring about" the development of our teen's sense of morality is by letting them know how we feel. It is a way that we express our expectations. Dr Berkowitz suggests parents consider the following 3 actions:

- We have to tell our child (clearly) how *we feel* about what they did. Not about them as a person but about what they did ("I am so frustrated with how you..."). "Frustrated" is how their actions made us feel.

- We have to *explain why* we feel the way we do and do it in a way they can understand. ("I am so frustrated with how you...because..."). The "because" is the key; we are not leaving them hanging—they know why we feel as we do. It is also clear that an action created the feeling, so it is not how we view them as a person.

- We need to highlight *the effects of their behavior* and how their behavior made *someone else feel.* ("I am so frustrated with how you upset your brother by picking on him because it's something he already worries about. And this family is about supporting each other.") This last step underscores what moral behavior should—and should not—look like.

Modeling

In imagining themselves as adults, the first thing children do is look at how we are leading our lives. How we behave is much more meaningful than what we tell our teens to be and to do. Dr Berkowitz points out, "It is not a matter of deciding to be a role model. We are all role models, whether we like it or not. There is no off switch. Rather, the only choice is whether to be a good role model or not." We don't need to be perfect or paragons of virtue. Being human is about wrestling with impulses and working hard to do the right thing. Sometimes we parent best when we hold meaningful discussions about why we do what we do and the process we went through to get there. And remember, teens are always watching us.

Supporting Our Teens to Be Caring People

The ability to care is the foundation of being a good person. It ensures we'll use our talents for good. Caring is different than empathy. Empathy enables us to understand another person's perspective, but it does not ensure kind behavior. For example, someone who can read people well could use their skills to manipulate them, whereas someone who is caring would not do something that would intentionally take advantage of another person. Let's apply the DENIM model to caring.

Demandingness

Although we can't demand that our teen is caring, we *can* let them know what we value and hope to expect. We do this by prioritizing caring and kindness as opposed to their achievements or success. Many loving parents will say, "What matters to me most is that you're happy." Those well-intentioned words send the message that what is valued most is personal happiness. Instead, you might say, "Because I want you to be a genuinely good person throughout your life, I want you to know how you must treat other people. You should treat them as you would want to be treated yourself. If you do this throughout your life, you will be rewarded with healthier relationships and feel good about how you treat others." This is the golden rule central to so many traditions. This philosophy also carries into how you might interact with the "evaluators" in your teen's life. Will you ask their teachers to first tell you about their grades or about how they treat their classmates? Will you first ask their coaches about their playing or team-building skills? Your teen is listening and learning what they believe you value.

Empowerment

Caring seems to be inborn in many children, but, like any strength, it can be further developed. Engage your teen in thoughtful conversations.

- Talk about other people's needs and feelings.
- Grapple with how we sometimes must sacrifice our own immediate pleasures to offer others what they need and deserve.
- Speak of the courage it takes to care for others' feelings when they are feeling belittled.
- When your teen has their feelings hurt, help them understand how much a supportive person can make a difference. Talk about what it means to pay that forward.

Young people also need ongoing opportunities to *practice* caring. Young people can

- Choose how to support charitable organizations.
- Pitch in around the house and see how a small investment of their time makes a difference in your life.
- Help a friend with homework and notice the friend's growing confidence gained through their support.
- Volunteer for an organization that uplifts the vulnerable or protects animals.
- Read about climate change and commit to protecting the environment.
- Welcome a new student to the class and help them settle in.
- Commit to making school a safe place for everyone, and ensure that upstanders make bullying unacceptable.

Your teen will feel most empowered when they have a choice in how to develop their caring muscles. Our role is to model caring ourselves, help them think through their values, and let them know how much it means to us that they are good people.

Nurturance

In Chapter 25, we discussed how empathy is something we don't dictate. Rather, we model it and allow our children to experience our empathy toward them. Here too, caring deeply about your child enables them to learn firsthand how much of a difference it can make in a person's life. In fact, your teen knowing how deeply they are loved by you will make it more likely they will see the world as a place that is loving and secure rather than threatening. Set aside time for meaningful conversations that include their thoughts and feelings. They'll know you care when you really hear what they have to say and remain fully present as they express their emotions.

Induction

The Making Caring Common Project found young people were 3 times more likely to agree than disagree with this statement: "My parents are prouder if I get good grades in my classes than if I'm a caring community member in class and school." It is through induction that we help our children understand what we really value. At the end of a school day, is your opening line, "What'd you get on the test?" or, "Were you able to help your friend better understand her math homework?"

When you hold meaningful discussions that empower your teen, let them know what it means to you that they are thinking through such important issues. Don't hold back your pride when you see them caring about issues that support those who are vulnerable or when they stand up to make school a safe learning environment for all.

The wonderful thing about raising our children is that we don't have to wait for "big events" to let them see that we are noticing their goodness. They likely display acts of caring and loving-kindness within your home. Helping a young sibling. Holding the door open for an elder. You don't have to shower them with "oohs" and "aahs," but a smile or a wink or a pat on the back and a "thank-you" can speak volumes. Take it to the next level by helping them understand what it is they did that pleased you so much.

Also notice when your teen is not being caring. Your displeasure should be clear and focused. Remember, you are not liking the behavior while still loving the person. "Your little brother looks up to you as a hero. He is having a really hard time with some kids at school, and he needed you to make him feel special. Instead, you teased him about the exact things he is most sensitive about. This was not like you, and I expect you to make it right with him."

Modeling

Teens need strong moral role models. If you want to support your teen being a caring person, it is important that they see you set it as a priority in your life. Our teens don't need us to be perfect people. We are sometimes the best role models when we don't have all the answers and are grappling with our own flaws. It gives them permission to be OK with being a work in progress. Our mistakes open the door for our sincere apologies and pledges to do better—another great thing to model for them.

Being caring toward others enriches our lives and can make us feel genuine contentment. But it also sometimes means putting other people first or sacrificing something for the greater good of the family or community. Sharing your thought processes as you make these decisions offers your teen real-world strategies to help develop their caring muscles. And it increases the likelihood that the message they receive about what you did will be the message you intended to send.

Addressing Issues With Cultural Humility

While all cultures share universal values, each approaches issues of values, morality, and character in its own way. We harm people when we fail to respect their cultural viewpoints or traditions. A good starting point is to recognize that each culture's standards exist to build strong communities and to strengthen families.

There is a long history of dominant cultures suggesting that other cultures' approaches are somehow faulty. For example, the dominant view in America centers around the individual and assumes that if an individual works hard enough, life will work out for them. It defines success as tied to material trappings. Other American cultures strongly value families and collective wellness. This worldview has deep and enduring strengths that have ensured communities' survival. When we consider the character strengths that lead to success, we must be careful not to imply success *only* comes from personal achievement. I, for one, celebrate families and cultures where success is tied to collective well-being.

My goal is for you to consider how topics I raise fit into *your* goals for your child, *your* values for your family, and *your* hopes for your community. All of this is strengthened by *your* cultural values.

Part of cultural humility, however, is being transparent about our own biases. Cultural humility does not suggest we don't have biases but insists we understand them and allow others to know the perspective we bring. My biases: I am a dreamer. To separate my aspirational nature from the science that I will be translating for you in this part on "bridging," the following statements begin with the phrase, "I believe," so that you are clear about my values and my biases:

- I believe it is a moral imperative to work toward equity, fairness, and inclusion.
- I believe a commitment to take care of one's family is at the center of human existence.
- I believe our culture has made a tragic turn over recent generations by no longer venerating its elderly. I believe in honoring our elders and drawing from their earned wisdom.
- I believe children are sacred beings. (This is a term I borrow from our Indigenous nations). They deserve protection and enrichment and to be nourished in every way that enables them to reach their potential.
- I believe adolescence is an unparalleled opportunity to shape the generation we hope will wisely and compassionately lead us into our collective future.

Recommended Resources

The Center for Character and Citizenship engages in research, education, and advocacy to foster the development of character, democratic, citizenship, and civil society. Its site includes a parent toolbox and resources for communities and teachers (https://characterandcitizenship.org).

Character Lab turns scientific discoveries about the mindsets and skills that develop character into actionable advice for parents and teachers. On this website, you'll find Playbooks, organized by character strength, with information and activities based on rigorous research studies. This site has a playbook on character strengths of the heart, mind, and will (https://characterlab.org).

The Center for Parent and Teen Communication offers practical strategies rooted in what is known to work to strengthen family connections and build youth prepared to thrive. It includes content on strategies to build character strengths (https://parentandteen.com).

The Making Caring Common Project stated vision is "a world in which children learn to care about others and the common good, treat people well day to day, come to understand and seek fairness and justice, and do what is right even at times at a cost to themselves." The site offers parenting materials (https://mcc.gse.harvard.edu).

CHAPTER 32

Nurture Meaning and Purpose

L iving life with a sense of purpose enriches our existence, and, therefore, we hope our teens find theirs. Parents cannot instill a sense of purpose in their teens, but they *can* support young people to find their own. Finding a purpose is a process that bubbles up slowly within your teen and is likely shaped by meaningful conversations you will hold and thoughtful, and sometimes fortuitous, life exposures your teen will experience.

Much of this chapter is driven by the work of William Damon, PhD, director of the Stanford Center on Adolescence and professor of education at Stanford University. Dr Damon has written numerous books, including *The Path to Purpose: How Young People Find Their Calling in Life*. To paraphrase Dr Damon, **purpose is the intention to accomplish something that is personally meaningful and, at the same time, leads to engagement with an aspect of the world beyond oneself.** For this reason, think of gaining a sense of purpose as something that not only will bring meaning to your teen's life but will also drive them to make meaningful contributions to others. It will help them to live well.

Working Toward a Purpose Is Different Than Achieving a Goal

Not everything people do is about their purpose or achieving a sense of meaning. However, these may be the *whys* that fuel our efforts. Living life and experiencing pleasure brings meaning to life, even when it does not transcend into a driving purpose. Teens might invest a lot of energy into goals unrelated to their purpose. For example, a young person might work hard at a job because they want to save to buy a car, earn enough money to buy nice clothes, or go out with friends. These are all valid goals that will bring pleasure to their life. The same teen, however, could be working hard at a job to help support their family, and supporting one's family undoubtedly fulfills a life purpose. That same teen could invest heavily in schoolwork because they plan to become an immigration rights lawyer. Driven by that sense of purpose, they work hard toward meeting their near-term goals (eg, good grades, increased knowledge) and may derive meaning in doing so. Note: they also might apply increased pressure on themself and, therefore, need parental support to learn to achieve balance in their life. In other words, if they expend an enormous effort, they must be also do something for themself that offers them energy, including enjoying hobbies; maintaining adequate exercise, sleep, and nutrition; and leaving room for relaxation. It is this balance that ensures that they will maintain the energy to work for others' well-being.

How a Sense of Purpose Benefits People

Young people with a sense of purpose are better able to work toward their goals because they know that what they are doing *matters*. In an interview with the Center for Parent and Teen Communication, Dr Damon stated, "Developing a sense of purpose...prevents people from being self-absorbed. People who see beyond themselves tend to stay out of trouble." Working toward a meaningful goal also prepares a person to contribute to the world. Not everyone operates from a sense of purpose, but people who do benefit in many ways, such as

- Having greater physical health and lower levels of stress hormones
- Being happy and having a greater sense of satisfaction
- Being driven by optimism and maintaining hope
- Having greater resilience, including being able to navigate different environments or circumstances
- Improved academic outcomes, such as grade point average, perseverance in studying, and completing homework
- Better self-regulation
- Improved grit

A sense of meaning and purpose can be found through positive exposures. In fact, however, a sense of purpose can arise from even the worst circumstances. The originator of the idea behind purpose was Viktor Frankl, who wrote *Man's Search for Meaning* in 1946 after surviving several death camps, including Auschwitz. Frankl believed meaning came from 3 possible sources: purposeful work, love, and courage in the face of difficulty. He stated, "Those who have a 'why' to live, can bear with almost any 'how.'"

He noted that just as he witnessed the worst of humanity, he also saw the finest of humanity—"We who lived in concentration camps can remember the men who walked through the huts comforting others giving away their last piece of bread.... They offer sufficient proof that everything can be taken from a man but one thing: the last of the human freedoms—to choose one's attitude in any given set of circumstances, to choose one's own way."

My in-laws, Regina (Schwarzova) Pretter and Eli Pretter, also Holocaust survivors, lived purposeful lives, fully rooted in the most fundamental understanding that each person has value. This powerfully earned belief derives from surviving a concerted and well-planned effort to dehumanize them. Universally respectful, they always spoke of what it meant to be a real human. It was about loving and seeing the goodness in each person. It was about living a life with integrity, committing to never look down on another person, always standing ready to lift them up, and refusing to avert their eyes to injustice. (Regina, at 96 years of age, is one of the last survivors of the first transport of Jewish women into Auschwitz. Eli escaped the Majdanek death camp and then lived in a hole in the woods for a year, struggling to keep the only remaining members of his family, his 2 sisters, alive. Only one survived.)

In my career, I work with many youth at Covenant House Pennsylvania who have endured hardships beyond measure, such as poverty, exposures to violence, and abuse. Many of them have also needed to navigate oppressive forces, such as racism and homophobia. I work with the finest humans on the planet. Precisely because they know how inequitable the world can be, they yearn for fairness. Precisely because they have not always experienced compassion, they are among the most compassionate people I know. Many of them are still learning how to survive day by day, but nearly all also yearn to repair the world—to give to others what they needed. They are driven to become healers or social workers, to work in criminal justice reform, or to share inspiration through the arts.

I'm not celebrating that purpose can be derived from the darkest forces in our lives, and I'm not suggesting that adversity is good for you. Every child, every person, deserves to feel safe and valued and to be surrounded by adequate resources and loving people. However, the aforementioned examples show that a sense of meaning and purpose *can* arise from the worst circumstances. In these contexts, a sense of purpose may bestow the greatest of all benefits—survival. In fact, Frankl once said, "Man is originally characterized by his 'search for meaning' rather than his 'search for himself.' The more he forgets himself—giving himself to a cause or another person—the more *human* he is. And the more he is immersed and absorbed in something or someone other than himself, the more he really becomes *himself.*"

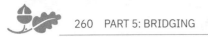

Teens Need to Find Their Purpose: Determine What Has Meaning

We mustn't allow "finding your purpose" to become the new version of the tired mantra of the last couple decades—"Find your passion." Teens experienced that slogan not as intended but as a strategy to write a good college essay. It turned the high school years into cauldrons of stress for too many students. Your teen will not find their purpose on demand, as they need to set their own pace. In fact, you can support the process by reminding them that meaningful decisions take time and that life allows us opportunities for reflection and growth.

Ultimately, if a sense of purpose doesn't arise from within them, it is not truly *their* purpose. So be careful not to suggest to them what *you think* their purpose should be. Although you'd likely never directly say, "Your purpose is _____," be careful not to inadvertently pressure them by making it clear what would make you proudest. This could create internal conflict within them because they want to both please you and forge their own path. Further, they may resent the effort it takes to work toward what they see as *your* goals. This can be a difficult line to not cross for parents, because sometimes we may see within our teen what they are not yet ready to see in themself. Hold on tight because you can support your teen in *their* journey toward finding their purpose.

A Parent's Critical Supportive Role in a Teen Finding Their Purpose

Members of the Adolescent Moral Development Lab at Claremont Graduate University, led by Kendall Cotton Bronk, PhD, reviewed the science behind the development of purpose and concluded that there are 3 ways parents can help teens find their purpose. First, they can help their children develop a sense of gratitude. Second, they can introduce their children to potential sources of purpose. Third, they can engage them in conversations about the things their children hope to accomplish. Let's think through how you might engage your teen in each area.

Helping Your Teen Reflect on Gratitude

Experiencing a sense of gratitude seems to have multiple benefits for young people. It makes them more likely to feel satisfied with their lives and to foster better relationships with others. Research has shown that expressing gratitude improves mental health. Joshua Brown, PhD, and Joel Wong, PhD, at Indiana University, found that people who wrote letters of gratitude to others, whether or not they actually sent them, reported better mental health. This was true both for people who were already feeling emotionally healthy and those who were experiencing mental health concerns.

Parents who discuss what they feel grateful for set the tone for their children to reflect on what they feel grateful about. Experiencing and expressing gratitude contributes to a teen's desire to want to contribute to the world. It may be that as they more fully experience the blessings in their own life, they will want to pay that forward.

Support Your Teen to Be Exposed to Purposeful People and Activities

Young people deserve to experience how much people can make a difference to others or to our world. They can watch you or others matter or learn for themselves how much they matter when they share their talents and offer their energy.

WHAT YOU DO MATTERS TO YOU AND TO OTHERS. Share *why* you do what you do. Talk about what you hope to accomplish. Discuss how it brings meaning to your life. "I volunteer at the food distribution center because there are people in our community who do not have enough, and with my free time, I want to make the world a bit fairer." Or, "When I was growing up, I saw too many young people who did not receive the guidance to reach their potential, so I decided I would be a teacher in our community." Or, "I realized when I was growing up that the elders in our family held us together. I decided then that my focus would be on family." As you model what gives you meaning, share any setbacks along the way and why being driven by your purpose strengthened your resolve to overcome obstacles.

PROVIDE OPPORTUNITIES FOR EXPLORATION. Encourage your teen to step outside their comfort zone. This could involve traveling across their own town or being exposed to topics affecting the world by listening to the news or watching documentaries. They can read about people who work on topics that intrigue or worry them and find opportunities to meet adults who work or volunteer in these areas. Joining after-school activities or taking on a part-time job may offer exposures that will foster their imagination or stoke their sense of purpose.

ENCOURAGE VOLUNTEER WORK. Guide your teens to spend time doing something meaningful to them. They will gain personal satisfaction and likely will solidify their values. Remember from our discussion about contribution, they will also earn others' gratitude, and that is protective to their well-being and will motivate them to want to continue to do the right thing.

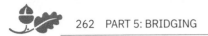

Engage Your Teen in Conversations About What They Want to Accomplish

Every young person possesses their own unique strengths, talents, and potential. Having conversations about these will help your teen better understand themself. Also, your teen will value having real discussions about what they care about, how they might want to make a difference, and what they hope to accomplish. Not enough teens hold these types of conversations with caring adults, and your child will feel gratified that you see their potential and want to hear how they might use it.

HOLD REGULAR CONVERSATIONS. We don't want these conversations to feel like a BIG event. **Hint:** don't start with, "So what do you want to do with your life?" Instead, start with questions like, "What did it feel like when you helped the neighbor the other day?" or, "What do you think you're best at doing?"

HIGHLIGHT YOUR TEEN'S STRENGTHS. Sometimes people's strengths feel so natural to them that they don't even recognize them as strengths. Another person's perspective can help them realize what might be their unique contributions.

IF THEIR ACTIVITIES MAKE SENSE, SAY IT. Sometimes adolescents will be involved in an activity that just fits. It involves an interest they have always had but moves it to a new level. Notice that and reflect on it. "I'm not surprised that you volunteer at the animal shelter. You have made me stop for every lost animal since you could talk."

CELEBRATE UNEVENNESS! Remember when we talked about success in Chapter 22? Noticing unevenness creates a road map for our children. It helps them find their "spikes" and imagine that they can strongly focus their energies in a way that both engages their skills and talents and fortifies their interests and love of learning.

Mentors and Heroes

Sometimes, we parent best by drawing from the strengths of other people in our teens' lives. We hope they find close and meaningful relationships with extended family, teachers, community members, and coaches, among others. These people see your teen in a different setting and may help them recognize their talents and skills. Exposure to other people also makes it more likely your teen will see someone doing something that captures their enthusiasm. That person can then become a mentor to them, not only by shaping what they hope to do but discussing the paths to get there. If your teen hears discouraging words or messages, the mentor can champion their dreams and prepare your teen to overcome barriers they may encounter.

There are people who your teen might not have close contact with but who still expose them to possibilities and noble purposes. Let's call these people *heroes*. They can be examples of the kind of moral beings people dream of becoming. However, discuss with your teen that they should not equate hero status with perfection. There is a harmful element of our society's culture, where heroes are built up to almost superhuman status, only to be torn down when they've made a mistake. In an era of personal destruction, social media conversations imply that these fallen heroes can no longer make valid contributions. If we bring down our heroes for all-too-human imperfections, there will be no heroes left. Heroes exist for a reason: they give us something to dream about and strive toward. But your teen might see that every time their hero achieves a certain height, it is only a matter of time before they are taken down. That might make your teen fear putting themself out there.

Our teens must know that all people, heroes included, have their own complexities and inner conflicts. This will help our teens know that their own imperfections neither invalidate the sincerity of their drive nor their inherent goodness. We must help them understand that they can accept every bit of their humanity—including their imperfections—while in pursuit of their purpose.

Recommended Resource

"The Psychology of Purpose" is a comprehensive assessment of the science of purpose. Created by the Adolescent Moral Development Lab at Claremont Graduate University for Prosocial Consulting and the John Templeton Foundation, it is accessible at https://www.templeton.org/wp-content /uploads/2020/02/Psychology-of-Purpose.pdf.

CHAPTER 33

Support Lifelong Learning, Foster Curiosity, and Encourage Humility

I was raised to believe that a person who loves learning could live to be 120 years old while growing every moment. I realize now that the conversations I overheard among my elder relatives were held within my earshot for a reason. They talked about their voracious appetite for new knowledge, discussed the adult learning opportunities they pursued, and held (sometimes heated) debates about newsworthy topics. They spoke about how people who loved learning would always look forward to the next day when they could grow a bit wiser. They made it clear that as long as life still held mysteries, they would strive to uncover them. Inevitably, one of their gazes would meet my eyes and they'd share a piece of cultural wisdom—"Knowledge is something you own that can never be taken away from you."

I suspect, however, that new knowledge is not the only reason love of learning brings people satisfaction into the elder years. People who love learning interact with others differently; they're always seeking new ideas. People open to new ideas, almost by definition, are less likely to be rigid. They are aware they don't know it all and relish hearing others' ideas. In other words, people who cherish learning will possess not only a growth mindset about knowledge but *also* about developing new relationships and deepening existing connections. This makes people of all ages want to engage with them. And human engagement is an invaluable source of contentment and well-being.

If we can nurture our children to love learning, they'll have a more interesting life, hopefully filled with meaningful human connections. While we cannot inject a love of learning into our teens, there is ample opportunity to nurture it. Adolescence is a phase of endless "whys" and hands us ways to support teens' innate curiosity. Hopefully, if we attend to their curiosity well, this will not be a passing developmental stage but a lifelong strength. The other strength we hope to encourage is humility. If they remain aware of their own limitations and open to others' wisdom, their continual growth is ensured.

Adolescence: The Second Age of "Why?"

Our younger children had a voracious appetite for discovery. They wanted explanations for...everything. According to Susan Engel, PhD, author of *The Hungry Mind: The Origins of Curiosity in Childhood,* 3- to 4-year-olds ask a question every minute! Exhilarating. Exhausting. "Why is the grass green? Why do clouds float in the sky? How did the people get inside the TV? Why don't cows speak English?" We answered as many questions as we could. We knew intuitively that if they felt good in seeking answers at 3 years old, they might never stop asking the important questions. It was also so darn cute, but did I mention that it could be exhausting?

As we discussed in Chapter 11, cognitive development drives teens to ask a whole new set of *deeper* questions. They don't want to know how the person got into the TV; they want to understand how digital signals cross the globe. They want answers to some questions long ignored but in urgent need of a response, such as how we can help endangered species. Some of their questions are challenging, perhaps making them less adorable (but impressive!) but no less deserving of a thoughtful response.

Just as in early childhood, how we respond to their questioning nature may make the difference in how they feel about the pursuit of knowledge. Will they see their innate curiosity as an integral strength? Will they feel a genuine thrill at asking challenging questions? If so, they are more likely to find the innovative answers. Will they feel safe in asking the hard questions? If so, they are more likely to contribute to desperately needed solutions.

Love of Learning *Should* Develop in School

Extraordinary human beings, also known as teachers, devote their lives to helping young people think. I don't remember in great detail the teachers who taught me spelling or multiplication tables. But the ones that sparked my imagination shaped my life. They drew me in when they helped me grasp that much of what seemed inexplicable could be explained through science. The English teacher who helped me find hidden meanings within literature forever shaped the way I refuse to accept the surface meaning...of anything.

Adolescents have a newfound appreciation for complexity and nuance. Because adolescents are hungry to seek understanding and to uncloak mysteries, good teachers can ignite their interests and solidify their passions.

Unfortunately, school settings do not always nurture curiosity to the extent we'd hope. Dr Engel points out that we'd expect curiosity to wane a bit with age, as our appetite for many basic questions have been satisfied. But she points out that even children who remain curious at home ask few questions at school. She suggests that this may be because many schools focus on disseminating knowledge rather than fostering deep inquiry. This may be a lost opportunity for young people to explore uncharted territories in areas they find most interesting. It is beyond the scope of this book to address educational settings. The Character Lab works with schools, and you'll find recommendations on their site. Additionally, Marvin Berkowitz, PhD, synthesized optimal practices for school settings in *Primed for Character Education: Six Design Principles for School Improvement.*

Nothing quite says buzzkill more than when a parent says, "It's really important that you study for this test because it will determine the rest of your life." We want our children to engage academically, but if we convey that success is solely determined by the immediate steps during and after high school, this pressure can prevent students from using these years to explore the large questions that could shape their lives—"What do I care most about?" "How can I uniquely contribute to the world?" It can prevent them from exploring those unanswered questions that will ignite their passion for further inquiry. Remember this: the most innovative thinking rarely earns an A the first time around.

I am not suggesting your child should care less about their education; I am hoping they will draw everything from the opportunity schooling offers. It can be helpful to think of raising your teen to be ready to get a great second job. Whaa-a-t?! Young people often stay at their first job for less than 2 years. What gets them the second job? Does that second boss call the first boss for a reference and ask how the employee scored on standardized tests or about their grades in high school? They ask questions like, "Do they get along with other people? Do they take constructive feedback well?" And they ask, "Do they grow on the job—are they able to continue to learn?" Once you realize you're raising your teen to have the skill sets needed to land that second job, you'll let out a deep breath of relief and begin parenting about the things you care about: social and collaborative skills. Love of learning. Curiosity.

Your role? Dial down performance pressure. Ask what excites your teen. End the day by asking what they've learned, not what they achieved. When you see that they're excited, ask them to teach you!

Curiosity

Who's going to come up with solutions no one else can find? Who's going to pay attention to problems others view as unsolvable? Who's going to seek wisdom from people with different life experiences than their own? Who is going to want to better understand why someone disagrees with their point of view? The answer to all these questions: curious people.

Curiosity is about wanting to know more. If anything can drive a lifelong love of learning it is the desire to satisfy our curiosity. Surface-level answers rarely satisfy someone driven to know more; they just pique their curiosity to keep learning. Curiosity drives us to invest the time and energy to uncover meaningful answers. It's not surprising, therefore, that highly curious people also have a greater sense of purpose in life.

We don't need to be curious about everything. We are uneven in our talents and interests. Your teen will thrive when they're pursuing their purpose and satisfying their curiosity. Dr Engel underscores that young people need the opportunity to be curious about what they're interested in. We adults should expose our children and teens to a wide variety of possibilities and then, when their spark is ignited, continue to create more opportunities for them to pursue their interests.

The Parent's Role in Fostering Curiosity

Dr Engel points out that studies of curiosity demonstrate what we might assume: children who ask a lot of questions and receive satisfying answers go on asking more questions. The fact that you intuitively knew this is likely part of the reason you took so much pride in your small child's curiosity and responded, as best you could, to their relentless inquiries. Don't stop now! Families where questions are encouraged are families where curiosity takes hold. The following are tips on encouraging curiosity:

- **Notice and celebrate inquisitiveness.** If your teen asks a question that sparks your interest, tell them! Let them know how pleased you are that they're an explorer.

- **Say "I don't know" a lot.** If our teens think we have all the answers, they'll just expect us to hand them what we know. If you pretend to have all the answers, they might feel ashamed of their own knowledge gaps. Instead, we want them to recognize what they know and what they don't know and be curious enough to fill the gaps.

- **But be a model. Follow "I don't know" with, "I'm going to find out!"** Let them see that you're willing to do the work. Model being a person who's always willing to grow. Let them see that when you don't know something, you'll search for accurate information from trusted sources.

- **Share your interests.** If you're excited about something, show it! Let your teen know where you found new ideas to ponder—TED talks, podcasts, or documentaries.

- **Explore together.** It may not surprise you to learn that youth who ask a lot of questions tend to have inquisitive parents. When you have common interests, explore them together. When they have a question you can't *yet* answer, figure it out as a team.

- **Ask open-ended questions.** You'll never know what issues your teen is grappling with if your questions can all be answered with a "yes" or "no." Learn to ask "how" and "why" questions.

- **Don't just turn their questions back on them.** Many adults think that the way to keep conversations going is to respond to questions with, "Well, what do you think?" If a teen asks you a question, they want to know your thoughts.

- **Provide good answers to questions (or find someone who can).** Your teen will continue to ask new and deeper questions when they hear interesting or satisfying answers. If you respond with simplistic answers or somehow minimize or belittle their curiosity, they'll stop asking. Remember, you're not supposed to know everything. Just encourage them to continue seeking the answers.

- **Appreciate mistakes!** Every failure is an opportunity for growth. For people endowed with a curious nature, every attempt to find an answer that misses the mark moves them closer to getting it right next time. Let your teen know that you are proud of their efforts and ask what they've learned.

- **Ask all family members (including you!) to share something they learned that day.** At the end of the school day, ask your teen what they've learned, not just how the test went. Create a family routine where you discuss what piqued everyone's interest that day.

- **Don't give up on the mystery.** Curiosity in its best form explores topics without readily available answers. The future will have more answers than we have today. Your teen might supply some of those answers! Enjoy imagining what the answers to the toughest questions might be. Guess! And then encourage them to think through how the best answers can be uncovered.

Intellectual Humility

Wise people listen more than they talk. They understand that wisdom is often earned from life experience and defer to those with firsthand knowledge. They respect the wisdom of years and venerate the elderly. They also cherish the purest wisdom, that which flows from the youngest among us; children see what we have forgotten to notice.

Mark Leary, PhD, professor emeritus of psychology and neuroscience at Duke University, synthesized key findings on intellectual humility for the John Templeton Foundation. He describes *intellectual humility* as "...a mindset that guides our intellectual conduct. In particular, it involves recognizing and owning our intellectual limitations in the service of pursuing deeper knowledge, truth, and understanding." He explains some of the reasons it can be critical to good citizenship, and, I might add, to healing our society. "...It promises to help us avoid headstrong decisions and erroneous opinions and allows us to engage more constructively with our fellow citizens."

People with high levels of intellectual humility tend to be more tolerant of varied views and are less likely to belittle those with whom they may disagree. They are more likely to be agreeable and less likely to get into contentious arguments. This doesn't mean they are wishy-washy. Rather, they are open-minded and willing to grow. They are better listeners and, therefore, I would propose, better teachers and more effective influencers. People are more likely to learn from those who are, themselves, open to learning.

As Tenelle Porter, PhD, explains in the playbook on intellectual humility on the Character Lab website, there is a connection between growth mindset and intellectual humility. This makes sense because if your mindset is that intelligence is something to be developed, you are both open to new knowledge and willing to state the current limitations of your own. Admitting what you don't *yet* know does not imply a lack of intelligence; it conveys an openness to growth.

The Center for Parent and Teen Communication conducted an in-depth interview with Eranda Jayawickreme, PhD, from the Department of Psychology at Wake Forest University, who has extensively studied intellectual humility. He revealed the following top strategies he recommends to encourage intellectual humility in both adults and youth:

- View your behavior from the perspective of others. Adopting a more "impartial" point of view can help reduce the impact of biases we may have.
- Resist seeing people you disagree with as inferior or less than.
- Reframe conversations with those you disagree with as opportunities for learning about others and their unique outlook on the world.
- Acknowledge the limits of your own knowledge. The more we learn, the less we realize we know.

- Pay attention to the feedback you receive. Ask yourself, "Are people unlikely to challenge me because of a position I may hold?" If you're in this position, encourage people to challenge you. (I would add that parents can demonstrate intellectual humility by allowing our teens to offer us feedback.)

The Parent's Role in Encouraging Intellectual Humility

Our children watch us from the very early years and do so with much more intensity when they are teens. Intellectual humility is not something that can be taught, but it can be modeled and reinforced. For each of the following, we have the opportunity to model these behaviors and the privilege to notice and reinforce them when our teens display these strengths:

- **Be curious.** All the strategies previously described to foster curiosity in your child will also contribute to them developing intellectual humility. Curious people are always searching and, therefore, will continue being exposed to others' ideas.

- **Remain open-minded to new ideas.** Teens watch how we interact with others and respect when we are open to the possibility that we also make mistakes. People are continual works in progress. Share when your thoughts have expanded or positions have shifted because you sought out new views.

- **Don't be certain if you're not.** Know what you know and what you don't know. Talk through how you seek information to inform your opinion.

- **Be flexible.** Don't express certainty in your beliefs when they are opinions. Remain willing to change your mind when new (or better) evidence presents.

- **Reflect on your biases.** We all have biases. This does not make us bad people; it makes us human. What makes us act with humility is when we admit that we exist with biases and confront them to make thoughtful decisions.

- **Share when your thoughts have expanded.** Say, "I used to think _____, but now I understand _____." When you notice growth in your teen's thinking, celebrate that. "I love seeing that you shifted your opinion after you heard someone else's viewpoint."

- **When your teen was a change agent, let them know!** Appreciate your teen when they make you reconsider a position you hold. Credit them for your growth—"I've never thought of it that way; thank you!"

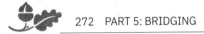

. . . .

Recommended Resources

Leary MR. *The Psychology of Intellectual Humility.* John Templeton Foundation; 2018. https://www.templeton.org/wp-content/uploads/2020/08/JTF _Intellectual_Humility_final.pdf

Challenge Success partners with schools, families, and communities to embrace a broad definition of success and to implement research-based strategies that promote student well-being and engagement with learning (https://challengesuccess.org).

CHAPTER 34

Appreciate Idealism and Experience Wonder and Awe

When we elevate rather than extinguish our teen's keen sense of wonder, we build their capacity to be change agents. When we expose them to the kind of things that help them experience awe—that indescribable connection to something larger—they often want to join with others in a shared experience. Wonder and awe can stoke idealism because they involve dreaming and move us to connect with others in a mutual effort.

We rely on the idealism of adolescents to inspire us to address problems long ignored or assumed to be unyielding. Their presence in our lives can serve as the catalyst for needed change! However, we are not just focused on their contribution to the world. We care that they have full, rich, joyful lives. We hope they will never forget to appreciate the simple pleasures of life while always remaining open to inspiration. So, while we care about how a sense of wonder and the capacity to be awed foster their idealism, we also want them to possess these character strengths so they can get the most out of life.

Honoring the Idealism of Youth

There is nothing you need to do to allow your teen to envision building a better world. The desire to do so seems to be integrated into their DNA. The greatest role adults can play is to choose not to shelter their older children and adolescents. Let them see the news and help them interpret it. Let them see the problems that exist within your own community. Share with them that you do not believe that we need to remain stuck in practices just because they "have always been this way." Let them know you care about the world you share today and the world they will inherit.

Idealists Benefit Our Daily Lives

An idealist believes it is worth putting in the effort to improve current realities. We need idealists in our lives. They do much more than ponder grand ideas. They put in the work to strengthen relationships. They are the kind of people who will lift up neighbors. We live in a time with too much division. It is said that the best way toward healing our communities is through well-worn paths between neighbors. It is idealists who will take the first steps.

Self-centered? Are You Kidding Me?

It is an unfair and dangerous myth that adolescents are self-centered and selfish. *The truth is that adolescents are driven by idealism and committed to repairing the world.* How could the total disconnect between reality and this myth originate? I believe it is because idealists create discomfort in those who have grown comfortable with the ways things are or who have given up on progress. It is hard to see problems such as poverty or to imagine the havoc that climate change may bring. It becomes more difficult when you realize that something could and should be done about these problems. One way to avoid that discomfort is belittling the messenger and calling their vision unrealistic or naive. When people create a false narrative about teens' self-centeredness, it becomes easier to ignore concerns youth bring to our attention. (Adolescents being self-conscious does not mean they are self-centered!) We need to set aside this myth and listen to our children. They will inherit our world and are highly motivated to improve it.

Young people are used to having their thoughts set aside by adults who want to silence their views, so we need to choose our words carefully.

Say This (to honor and elevate idealism)	Not This (to diminish or belittle dreaming)
Tell me what you think could be the solution here.	I think...
Tell me the first step you would take to address this issue.	We've tried that.

Say This (to honor and elevate idealism)	Not This (to diminish or belittle dreaming)
You always think about possibilities. I appreciate that you are a dreamer.	You're such a dreamer (stated sarcastically or with condescension).
The world will improve when people like you notice what needs to change.	This problem has lasted forever and will never change.
You are developing a lot of wisdom. You will learn how to develop strategies to turn your thoughts into actions.	You are naive.
Young people today care so much about the future.	Young people today are self-centered.
Say This (as you witness problems)	**Not That**
There's got to be a better way. The world doesn't need to be like this.	It's always been this way.
I wonder what happened to that person?	What's wrong with that person?
Strong communities must figure out how to support each of their members.	That person doesn't care enough to improve their life.

A Note of Caution

If your teen is a seeker, make sure they are vigilant to how radicalizing forces look to indoctrinate deeply caring young people. As we discussed in Chapter 21, the nature of search algorithms can expose dreamers to radical views. Therefore, we need to have clear and frank conversations with our teens about consuming internet information. Consider saying something like, "I value and admire your commitment and idealism. And I am glad that you can amplify your voice and learn more through the internet. Be aware, however, that fringe and dangerous elements are seeking idealistic young people to join them. Sometimes it is not obvious, at first, who are the real idealists and who are the radicals. They often draw teens in with ideas that make perfect sense and that match their passions. Just pay

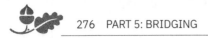

attention if they are spreading misinformation or if the chat spaces seem to be drawing people into beliefs or unacceptable actions that are divisive or dangerous."

Wonder

At the very core of curiosity is maintaining a sense of wonder. Wonder allows us to see the *extra*ordinary in the ordinary and to find joy in our everyday lives. It also allows us to connect with others in an organic way by inviting them to share our experiences.

Do you know anybody whose openness to people makes you endlessly proud but whose actions simultaneously remind you that you are a bit shy? That's my wife, Celia Pretter. She's the most open, loving, and respectful person I've ever met. She is a true extrovert who contrasts with me (a guy who talks a lot but has a quieter nature). When away from home, we prefer to people watch than look at monuments and, therefore, tend to find where the townsfolk hang out. I sit on a statue or a bench and just observe. My wife goes into the center square and begins blowing bubbles. Immediately, the grade school kids gather around and blow the bubbles back into the air. When the parents of the younger children see that it's safe, they give them permission to join in. The teens, at first, feign indifference and then predictably become the most enthusiastic participants. It's only a matter of time before she's handing out bottles of bubbles to strangers and has created a common space where everyone is enjoying a shared experience of wonder. There's so much to see and to learn through something so simple. I'm not sure how much time you've spent with bubbles since you've grown up, but they are breathtaking in their simplicity and stunning in their beauty. Celia takes the same approach working on the streets with people who have had very hard lives, many of whom experience substance use disorder. She blows bubbles or hands out lollipops to start conversations. Sharing common, joyful experiences that embrace our commonality—that is the gift of wonder.

To describe the benefits of wonder, I interviewed the greatest expert I know, Celia, on eliciting wonder to elevate our shared humanity.

The Benefits of Sharing Wonder

- Wonder brings out the common humanity in us. We experience joy and amazement together on the same playing field. It's not about you or me; it's about us.

- Wonder gives us an opportunity to share what excites us. We don't have to offer an opinion or commentary just to point out what is there. A rainbow. A blue heron on the water. A child tasting cinnamon or a spicy food for the first time. (Seriously, have you ever seen that?)

- Wonder guides us to seek answers or explanations for bigger life questions. On the other hand, it allows us to enjoy life without always needing to find an answer. When one seeks new experiences, sees everyday beauty, or ponders unanswerable questions, it creates a lifelong quest to want to grow and learn and evolve.

- You are sharing something you notice, not something you've created or believe. It is not yours; it is ours. You have no personal stake in altering another person's experience; therefore, it is naturally and authentically generous.

- Sharing wonder is nonjudgmental. It is about offering something new to another human and being thrilled to do so. It is not about gaining influence; it is about sharing something special. For that reason, it builds bridges with little effort.

Allowing Wonder to Exist

To elevate the sense of wonder in your children's lives, just choose to not extinguish the natural wonder of childhood. Have you ever followed a toddler as they explore the world? Seen through the eyes of a child, the whole world is a mystery waiting to be understood. The first time they look at an insect and see its unique eyes they feel as if they've discovered a new continent. When they see the beauty of a flower, they appreciate it in ways we've long forgotten. I'll never forget my girls' first ice cream cones. They weren't yet talking, but the looks on their faces told the whole story. They seemed to say, "How long have you guys been holding out on this stuff?" They literally dove into the cones. Then life becomes rushed, and there's so much to learn. Our children spend so much time with books that they ignore the science experiments and miracles of nature they walk past every day. There is a reason why the expression. "Take time to smell the flowers" exists. If we all slow down and experience what surrounds us, we'll show our kids that they don't have to give up their desire to do the same.

I'm going to tell you once again to be a role model, but I hope my suggestion feels like a gift. If you slow down, smell the flowers, blow more bubbles, and go out after storms pass in hope of finding a rainbow, your teen will more likely see basic experiences of joy as their birthright. Open yourself up to what surrounds you and let the little child within you out.

Awe

Wonder is something experienced in everyday life and awe is something larger; you almost have to allow yourself to be taken by awe. For millennia, awe was something most associated with religious or spiritual experiences, and it still can be. But it also can be experienced by feeling overwhelmed with something as breathtaking as a canyon or by the miracles that happen in front of us, such as the leaves unfolding glorious colors as the seasons change or a caterpillar transforming into a butterfly. Awe also can be inspired by witnessing and elevating the acts of loving-kindness that surround us. And, as you read moments ago, I am in awe of my wife's connection to people.

The Greater Good Science Center (GGSC) produced a summary paper on "The Science of Awe" for the John Templeton Foundation. Much of the work it cites flows from the work of Dacher Keltner, PhD, professor of psychology at the University of California, Berkeley and GGSC founding director, and Jonathan Haidt, PhD, social psychologist at the New York University Stern School of Business. The paper describes awe as an emotion that can help us feel as if we are part of something greater. In so doing, it can shift attention away from ourselves in a way that can be both healing and inspiring.

Drs Keltner and Haidt say that a sense of awe first involves a person having an experience of "perceived vastness." The GGSC describes awe as "the feeling we get in the presence of something vast that challenges our understanding of the world, like looking up at millions of stars in the night sky or marveling at the birth of a child. When people feel awe, they may use other words to describe the experience, such as wonder, amazement, surprise, or transcendence."

It is the perspective we gain while experiencing awe that explains why this idea fits so nicely into our thinking about teens being a bridge to the future. Experiencing "vastness" makes us see ourselves as part of something greater. In the very act of making us relatively smaller, we can lose our self-centeredness and reimagine our role in the universe. It makes people want to join in a shared experience. Awe has been shown to make people more generous. That may be because the experience of awe makes people see themselves as part of something larger and that, in turn, can have them connect more deeply with others to share that experience.

The Benefits of Experiencing Awe

According to the GGSC,

- Awe makes us feel good. People tend to feel many other positive emotions when they experience awe, such as joy and gratitude. These feelings are linked to improved health and well-being.

- Awe makes us happier. People have higher well-being when they experience awe.

- Awe encourages curiosity and creativity.
- Awe makes us more generous, encouraging us to help others even if we gain no personal benefit.
- Awe helps us gain perspective. Feeling smaller can increase our humility and relieve us of pressure.
- Awe is linked to better physical health.
- Awe allows us to immerse ourselves in the moment, offering an "instant vacation" from routine concerns or worries.
- Awe encourages critical thinking.

Raising Our Children to Experience Awe

As a pediatrician and child advocate, I suggest that if you want to get back in touch with your own ability to experience wonder or awe, then spend more time with children. See the world through their eyes. You'll experience joy, unlock the mysteries that surround you, and be *awed* by their developing brilliance. It is hard to persist in taking anything for granted when you've seen the world through a child's eyes. Personally, I also think seeing the world through a teen's eyes is pretty awe-inspiring as well. They're not necessarily as cute chasing a butterfly, but their newfound capacity to seek a deeper understanding of the universe is astounding. Their capacity to care so deeply about others and to remain idealistic should be an inspiration to us all.

The following are some other ideas on sharing moments of awe with your teen:

- Talk to your teen about what kind of actions inspire them. Then help them find a biography or documentary about someone they'll find inspirational.
- Search online for awe-inspiring videos.
- Think of an idea about how a person could lift up another person through an act of selflessness or generosity. Search online for cases where people have done just that. Be inspired alongside your teen by the capacity of people to care for one another.
- If you attend a religious or spiritual service, don't let it be routine. Follow up with a discussion of what values were taught that day.
- See nature. Be amazed at the diversity of life on this planet and commit to protect it.
- Visit local museums and allow yourselves to be blown away by history, art, or science.

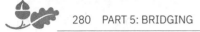

Recommended Resources

Greater Good Magazine is published by the GGSC at the University of California, Berkeley. The GGSC explores the roots of happy and compassionate individuals, strong social bonds, and altruistic behavior—the science of a meaningful life (https://greatergood.berkeley.edu).

The John Templeton Foundation. The Science of Awe. A White Paper Prepared by the Greater Good Science Center at UC Berkeley. 2018. https://www.templeton.org/discoveries/the-science-of-awe

CHAPTER 35

Advocate for a Better World for All Teens

I f we are serious about building a bridge to the future, we must make sure it is wide enough for the entire generation to cross. Your role as an advocate—especially when joined with other committed parents—is a game changer. Alongside being your teen's biggest supporter, this chapter covers how important it is to be an advocate for teens in your community and school settings.

We must ensure that every young person is prepared to lead us into a better tomorrow. Some will be activists or innovators and inspire others on a grand scale. Others will use their collaborative skills or supportive natures to build strong families and communities. We hope they all live a life of integrity committed to caring for and about others.

We cannot leave our collective future to chance. The best way to guarantee a better world is to invest in our youth today. Every teen deserves the security that comes from adults who believe in their potential and see their strengths. Every teen deserves the resources to enable them to stake a claim in the future. Ask yourself (and policy makers!), "What is this community (and nation) doing to support youth to reach their potential?"

Committing to Positive Youth Development

Richard Lerner, PhD, director of the Institute for Applied Research in Youth Development at Tufts University, and author of *The Good Teen: Rescuing Adolescence from the Myths of the Storm and Stress Years,* states, "Imagine if you viewed all teens, not just your own, through the lens of positive development. If all teens are thought of as assets in the making, rather than problems waiting to happen, then not only our own families but also society as a whole could be transformed."

As advocates for a better future, we must reject the notion that adolescence is an inherently risky time and that it is good enough if our teens just get through problem free. No! "Problem free is not fully prepared." This crystal-clear message was first stated in the 1980s by Karen Pittman, former president and CEO of the Forum for Youth Investment. Her call has been echoed by others, including Dr Lerner, who says, "A child free of problems... is not necessarily a child who has the knowledge and skills to compete successfully in the global marketplace. Educators and employers will want to know that young people are not engaging in harmful behaviors; however, they also will want to know that young people are prepared to fully participate in school and career."

Ensure Youth Receive Positive Messages

Young people *are* impressionable. Because teens endure so many changes, many of them worry about if they are "normal." They seek clues about what normal looks like and may model themselves to match how they think "normal" adolescents should look, feel, and behave. But where are they finding their input on what a normal teen is? And what do those portrayals look like?

To protect young people, we must reshape the way the teen years are portrayed by painting an accurate picture of adolescence that highlights the great majority of adolescents who display healthy and wise behaviors. As long as adolescents are routinely described as self-centered, impulsive, incapable of rational thought, inherently risky, or even dangerous, too many teens will believe their behavior should match these inaccurate portrayals.

Teens need people who will speak the truth about them. Rather than laughing or remaining silent when other adults repeat a stereotype about teens, choose to calmly state the truth. You might say, "Actually, I have found many teenagers to be some of the most thoughtful and caring people I know." Or, "I find their energy and commitment to friendship (or to social causes) inspirational." Sometimes, however, your advocacy work will need to move beyond one-on-one conversations. Teens deserve adult advocates who will address media coverage of teens or speak up when community programs miss the opportunity to elevate youth to their potential.

Make it more likely that teens will be surrounded by positive messages by

- Noticing the acts of generosity and compassion shown by young people and sharing these stories among your friends and neighbors.
- Advocating for the positive portrayal of youth in the news by asking them to present an accurate and balanced view of young people. Media coverage focuses on the highest achievers and youth who commit crimes. We have to celebrate the everyday kids who perform acts of loving-kindness, protect the vulnerable, work to build a better community, and take action

to protect and preserve the environment. These newsworthy stories paint a very different picture of adolescence.

- Advocating for public health messages that go beyond telling youth what *not* to do. Messages that solely tell youth not to do drugs, for example, can miss the mark in 2 critical ways. First, they may inadvertently suggest that it is expected that teens will do drugs when, in fact, most will not. Second, not doing drugs (or not becoming pregnant) is not an inspirational message! We have to help teens dream of a future in which they can have a fulfilling life and make a meaningful difference to others. We have to let them know what they *can* do. Then, critically, community programming must support youth to realize their potential.

Listen to Teens

As you advocate for teens, have the real experts stand by your side: teens. Nobody knows better what they need to thrive than teens themselves. Allow their energy to fuel your efforts and take advantage of the lens youth bring to key discussions. As we discussed in Chapter 34, teens recognize problems in need of solutions for issues adults have long ago chosen to ignore. Involving teens in community advocacy efforts can help you envision programs that will lift and empower teens. Giving them a voice now will encourage them to stay involved in projects that can create lasting change. As you stand next to a teen today, realize you may be standing next to a leader of tomorrow.

A Culture of Noticing, Mentoring, and Role Modeling

Noticing

Young people benefit when they have touch points with many adults. Too many of us assume that teenagers would rather be hanging out with peers in a parallel universe. This perception of teenagers is linked to the myth that adolescents don't like adults. They do want peer time, but they also value time with adults. A simple hello reminds teens that you are noticing them. Even better, take the time to sit down with your young neighbors and ask them how things are going for them. You may find that you have a special role being an adult guide for some of your own teen's friends.

Young people noticed by adults are more likely to find role models and to glean wisdom from elders. They are also less likely to fall through the cracks. Each adult they interact with serves as a level of protection who can notice changes in their behavior or mood. There is great power in an adult saying, "I've noticed you seem to have something on your mind. Anything you want to talk about?"

Mentoring and Role Modeling

The more exposures teens have with adults, the more likely they are to find inspiration. The best chance for them finding something that sparks their interest is to see someone else pursuing their passion first. Every adult can inspire a young person if they're willing to talk about what they do. Young people need to know what the real world looks like so that they can imagine the possibilities of how they might contribute.

Some adults can take the next step and change a life direction by becoming a mentor. Mentoring relationships prepare youth for the journey toward a satisfying career and may include frank discussions about barriers that need to be overcome. There may be formal opportunities in your community to be a mentor. If you don't know how to find them or want to explore this on your own, visit MENTOR at mentoring.org. This organization expands mentoring initiatives around the country. They identify and link youth with adults in local communities who are willing to guide and spend time with youth.

The benefits of role modeling and mentoring are a 2-way street. It is easy for our work lives to become routine. It is energizing to look at our lives through fresh eyes. We can become rejuvenated with the knowledge that what has become mundane to us remains a dream for a young person.

Refuse to Give Up on Anyone

The motto of Kids at Hope, a youth development organization, is, "All Children are Capable of Success, No Exceptions!" Such an aspirational vision is possible with a sustained commitment. Too many communities invest in only those youth who are easiest to reach. Advocate for your community to leave no one behind, by joining with other parents and making it clear that communities thrive when *all* youth are given the opportunity to contribute. The following thoughts may help you change the hearts and minds of those who give up on the potential of every youth too easily:

Youth Who Have Endured Hardships Possess High Levels of Compassion

Some young people who have had the hardest lives may be less likely to initially engage with adults. They've earned the right to be suspicious and to withhold trust until we have passed their tests. Much of my work in the last 4 decades has been with youth who have experienced childhood traumas. I work with some of the finest human beings on the planet. Although it may take time until these youth feel safe, once they do, their truest selves are revealed. They are often deeply compassionate and caring young people, committed to repairing the world.

Young people who have endured hardships have a particularly well-developed emotional and reactive part of their brain. This is precisely what allowed them to sense danger in their childhood and to avoid it whenever they could. These young people have "protector's brains." They seem to be wired to protect themselves and others they care about. When they sense danger, their emotional reactive brain dominates over their thoughtful and compassionate selves. On the other hand, when we create safe settings for them, that same part of their well-developed emotional brain taps into its potential. This part of the brain is also the root of human compassion. When they feel safe, it is as though they have protection to spare. Their empathy—their desire to see others' needs and to keep them safe—is elevated.

Brain science does not do justice to this topic. There is something much deeper on a spiritual level that explains the profound potential of youth forced to be resilient. The takeaway is that we should never allow their initial mistrust or reactivity to diminish our engagement. They deserve our investment, protection, and nurturing now. In turn, they will lift others up over their lifetimes.

Youth Who Push Us Away

If we're going to live by the mantra of no exceptions, then we also must consider what to do with those young people who say they do not want our involvement in their lives or who even push us away. Remember, many youth have earned the right to test us before trusting us. But many youth work hard to pretend they don't care or don't want our involvement *precisely because the opposite is true.* It may be that their sensitivity is so overwhelming to them that they feel the need to pretend they don't care to shut away the intensity of their feelings. They may even engage in behaviors counter to what adults hope to see teens doing. For example, young people who use drugs may act as if they do not want our involvement and behave as though they don't care about their future. In many cases, their desire to shut down the depth of their emotions led them to the problem behavior.

We must give every young person—no exceptions—the opportunity to reveal how much they do care. They'll only allow themselves to be vulnerable in this way if we let them know we stand by them, hear them, and support them through their struggles. Again, we must stop telling these kids what *not* to do and instead tell them what they *can* do. It starts by seeing them as they deserve to be seen and not through the lens of the problematic behaviors.

Working Toward Equity

While teens are generally held to relatively low expectations because of common myths and misperceptions about them, some youth get double the dose of lowered expectations. These undermining expectations may be as a result of "isms" related to race, gender, gender identity, sexuality, poverty, or immigrant status. Youth in varied settings also may receive fewer resources than other youth and, therefore, draw a conclusion about how society values them. For example, youth who live in rural or urban settings often receive fewer resources than their suburban counterparts.

Working toward equity is about promoting and creating the conditions in which *all* young people can participate fully and reach their full potential. In other words, equity is about everyone having what they deserve to be successful and to thrive. A commitment to equity raises every young person and builds a better world for all of us. Everyone gains.

When efforts at equity are viewed as something one person must give up to benefit another, we miss the opportunity to build a more just and better world for us all. Equity is about giving the opportunity for every young person to be their best self and to illuminate those barriers that might get in the way for some people to achieve. People who have had the cards stacked against them for whatever reason are deserving of extra supports, nurturing, and resources. In a world in which every young person can strive to be their best self, we all rise together.

Preparing Youth-Serving Professionals to Use a Strength-Based Approach

We all must be grateful to those youth-serving professionals who devote their lives to building the next generation. To support youth-serving programs' capacity to serve youth with strength-focused practices, I created and edited *Reaching Teens: Strength-Based, Trauma-Sensitive, Resilience-Building Communication Strategies Rooted in Positive Youth Development,* a professional multimedia toolkit published by the American Academy of Pediatrics. It offers a comprehensive, strength-based set of strategies to serve youth. Its contributors represent a diverse group of more than 120 youth-serving professionals from multiple disciplines who offer practical guidance on optimal communication strategies. It also includes scores of youth sharing what engages versus alienates them.

At its core, *Reaching Teens* is about preparing professionals to be the kind of adults young people deserve to guide them to be their best selves and to change course when necessary. It addresses key challenges in young lives but always views them through a strength-based, trauma-sensitive lens and has a goal of building their resilience while preparing them to develop to their potential.

PART 6

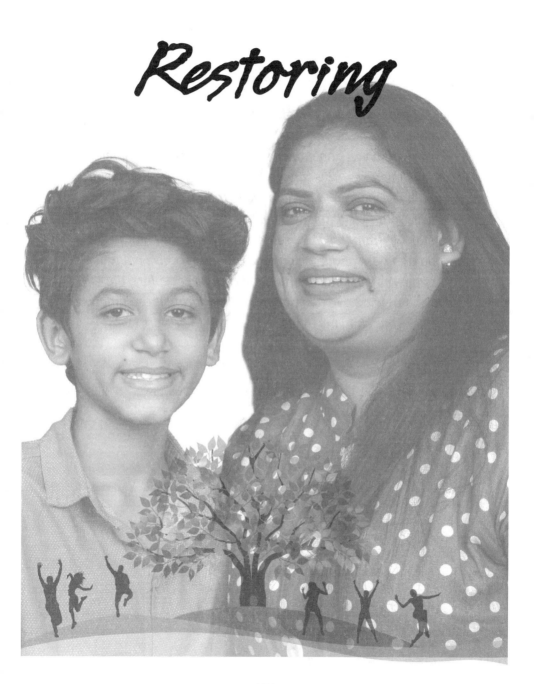

Restoring

Relationships are complicated. And adolescence will include some bumps and bruises. Your child may pull away from you and make some unwise choices or even serious mistakes. You can work to restore your relationship and bring your child back to being their better and wiser self. Your best chance of successfully achieving this is starting from the deep-seated knowledge of all that is good and right about your child. You may receive guidance from professionals, but nobody can ever replace the love that you have for your child. It is during these times that your child most needs you to be their North Star.

CHAPTER 36

Strengthen (or Restore) Your Relationship

Adolescence is a time that simultaneously challenges and strengthens families. There is a natural tension between a parent's need to keep their child safe and an adolescent's need to stretch their wings. That tension can sometimes boil over in even the strongest and most functional families. Furthermore, precisely because children feel secure in our love, they may release their frustrations over school or peers within our homes. Enduring these challenges can seem to threaten our relationships. But resolving these tensions while demonstrating that our love is unshakable makes our relationships more secure.

Families are complicated. It is within our homes that we learn that you can have conflict and recover. Too often we focus on our adolescent's heightened emotions as driving the tension in the home. That is unfair because all of us behave badly at times. Life isn't supposed to look like a greeting card. It is real. When our families are under strain, and we never stop caring about each other and continue to draw support from one another, we show what unwavering love is *really* about.

This chapter starts with a recap of key strategies that create the secure, loving relationships that enable families to weather life's inevitable storms. Then it will be divided into 2 parts: securing the foundation of strong parent-teen relationships and restoring your relationship after it has been challenged. However, our lives are not neatly divided in that way. Rather, we live life with both things occurring simultaneously: we are always working on strengthening our families and we are always working to grow stronger from resolving inevitable tensions.

The Foundation of Strong Relationships

This entire book has presented strategies that foster open communication between you and your teen and create the kind of relationship that will lead to *inter*dependent lives far into the future. In the following, I underscore just a few points:

- The knowledge of who your teen *really* is enables you to see the best in them even when they are not displaying their best self. You, in turn, serve as an ever-present reminder of their very best self.

- Knowing how much you matter drives your presence. You understand the truth: adults are the most important people in the lives of young people, and teens like adults. In fact, adolescents care more about what their parents think than they care about anybody else's opinion. Knowing this, you see adolescence as an opportunity to guide your child as they prepare to launch into adulthood.

- Lighthouse parents have the best relationship with their adolescents and are more likely to have emotionally healthy teens who have the best academic success and lowest behavioral risks. At its core, lighthouse parenting is about achieving that balance of expressing our love for our children while setting and monitoring the boundaries that keep teens safe. Communicate: "Because I love you, I insist that _____ to keep you safe."

- Families thrive when they are *inter*dependent on one another. To develop these healthy relationships, parents honor their adolescent's need for growing independence. Parents who hover or overprotect their teens end up installing "control buttons," which may cause their young adult children to reject their continued close involvement.

- Parents who see adolescents as experts in their own lives honor their teen's growing developmental capabilities and seek to learn more about their lives. When parents listen more than they talk and learn to withhold their reactions, teens are more likely to share.

- Teens appreciate parents who keep them safe and hold them accountable. When discipline is about teaching with the goal of adolescents developing self-control and wise decision-making capacities, it works well. When parents, instead, view discipline as control or punishment, families can suffer, and teens often resist their parents' demands.

- Families thrive when all its members work to develop a growth mindset and a willingness to learn from each other. This means that parents recognize that honoring the wisdom and idealism of youth and capturing their sense of wonder can contribute to their own lives.

Continued Growth in Our Relationships

A starting point to continuing to strengthen our relationships is to create the space for enjoying one another and allowing thoughts and feelings to surface. This means backing away from thinking your limited time together should always be "productive," by focusing on high-yield subjects such as grades, performance, or reprimanding about behaviors. These topics are important, but if your relationships are limited to discussing only those, you'll miss the ongoing miracles of development. Create spaces where you can genuinely and deeply listen. If you do, talking and sharing from your teen will happen. Nothing says, "I respect you," more than creating a nonjudgmental space where a person can truly be themselves. When teens feel respected, they safely reveal themselves. Create spaces for sometimes doing nothing and other times having fun. You'll laugh and share interests. You'll learn what they care about and witness their developing values. You'll know who they are. What could be higher yield than that?

The Importance of Knowing and Valuing Each Other

Teens need to understand that parents can only focus on what they know. If teens share only what they are doing (eg, grades, activities), parents may not know what their teens are feeling. If parents only learn about their children's lives when they get into trouble, then how can parents catch all of the good things teens are doing? **Your teen may lack insight into the fact that they determine what kind of things you discuss as a family**. Tell your teen that you want to be supportive in all areas of their life and take interest in what they care about but that the only way you can do that is when they share with you what matters to them. This is the way they'll earn your compassion and enable you to shape your parenting to meet their needs.

Adults often forget how much teens *need* to know who *we* are. Remember, they're trying to imagine what it means to be an adult. They don't want deeply private details of your life (relieved?), but they want to see more of you than many parents choose to display. They want to know what you enjoy and how they can bring pleasure into your life. Don't get me wrong, they don't need you as a friend, but they do need you as a guide. They want to know what you care about. They want to see you reconcile your values with your realities. Role models are not perfect; they are humans learning to live with their imperfections. Remember, teenagers don't want to see their parents as ducks gliding effortlessly on the water; they want to know what your little feet are doing underneath to stay afloat.

Teens want to know they are adding to your life. If you focus only on grades and good behaviors, then many teens apply too much pressure on themselves to fit into a mold of your making. When, on the other hand, you genuinely cherish watching them develop their interests and hone their values, they'll know they please you by being their best selves. When you appreciate their sense of wonder and the rapid pace at which they are learning, you can allow them to be your teacher. They will relish knowing they are contributing to your growth.

Understanding Development Can Prevent Your Relationship From Being Derailed

It is an active decision—and one that preserves our relationships—to choose to place certain challenging aspects of our parent-teen relationships in the context of development. For example, their occasional moodiness is less likely to throw you for a loop if you grasp that it is the flip side of the very brain development that ensures their growing empathy and sensitivity. Perhaps the most painful aspect of the parent-teen relationship is when our teen stops sharing as much of their life with us or sends us clear signals that they want us to be invisible (or at least silent) in public. Knowing that this is a typical developmental process on the road to independence can allow you take it less personally. The reason your teen may push you to the sidelines is that they are self-conscious and, because you are so similar, they feel as if you are representing them when speaking. They don't want to be on display and feel they are being scrutinized when you speak. The greatest issue for them, however, is that they love you so much and know, in time, they'll need to separate from you. That is too much to think about, so rejecting you allows them to ignore those feelings for a bit. Knowing that pushing you away is really about loving you makes it hurt less, doesn't it? Hurting less allows you stay near—at an appropriate distance that allows growing independence—even if it feels like you are being asked to stay far away.

Restoring Your Relationship

In Chapter 38, we discuss the things you might say after your relationship has endured some bumps. In this chapter, we discuss setting the tone in your home that allows relationships to be repaired.

Back to High-Yield Time

The air in your home can feel laden with intensity, especially after you and your teen have engaged in a heated discussion or you've needed to dive in deeply to avert a crisis or manage a behavioral concern. It puts pressure on your relationship. People fear the deep discussions that are needed to restore calm in the house and regain trust. Above all, your child wonders whether your love, in fact, is unconditional or whether they have lost it. Because of how much intensity is present, set the problem aside for a while.

Get back to just being together. Enjoy each other. Your teen may fear that every time they're with you, the big topics are going to come up. They need to understand there will be a time and a space for that, but first, you need to just be together to remind each other that no problem is greater than your love. In fact, explicitly say, "Let's go out and _____. I promise not a word out of my mouth about correcting you. I just want to be with you."

Maintaining (Unconditional) Love

It's not easy to be unconditionally loving when you're worried out of your mind or bursting with anger over a particular situation involving your teen. It is in these very moments that you need to draw in that deep breath and be intentional about taking no action. Your goal is to move past this temporary feeling and ensure that your relationship is maintained during the toughest moments and ultimately strengthened because you have endured them. Your teen needs your love as the most protective force in their life. Knowing that you know who they really are is the very best chance your teen has to return to their better self while managing the stressors driving their behavior. Knowing how badly your love is needed by your teen may not make it initially easier to move past your justified feelings of fear or anger. But your love will remind you that there is no other path than to show up for your child when they desperately need your presence. Parents whose anger takes such a deep hold that it prevents them from engaging with their teens in crisis may lose the opportunity to steer their children back toward safer, wiser behaviors.

As you are taking that breath, fill yourself with the knowledge of why you feel so strongly. Your feelings are valid and your emotions are earned. Remember, it is the depth of your love that makes you feel so fully. I know this sounds a bit like poetry while you have to parent in prose. But I hope it reminds you why you are so committed to getting this right. You can forcefully reject your teen's misbehavior while simultaneously never giving up on them.

You may need a reset button. Remind yourself why you care so much. You might do this through talking to your teen's other parent. Your child might be a teen now, but inside of them is the baby you swaddled and the child you reluctantly dropped off on the first day of school. Your teen might occasionally make you want to tear your hair out, but your teen is the same person as the toddler who ran to greet you at the front door. Remembering this may be what you need to reach the calm and loving state from which you parent best.

294 PART 6: RESTORING

It's not just the memories of yesteryear that should remind you of how completely you love. Reflect on all that is good and right about your teen now. A first step can be considering the whys beneath the behaviors. Sometimes it is how much they care that makes them invest heavily in pretending they don't care at all. It may be maddening that your teen no longer accepts all of your rules, but hasn't it been awe-inspiring to watch your teen learn to think for themself? Launching from this place of love, you can handle the challenges...together.

On the other side of this crisis may be a stronger relationship with a child who has once more learned to turn to you. Your steady presence might be the key ingredient that will endow them with the confidence to right themself.

Rebuilding Trust

Teens know when their parents' disappointment and anger overwhelm them. Countless teens have explained their behaviors to me as actions they took once they realized they had nothing left to lose. They have said, "My parents don't trust me anyway. I may as well live my life and have fun." I have heard this used as justification to use drugs, cut classes, and stop following household rules. I have seen teens who were deeply depressed because they felt as though they had lost their parent's love and others who were highly anxious for fear that they could never get it back. Many other teens have escalated their behaviors so that they could still get a rise out of their parents. They learned their parents stopped paying attention to the smaller issues, and they did what they thought it would take to get the only kind of attention they knew how to muster.

We must avoid having our teens believe they have nothing left to lose. We must never lower our expectations, because our adolescents will continue to strive for those standards. You never want your child to feel they have already lost your respect or belief that they are a good person. We must always ensure our teens understand that it is our job to discipline them appropriately, and sometimes that includes restrictions to keep them safe. And yes, it is OK to admit that sometimes our confidence in them is shaken and our trust is tested. But we always leave a path open for them to fully regain our trust. "My goal is for you to become the wonderful person I know you are destined to be. To get there, you will make mistakes. These mistakes do not define you or make me love you even the slightest bit less. But it is my job to protect and prepare you. Privileges are earned with responsibility. You have temporarily lost a privilege because of your behavior. Let me be clear about what I need to see to believe that you are ready for this privilege again."

There is a decent chance your teen's other parent or guardian may not (initially) be on the same page with you. Especially during behavioral challenges, you must come together because the stress of the situation could easily push you apart. Otherwise, one parent will become labeled as "nice" while the other one is seen as overly controlling. This is how families break apart. It's also a starting point for adolescents to learn manipulative behaviors.

Present a unified plan to your child that covers both your expectations and the path toward rebuilding trust. You both

- Love your teen and want them to be safe.
- Care that your teen has character strengths that ensure happiness and success in the future.
- Disapprove of the current mistaken behavior.
- Agree on a consequence.
- Continue to see your teen as a wonderful person, and this mistake does not change that.
- Know that they will fully re-earn your trust and will share together how they can do so.

Tell your teen that, to regain and hold your trust, it will have to be earned. The best way for them to do that is to demonstrate responsibility moving forward. Let them know you will watch them closely and expect to see them doing the right thing. Trust will be regained when their behaviors prove they are learning to be more careful or responsible. It is not good enough to let this general idea float in the air; help them imagine what they might do to demonstrate they have learned a lesson. Ideally, you can facilitate their thinking. For example,

> **Parent(s):** You know that coming home late and drunk was unacceptable. Of course, we took away the car keys because, as long as you are drinking, we have to be certain you'll never drive.

> **Teen:** But I wasn't drinking and driving. I parked the car at my friend's house and walked home and that's why I was late.

> **Parent(s):** Drinking is illegal at your age, and you could put yourself at risk even if you weren't driving. But because you weren't drinking and driving, you'll have an opportunity to get your keys back. If you were driving while intoxicated, you would never get those keys back. You did the right thing in not driving but made a mistake by not letting us know where you were or involving us. What can you do to earn our trust back?

> **Teen:** I'll call you if I ever find myself in any risky situation again. I'll also let you know where I am ahead of time. And if I am ever going to be late for curfew, you'll know why.

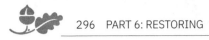

Parent(s): In this case, we could have arranged for you to get home. Assuming you show us you'll always be on time for curfew, and that we know where you are, you'll get your keys back. But there's one more thing.

Teen: Let me guess, I'm about to get a lecture on alcohol.

Parent(s): Not a lecture. But it is our responsibility that you understand how alcohol can put you in danger. It's a lot more than about driving, it's about how you make decisions. And, as we said, it's also illegal at your age. We're going to talk about this after you've read through the materials at https://teens.drugabuse.gov/teens. Let's add all of this into our agreement and we'll look at how you're doing in 2 months (see Chapter 27). We love you and nothing matters more to us than your safety. Deal?

Teen: Deal.

Home Relationships Affect All Relationships

The relationships in our homes are training grounds for all human interactions. When I speak to teens about the importance of restoring a strong relationship with their parents, I discuss that it will influence how they generally respond to authority, arrive at decisions, and react to feedback. We talk about the fact that relationships will always be hard work and their willingness to forgive people of their human frailties predicts whether future ones will flourish through rough patches. We speak of how the health of their relationships at home will make a difference to how they interact with teachers and coaches now and their bosses, colleagues, and spouses later.

Frustration and anger are real. But because you deserve a good relationship with your teen, and because it will shape all others in their life, never question whether your relationship is worth the investment it takes to restore it to health. Nothing could matter more.

•••

Recommended Resources

The Center for Parent and Teen Communication offers materials written by young people to help other youth understand their parents' viewpoint and how to effectively communicate with them (https://parentandteen.com /category/talking-with-parents).

Raising Kids to Thrive: Balancing Love With Expectations and Protection With Trust contains a section entitled Rebooting: Moving Toward the Relationship You Hope to Have. It has 5 chapters for parents as well as "A Chapter for Young People: First Steps Toward a Better Relationship With Your Parents."

CHAPTER 37

Bringing Them Back
Seeing All That Is Good and Right in Them...Again

As a pediatrician, I have advised thousands of families over the years. The conversations often begin with the family expressing concerns about their teen's behavior or mood. As I listen to their concerns, I work hard to hear both their worries and the depth of their caring. I've witnessed teens trying not to show how upset they are that they've disappointed their parents.

It is my job to get families on the same page and to help teens understand they are in a safe place. I concentrate on the fact that the room is filled with caring people. I turn to the parents and ask them to tell me where the caring comes from: "Tell me who your teen really is. What makes you proud? Tell me about things you've seen from the time they were a toddler." More often than not, parents will cry as they describe their child's goodness. The tension in the room diminishes. Shame and defensive anger are lifted.

Now, the real work can begin. During moments where we feel the most challenged, we can draw from the knowledge of our children's strengths. Teens may question who they are. But *we* must never question who they are. Our clarity will move them through tough times and serve as the foundation to strengthen our families.

In Chapter 4, we focused on recognizing and reinforcing our teen's strengths as a central strategy to launch them into a secure adulthood. In this chapter, we use those same strengths to take the first steps in restoring our child to being their best self after they have strayed into worrisome behaviors or as a first step to address their emotional distress.

When Your Love May Count the Most

At some point, your teen may engage in self-destructive or harmful behaviors. They can feel so much distress that they may act out, blinding us to the fact that their irritability or anger is rooted in sadness. These trying times can challenge our relationships. We may love but have moments we don't like what they are doing or even like the side of themself we are seeing.

Your love matters more now than ever. Your unwavering presence serves as that beacon from the lighthouse, signaling that they can find their way home. We mustn't allow them to believe you've stopped caring or have given up on them—that there is no returning to the way it had been. Our teens sense what we feel. The frustration. Disappointment. Sadness. Powerlessness. Anger. Guilt. Therefore, **find your strength to feel hope**.

Despite the words your distressed child might be saying, your approval matters. When young people hurt deeply, they may feel they are not worthy of being cared about and push people away. Do not believe their actions; they are lying to themselves. Believe *your* love. Our teens need us to believe in them even when they've lost faith in themselves. If they've gone beyond the safe limits we've set, they need our reminder that there is security within our boundaries and they are welcome back. Once a teen knows they have something to turn back toward, they will more likely take the first steps.

Restoring Confidence: A Critical Step to Gaining a Sense of Control

It's easy to focus on a problem, especially when it won't let you turn away. It is harder to see beneath the surface to allow the strengths to reveal themselves, yet it is key to positioning you as a change agent. We must begin the process of moving our teens who are experiencing paralysis and inaction to confidence and empowerment. This can only happen if they realize that something they can do might make a difference. To regain a sense of control, they must believe that decisions they make and actions they take can matter. Therefore, the first step toward positive behavioral change may be gaining the confidence to start. A teen builds confidence through receiving and trusting the feedback that they have demonstrated the skills and attributes needed. Ultimately, they solidify confidence when they take those initial steps successfully.

A person's confidence, on the other hand, is undermined when they believe they are incapable. Sadly, as we discussed in the introduction, it is common for teens to absorb messages that they are impulsive, thoughtless, and even the source of problems. However, some adolescents have had a heavier dose of these undermining messages. They may view themselves as undeserving and view their destiny as out of their control. They may have tried to make changes but were met with repeated failure. Demoralization can set in, which can diminish their belief in the potential of progress.

The power to transform a life starts when we see a person as a whole human being rather than as a problem. A strength-based approach reinforces that a person can control their destiny. It reinforces strengths and skill sets that can be built on to change circumstances. Several times a year, I connect with a young adult (or, at this point, middle-aged person!) who I knew during their adolescence. They write to me or see me on the street and share that they were listening after all and that they have lived meaningful lives. When asked what turned their life around, they can almost always point to an adult who believed in them. **It is most powerful when they are describing a parent or caregiver.** "It was when _____ made me understood I was worth something." "It was when _____ stuck with me until I was ready to listen." "It never felt like anybody was on my team until then. It felt like _____ saw me before I was ready to see myself." Be the kind of adult who knows that love is more than a feeling. See your teen as they deserve to be seen, for who they really *are*.

Seeing People Through a Strength-Based Lens

If you are caught in the middle of a crisis or are managing a child in the depths of emotional distress, you may have, by necessity, taken on a problem-focused lens. Because teens often see themselves through the reflection in our eyes, we can't allow their identity to develop based on a problem they are struggling with. You may need a professional by your side, but you can still offer something no professional can: draw from the memories of who your child really is. When you remember all that is good and right about them, your memories will ground them in their true self. They'll remember who they have been and who they want to be. There are no perfect words. Even when you say little, while holding those memories close and remaining present, your teen will know that you care. And that is a gift only you can offer.

Using Those Strengths to Build Confidence

A teen's challenges must be addressed, but that is done best when seen among their strengths. This will lessen shame and promote action. This strategy is most effective when the strengths we recognize can be easily linked to the behavior we hope to promote within them. Confidence comes from knowing that success is possible. Remember to reinforce those strengths that are starting points toward progress. I am going to ask you to trust me here—even if you are hurting deeply right now—the youth who worry us most during adolescence also possess some of the deepest strengths that predict that they will have a rich adulthood. We must focus now, however, on moving them past this point safely.

Based on decades of my professional experience, the following are examples of strengths coupled with how they serve as starting points toward progress:

- **Sensitivity:** Young people in emotional distress often possess a deep sensitivity. They struggle in managing all their feelings, which can contribute to anxiety or depression. Teens may use substances to shut down their feelings to avoid the depth of their emotions.
  - We can affirm their sensitivity by reinforcing all the ways it will benefit them in the future, while supporting them to deal with how overwhelmed they are with feelings now.

- **Compassion:** Many young people who have endured hardships also have a remarkable ability to empathize with others' pain. Consequently, many of them see themselves working to support youth like them in the future.
  - Their intention to contribute positively to others' lives can be the starting point to commit to their own wellness. You can frame this as a critical step to become stronger now so they'll be stronger for others later.

- **Commitment:** Many adolescents wish for a better world. This may be especially true for young people who have led hard lives. They hope for a world that looks more like the one they wished they had experienced.
  - Support your teen to understand the power they will possess if they first strengthen themself by taking the steps to become emotionally healthier or to make wiser decisions.

- **Loyalty:** Many teen behaviors (positive or undermining) are intensified when with their peers. A person's loyalty to their friends is a great strength. They often possess a deep-seated sense of fairness and a strong desire to protect others.
  - This strength can be leveraged to help them grasp that, if they want to impactfully support their friends who engage in unhealthy behaviors, they can first heal themself and, in so doing, become a role model to their friends.

- **Respect:** It is remarkable how deeply many teens are committed to respecting others. The code is that if you offer respect, you earn it back.
  - Let your teen understand how much you admire their commitment to treating others respectfully. Support them in learning to treat themself with respect as well.

- **Perseverance:** Many teens who participate in undermining behaviors still possess a drive to improve themselves and others. Look and listen for their remarkable desire to never give up. For example, your teen might still be making it to school daily despite their severe depression.

  — When recognized, perseverance can remind a young person that the drive remains within them to complete a task or work toward returning to their best self.

- **Resourcefulness:** It is remarkable how teens can stretch their resources or make systems work for them. For example, does your teen still have the care and support from school staff despite their disruptive behaviors? When you notice that your teen most needs you, that reflects their ability to draw needed attention.

  — If you are grateful for this, it is an entry point to remind them of your care and of your intention to secure for them the resources they deserve.

- **Honesty:** If you are not liking what you hear, it is probably because your teen is willing to share their truth with you.

  — Admire this and reinforce for them that they can also share their story with professionals and/or advocate for their needs.

- **Insight:** If your tween or teen can describe to you the "whys" behind their behaviors, they likely possess insight beyond these years.

  — Leverage their understanding of themself to problem-solve and develop plans that will uniquely work for them.

- **Resilience:** It is inspiring to see how well your child has survived difficult times.

  — If you see this, name it. It will mean so much to them that their strength amid adversity has been noticed. It offers you an opening to join with them in continuing to build their resilience. It allows them to begin to reframe themself as a survivor.

Remember, your goal is to raise a child who will exhibit self-control and ultimately take control over their own life. Therefore, they must see their own strengths as skill sets to be accessed on their own. Remember how Dorothy from *The Wizard of Oz* became self-aware that the solution to her problems were always within reach? We must have your teen recognize their own "ruby slippers."

Using Your Teen's Strengths to Initiate Progress

After you've focused on uncovering your teen's strengths through active listening, you will be ready to share with your teen what you've heard and partner with them to move forward. The following approach recognizes, reinforces, and builds on strengths and then invites a collaborative problem-solving approach. You will recall this described in Chapter 4 as the "heart-belly-head-hands" approach. This active listening style allows you the freedom to *feel* rather than *strategize*. Focus on listening and pay full attention to your body. Sensations will flow and your body will send signals. Your heart melts and flutters as you are reminded how deeply you care, and your belly may tighten when you become worried. This approach gives you the structure to share what you feel while engaging your teen to start a healing process.

- **Heart:** Explain to your teen how you were reminded about how deeply you care. Recount what you see that reminds you of their core goodness. You are on their team—now and forever—and they are deserving of your love and capable of becoming their very best self.

- **Take a moment to reflect:** You might pause here or even take a deep breath. You are modeling how to re-center your thoughts.

- **Belly:** Share why you are worried. Despite all the strengths you see, you fear current behaviors (or their emotional distress) will undermine their potential (or cause them to sink deeper into despair).

- **Head:** Ask if you can create a plan together, recognizing that they are the expert in their own life but that you are a committed guide. Your life experience may mean you have ideas on where to start. Suggest that the behaviorally operational strengths that you've highlighted are critical starting points.

- **Hands:** Ask how you can best serve or support them to move forward. You are giving them control, but you'll stand by their side as they move through it. Now may be the time to share that they deserve professional support as well (see Chapter 39).

It is easier for adolescents to deal with our concerns if we first note their successes. It may be transformative for you to notice and elevate something wonderful within them. At the very least, it will diminish their shame enough to lower their defenses. Once we get permission to address a problem, we get buy-in and can offer them the kind of control and self-confidence they need to be willing to consider taking steps to change. This strategy also lets them know that we partner with them in the plans and will stay by their side in the journey.

But I Am Too Hurt and Angry to See Strengths

You've earned your anger and your frustration. You need to give yourself permission to experience that hurt and even forgive yourself for the frustration that makes you not want to give more of yourself right now. Anger is a safe emotion to feel. Safer than displaying your real emotion—fear. We are most angry when we are most worried, and we worry because we love. If you weren't so deeply connected you wouldn't feel so fully invested. Remember to separate the behavior from the teen. You can hate the behavior; you can despise what the emotional distress is doing to your teen. You can be angry at the distress, if not chaos, the circumstances have brought on you and others you care about. But you cherish your child. See their strengths, even though their behaviors are unacceptable.

A Professional's Critical Role

Your role in giving them the security to begin healing is irreplaceable, but it may not be enough. Your teen likely deserves professional psychological or medical support. Many conditions that endanger young people or bring them to the brink of despair have a biologic basis. Substance use and eating disorders, for example, start as behaviors but become brain diseases. Anxiety and depression and other mental health conditions are often associated with an underlying chemical imbalance in the brain. A professional offers an objective, caring person in their life. This objectivity is critical. It enables our children to unload without worrying that they are hurting or burdening us by revealing to us the depths of their distress.

Communication Is a 2-way Street

You are committed to open and respectful communication. You are working to focus on strengths as an effective strategy to address problems. But communication is a 2-way street, and you expect respectful communication in return. That is more than fair. Be aware, however, that a teen in crisis may need time and growth before they are able to offer you what you're able to give them. When they become better regulated, you'll get back some of the respect and compassion you've offered without condition. It will require some patience on your end with a healthy dose of optimism before you'll uniformly receive the communication you deserve. In the meantime, ask an involved professional to support your teen to develop the communication skills that will prepare them to better partner with you moving forward.

Let Them See the Good In You

Relationships are complicated, and what goes wrong is rarely based on what just one person does. It is possible that actions you've taken, or not taken, were hurtful to your child. It is possible that part of their behavior or emotional distress can be explained by a situation within the family. I cannot tell you whether anything you did or didn't do contributed to the problem. But I have noticed that caring parents always try to blame themselves. And I can tell you with certainty that you *are* part of the solution.

I can tell you something else with certainty. There is a lot of good and right about *you*. You deserve to have your teen see that. But remember, empathy isn't best taught by someone saying, "You should care about others (or me)." It's developed through personal experience of receiving empathy. Here too, your strength-based approach to your adolescent will pay off by the example you set. When you are deserving of empathy, we hope the script in their head will play something like this: "It has felt so good for someone who knows me this well to still see me as a good person even when I haven't been proud of how I was acting. They annoy me sometimes, but I know down deep that they are a good person. I'm proud of them."

Give it time.

CHAPTER 38

Listening and Talking
The Language and Mindset of Restoration

The mindset of restoration is about committing ourselves to returning to a previous (or improved!) state. But why are we requesting a reset? And where are we setting the bar? What is the standard we are hoping to reach? Throughout this work, we've talked about seeing all that is good and right in your child. That is the answer to these questions: you want your adolescent to be the person you know they're capable of being. You expect nothing more—or less—of them than to be their true self. We are not talking about perfection or even about what they achieve. When they go astray, you're asking them to restore themself to their better self.

You may be asking your child (or they may be asking you!) to invest in repairing your relationship. You're asking them to return to your family in its best light. It was never a perfect family, because such a family doesn't exist. Think about your family and reflect on what you value most. That is what you're inviting your child to be a part of again. If your family was never the model you hoped it would be, you're inviting your family members to grow together. Using the language of restoration, join with your teen and other members of your household and say, "We can be better...we can be stronger...we *must* support each other. The world may be unpredictable, but we can work toward peace in our home."

When Is a Reset Needed?

The first step in changing your parenting (or relationship) patterns is to realize you are not functioning as you should. That is **not** an admission of failure. You are modeling a growth mindset and demonstrating flexibility! You refuse to remain entrenched in ineffective cycles of communication.

You are looking at your teen and seeing that they are not thriving. Maybe they are stuck in a rut and can't seem to be able to dig themself out. They might be engaged in unhealthy or unwise behaviors. Perhaps they're feigning laziness, acting as if they don't care, because they care so much. On the other hand, maybe they're working too hard to be the "perfect" child, and you know the harm that comes from striving for the impossible. Maybe the way your family communicates is just not working. Perhaps too much of your time is spent nagging or yelling. You may find yourself wasting energy with other adults (eg, spouses, former spouses, extended family) arguing over how to parent. Perhaps you've grown frustrated that your family is always problem-solving instead of enjoying each other's company. What ties all these things together is that members of your family (maybe even you) have grown to expect these patterns.

You recognize that healthy relationships in your home are the bedrock of happiness and the key to your teen having a second chance to be the person you know they deserve to be. You need to reset the communication patterns in your family. And you're courageous and committed enough to know your family is worth investing in!

Getting on the Same Page as Other Key Adults

Your views on parenting may differ from other adults who are central figures in your teen's life. Reading this book may have brought your varied takes on parenting into sharper focus. No 2 individuals will ever agree on everything. But, for the sake of your teen and their relationship with each of you, try to portray a united front. If you are inspired to shift some of your parenting practices, don't take other key adults by surprise. Wrestle through ideas together and arrive at points you can generally agree on. The best strategy is to start by recognizing each other's parenting strengths and then invite people to add new skill sets to their existing strategies.

If you act before coming to a joint decision, you may set other adults up to look badly, which will undermine all your relationships. Suppose, for example, you believe your teen will benefit from being able to demonstrate that they've earned privileges, but another adult remains overprotective. You will appear flexible, and the other adult will look overly demanding. In this case, your desire to parent more effectively could unintentionally harm the relationship between your teen and another adult. It is better to approach with a unified compromise than to parent from opposite poles. When you share a position, you'll spare your adolescent from the anxiety that results from having to process mixed messages.

Launching From Existing Strengths

Your teen may have learned precisely which of their behaviors have gotten the most attention from you—and some of those may not have been the pleasant ones. To be willing to give up what—for better or worse—has worked for them, they must know what they're getting in exchange. If it's a better relationship with you rooted in your knowledge that they're a good person, they will eagerly make that choice.

To start, write down a list of everything you admire about your teen. If fleshing out that list right now is hard because you have been through too much recently, recall them as a child and fall in love again. And ask their teachers or friends' parents for their thoughts. It is likely they are seeing who your teen *really* is despite the behavior you might be witnessing at home. Keep the list as a touch point.

It makes sense to see the best in your adolescent as a starting point for moving forward, doesn't it? Now, apply the same approach to yourself and to your family. Think about all that you are doing right as a parent and your own existing strengths. It is too easy to feel inadequate, and too many parents feel guilty when things are not going well. Try to let that go. I don't know you, but I do know that you are a committed and caring parent. If you are struggling, **remember that self-forgiveness and self-compassion are critical resilience skills your teen can learn from you.** When they see you being forgiving of yourself for your all-too-human errors or missteps, they gain trust that you will also be forgiving of them. When they see that you continue to see your own strengths even when things are not going smoothly, they'll more confidently believe that you really do continue to see the goodness within them. These are starting points toward meaningful change.

Spaces and Places

We need to be flexible in timing our conversations with our teens and in choosing places less demanding of that eye-to-eye contact that makes some teens run for the hills. My book, *Raising Kids to Thrive: Balancing Love With Expectations and Protection With Trust,* includes the views of several hundred young people, but a small teen advisory panel offers detailed advice about key topics. They have strong views about how to hold important parent-teen conversations.

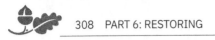

1. Keep conversations low-key, at least at the start. If you start out too emotional, it makes teens uncomfortable. It also makes them feel the need to take care of you, which makes it harder for them to problem-solve.

2. Never have these conversations in public.

3. Never have these conversations in front of friends.

4. Don't start these conversations when teens already have a lot on their mind or if they are already nervous about something, such as a big homework assignment. They'll just be angry when you approach them and may not regain their focus.

5. On the other hand, if they're finally relaxing after a long stretch of work, it's not the time to approach them either. (This admittedly makes it tough to find the "right time," but you are looking for a time that is more neutral.)

6. It is easier to talk with one parent at a time. Otherwise, teens can feel like they are being ganged up on. (This is another tough one because it remains important to stay on the same page with your partner. Nevertheless, this idea was offered repeatedly by teens.)

Finding the Right Tone

Change is hard. People can buy into the hard work of change or refuse to consider it. Let's summarize key points that set the tone that will more likely get your teen on board.

Align Your Words With Your Unspoken Signals

This is not a crash course in body language; it is a reminder to get yourself to a place where everything you say is rooted in your caring and that you genuinely believe progress is possible (because it is!). Why? Because, as we discussed in Chapter 19, your words will not be believed when your body and facial expressions don't match what you say. Believe in the possibility of change. Sincerely get there before words begin flowing out of your mouth to ensure your spoken and unspoken signals are in alignment.

Important but Not Urgent

Recall what we've learned about the adolescent brain in Chapter 8 and about co-regulation and dysregulation in Chapter 20. People can't think when they're running from the tiger, and they can't feel fully. So, as urgent as these conversations may feel, approach them as though they matter but not as though you are in a crisis. If you approach these talks emergently, you will activate the stress hormones that prevent the thinking and feeling needed to move forward. So, draw those deep breaths and remind yourself that there are going to be plenty of opportunities to slowly rebuild your relationship; it does not all ride on any one conversation. This will allow you to approach your discussions more calmly and, thereby, partner with your teen whose thinking skills will remain sharp and feeling capacity will remain intact.

Some Feelings Can Be Left Out of the Conversation

Teens don't like too much drama, and they'll withdraw when it becomes too heavy. Sharing the depths of your concerns and fears might not be necessary. In fact, it might create that previously described sense of urgency that can backfire. If you focus too much on how hurt you are, it can make the discussion feel like it is about *you* instead of *them* or your relationship. Further, if you make them feel too guilty or make them worry too much about you, they may begin to keep things from you to protect you and your feelings.

Be a Facilitator

Remember when we talk *at* young people it drives them away, whereas when we talk *with* them, they engage. So, speak from your heart but never forget your goal is to speak *to* the heart of your child. They, too, want to return to their best self and have a better relationship with you. They, too, miss your loving relationship. Avoid the dreaded lecture listing all they've done wrong and the problems they've caused. Instead, help them understand that the possibilities for change exist and that the solutions reside within them (see Chapter 27).

Trust

As discussed in Chapter 36, you will be giving your teen the opportunity to regain your trust, but you should begin your discussions with a different kind of trust. Trust that your teen *does* worry and *does* want what is best for them. The myth that adolescents think they are invulnerable has been widely disproven. We know young people worry a great deal and have a rich inner life in which they wrestle over decisions. They sometimes *behave* irresponsibly (especially in groups), but those behaviors are often a cover for far more complex feelings. When we trust they want to stay safe and have a good relationship with us, they'll more likely reveal their true selves.

Opening Statements

Your goal is to make the discussion feel important *without* making it feel like a big deal. How's that for a double bind? If you sit down and speak deeply from your heart, speaking the language of hopes and dreams and pain and anguish, the pressure might be…just…too…much. If you share a list of concerns, it might lead them to worry whether everyone sees their insecurities or problems with as much clarity as you do. If you make it about how much you believe their friends' parents are getting it wrong, they might stop the discussion before you separate them from their friends. If you share too much guilt or self-blame, they may feel they need to parent and protect you. This can feel like too much.

Instead, be clear that you both need to tackle a problem. Did you hear that? You *both* have to tackle a problem. Frame this as a partnership, and you're on your way. Let's try out some examples.

> *"I've been thinking that there is too much pressure on you and that it's hurting your ability to figure out what you want to do. Believe it or not, there's a lot of pressure on parents too. I feel like we never get it quite right. I have been trying to be supportive, but I may have just added more pressure. All I want is for you to find out for yourself what you want to do in the world. I need your guidance on how I can best support you to do that."*

> *"I've made it clear that I don't always like or agree with some of the choices you make. You must feel like I'm just yelling at you about one thing or another most of the time. This is not the kind of relationship I want to have with you, and I never wanted to be the kind of parent who yelled more than I listened. But here I am. I want you to know that I don't see you as a bad kid even though I might act like I do sometimes. I know what a good person you are, but I don't think I tell you often enough. I see you as a bright, highly sensitive person who has always taken life seriously. I've always loved that about you, but I worry that your sensitivity could be hurting you now. I'll make you a deal. You show me more of who you really are, and I'll work hard to stop focusing on your mistakes. I might need some reminders, so please tell me if I'm getting back to my old habits. How about we start with you telling me something I can do right now to be a better parent?"*

Don't be surprised if your teen hears your heartfelt words and responds with, "Why do you care all of a sudden?" Breathe. Respond with, "I care because I love you. I always have and always will. I just want to make sure I am being the kind of parent you deserve." If your adolescent turns up the heat with, "If you want to help me, just get out of my life!" say something like, "I'll step away to give us both room to think. But the one thing I'll never do is get out of your life. I love you too much." Are you remembering to breathe? You are being tested. You pass this test with your continued presence.

Listening and Talking

How you listen makes the difference in whether your teen feels that it is safe for them to share their vulnerable side. Kids don't talk if they think that they're going to get a quick reaction. They talk when the person listening makes them feel heard. How you talk makes the difference in whether your teen will listen to you. Supplying them with directives pretty much ensures that they will resent, if not ignore, your words. Engaging with them will encourage them to hear you and will keep them responding. This is covered in detail in Chapters 17 and 18.

Forgiveness and Apologies

First, forgive yourself. If you were overprotective, it wasn't because you wanted to be overbearing; it was because you chose to protect with every ounce of energy you could muster. If you haven't been a perfect role model, it was because you were highly stressed and working to deal with challenging times as best you could. If you haven't maintained your cool, it was because you felt a sense of urgency and made your points as powerfully as you could. We've all had plenty of opportunities to disappoint ourselves. To move forward, show yourself some compassion.

Next, forgive others. If you enter a conversation holding a grudge, it's not going to go well. You'll work to prove yourself right or teach a lesson more than you'll partner toward improvement. Anger defeats us and guilt paralyzes us, whereas forgiveness heals us.

Nothing earns a reset like an apology. Put it out on the table. You are asking for a do-over. You still won't be perfect but, by starting with acknowledging that something went wrong, you'll all grow together. An apology is not an explanation or justification. Telling someone why you think you may have done something might feel helpful to you but can be misinterpreted as an excuse. Just say you are truly sorry; it helps the other person realize you know they were hurt.

It may be that, from your perspective, you've done nothing wrong. But your teen may disagree. Nevertheless, model how to move past bad feelings. If you are not sure precisely what to apologize for, keep it general and say, "It is clear to me that my actions hurt you." If you feel tension that you cannot explain, try out an apology such as, "It seems like you're upset. Is there anything I may have done—or not done—that I could fix?" The humility you display models for your teen a way to move past communication roadblocks.

You Might Start With a Letter

Sometimes you want to get it just right. Or you might think, "They'll never listen long enough for me to get the words out." In either case, consider writing it out before you have a sit-down conversation. You might be thinking, "Nobody writes letters anymore." Exactly. That's why writing one is so powerful.

The following are thoughts about writing letters:

- Keep the drama down.

- Focus on the present rather than the past; don't dredge up anger.

- Focus on strengths; use this opportunity to give the details on all you see that is good and right about them.

- Letters can be the perfect tool to state how deeply and unconditionally you love someone. Add stories. Recalling antics from younger years that displayed the roots of their personalities will keep them reading.

- Make a clear statement on what you want reset and your commitment to moving forward.

- Letters are the perfect place to offer a sincere apology.

- Do not use the letter to criticize. Express concerns in general terms only. Avoid this communication trap: some people will focus on the one negative sentence in a 2-page letter and then use that single sentence as the reason to avoid further discussion.

- Consider having a trusted and objective reader review the letter before you send it. Have them check for anything that could be misinterpreted or any phrases that could trigger backlash. If there is even a small chance a thought will backfire, remove it.

- Remember, letters are not for arriving at solutions or for covering every issue; they are for getting conversations started.

Communication Pearls

Use "I" statements. The "I" statement gets your views across without escalating tension and draws out another person's empathy rather than defensiveness. Arguments tend to start with accusations of what somebody else has done wrong: *"You did this!"* Once a person feels blamed, they hold their position more rigidly and may escalate the tension by responding, "No! You did that!" Instead, the "I" statement draws out their empathy. It starts with "I felt..." or "I experienced...." This activates compassion and might trigger an apology such as, "I'm sorry you felt that way, I meant to...."

Don't bring up things from the past; focus on the current issue. It's so easy to justify your frustration by bringing up something from the past. This places people on the defensive and can overwhelm them. Overwhelmed people stop talking. When you pile up accusations or generate a list of problems, it also points out a pattern of behavior. The last thing you want to do is suggest that a behavior "is just the way you are" because that makes someone feel incapable of change. It is hard enough to change something in the present. It is impossible to alter the past, so there is no use in revisiting it.

Never minimize a feeling. We sometimes say things like, "Don't worry about it," or, "You can handle this, it's really not that big a deal." These well-intentioned efforts at reassurance may stop communication because people can feel belittled. Even if you do feel something is easily solvable, let your teen know that you hear their concerns and want to be supportive. It may be enough to say, "I hear how much this means to you." If it's a tough situation, then ask how you can best be supportive and reinforce that you have faith they'll get through it.

Never imply that a feeling is mistaken. Secure relationships allow feelings to be shared and solutions to be developed. You can believe that an emotion is undermining or destructive to someone, but the feeling itself is never wrong. Learn to respond with phrases such as, "I hear that you are feeling _____," or, "Thanks for trusting me enough to let me know you are feeling _____." Without thoughts and feelings on the table, real conversations don't get started.

Never say "I understand." You don't. An upset teen will respond, "How could you understand? You've never had _____ happen to you." Instead, try, "Help me understand," or, "This has really hurt you. Tell me what you're going through." If something is feeling overwhelming even to you, say, "I can't imagine all that is going on. I'm here to listen; help me understand." Ask for their guidance. "Tell me what I need to know to support you right now."

Check your assumptions. We all make assumptions about what others are thinking. We often assume that we fully understand the words they are saying. We also might believe our intuition is correctly interpreting unspoken cues. However, we are often wrong and can enter communication traps. For example, do your teen's folded arms and distant gaze represent anger at you, or are they replaying a difficult peer interaction and barely holding themself together? The wrong assumption leaves you feeling defensive, when what your child really needs is your support. Check your assumptions. "It seems you might be feeling _____, am I right?" Or stay more open-ended. "I sense something's troubling you. I'm here to listen—now or later."

Talk in a way that promotes a growth mindset. We need intellectual and emotional flexibility to break unhealthy interaction patterns. When we imply that our teens (or spouses!) *are* something, we set our expectations (and theirs!) that they will remain that way. You *are* self-centered. You *are* stubborn. You *are* thoughtless. When we instead comment on what they *do*, we remind them that they are capable of change and in control of their choices. "I felt awful when you behaved as though you were not considering how that would affect me. It wasn't like you."

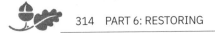

Leave With Solutions and End With a Plan to Talk More

You've invested in having a healthy and supportive family. It's likely your teen will be breathing a sigh of relief—they need you, and deep down they know they always have. It is important that you leave the discussion with some next steps—either solutions or a path toward finding them. Ideally the whole family will be part of the solution. If the solution proposes that only one person make changes, they'll assume the label of being "the problem" and that will end the partnership.

Before you approach serious conversations, think of actions or strategies that could make things better. Bring them to the table. Make sure the conversations include opportunities for others to add their solutions. If their input is included, they'll much more likely buy into the solutions moving forward. Don't suggest everything is solved; that would set people up to feel demoralized with inevitable backtracking. Communication takes ongoing work. Acknowledge this by ending your discussion with, "I feel a bit better. Why don't we talk about this again in 2 days?"

Will these strategies solve all my relationship issues? No. There are no perfect relationships, just those worth working on. Your teen is worthy of this investment.

CHAPTER 39

The Strength of Seeking Professional Guidance

It is neither a sign of weakness in our adolescents nor a result of poor parenting when our teens display human limitations. Invulnerability is neither an option nor our goal. Nevertheless, it is among the more challenging moments of parenting when we realize our support alone is not enough. But it is a genuine act of love—and good and responsible parenting—when we guide our tweens and teens toward professional help.

Your teen may feel ashamed they can't handle their own problems. They may worry that seeking professional help confirms that they are incapable, weak, or even "crazy." If your teen is questioning their worth during challenging times, your strength-based approach can make the difference in how they see themself. Your knowledge of who they really are, beyond the moods they may be experiencing or the behaviors they may *temporarily* be displaying, is the grounding they need.

How you frame the help-seeking process can make the critical difference toward their willingness to seek help. Discuss professional guidance as what they deserve, not what they "need." Let them understand that what they are currently experiencing can be temporary, and professional guidance can support them to be their better self and to learn to be more comfortable with their feelings. This will influence their investment in professional services and, therefore, the likelihood of its success.

Be on the Alert for Distress Signals

Ideally, our teens would speak to us openly whenever they are in distress. We have covered how being an effective listener and following a balanced parenting style make it *more* likely that your teen will tell you what they are feeling. However, they may withhold thoughts when their emotions are particularly distressing. Stay attentive to their signals. Even teens who can't summon the courage to tell their parents how they feel are relieved when their parents notice something is wrong.

- Look for **changes in behavior,** such as a sudden refusal to follow family rules or standards, a new circle of friends, or radical change in dress style. Any concerns about your teen turning to **substance use,** including cigarettes, deserves early intensive involvement.

- Many parents are very attentive to **signs of depression** but mistakenly believe adolescent depression looks the same as adult depression. Depressed adults may have sleep disturbances, become withdrawn, and experience a lack of energy. They have a harder time experiencing pleasure, may feel hopeless, and likely will acknowledge feeling sad. When teens exhibit these same symptoms, most adults recognize they are depressed. However, nearly half of depressed adolescents are **irritable** instead of withdrawn. They may have excess energy and act out with rage. They may not even feel sad. Because teenagers may have periods of heightened emotions normally, parents can miss a teen whose irritability is a distress signal. If your teen is irritable for a prolonged period, seek a professional evaluation.

- Notice increased signs of anxiety. **Excessive worry,** an inability to focus, catastrophic thoughts, or greater difficulty in participating in academic life or social circles are signals of increasing distress.

- Stress is often experienced through our bodies. **Frequent aches and pains,** including bellyaches, headaches, dizziness, muscle strains, and chest pain, may be signs of stress. Don't assume your teen is fak-ing these symptoms to avoid school or shirk responsibilities. Even when stress is the cause, the symptoms are very real. Teens (and many adults) don't always notice the connection between their emotions and their bodies' responses. Involve a health care professional to be sure there is not an underlying illness. Your teen will benefit from reassur-ance that healthy people can experience these discomforts from stress.

- Pay attention when your teen has frequent **complaints that prevent them from going to school.** Notice if symptoms are less frequent on weekends or vacations. That will be helpful information for a health care professional, who will consider the possibility of school being the triggering stressor. Again, this is likely stress related— not faking.

- Watch for **signs of fatigue** or **difficulty waking up** in time for school. Some adolescents who are troubled show signs of sleep disturbances— sleeping too much or having trouble falling and staying asleep. Many people are not aware that they are sleeping fitfully and, therefore, may not connect stress to their fatigue.

- Teens can reveal stress through **school performance.** Just as our performance at work declines with increasing stress, teens may find it difficult to focus on schoolwork. Anytime grades slip significantly, it should be a red flag for either general stress or academic worries.

People often think of teen problems as falling into one of 2 categories: emotional/mental health or behavioral. While it is true that you may seek professionals with different specialties to address these issues, don't separate these into 2 distinct categories. Drug use, for example, is a worrisome behavior, but the *why* behind the use is likely emotionally based. Your teen needs a professional with expertise in substance use disorder. But nothing substitutes for parents' presence, and seeing the sensitivities and anxieties behind teens' substance use is precisely what positions you to be most supportive.

Working Through Your Own Feelings

Many people have ambivalent feelings about mental health and social support services. And you likely will feel most dysregulated precisely when your loved one is most deserving of these services. It is important to work through your feelings so you can calmly and sincerely speak to your teen about why these services will benefit them. Let's briefly recap why your feelings need to be considered before you speak to your teen.

- Teens are highly sensitive to other people's social cues. This means they are very good at sensing insincerity and ambivalence.

- Even if your words are chosen perfectly, your body language and facial expressions tell the real story. You want all the signals you send to be aligned.

- When our teens are dysregulated, they rely on us to lend them our calm through co-regulation. This is hard to do when we are dysregulated ourselves.

When teens reach their limit, it's important that they do not need to also worry about you. If they see you feeling guilty about what they are going through, they may feel worse about their own hardships. If you experience your child struggling as your own failure, you may unintentionally transmit that you are disappointed, stressed, or angry. **Good parents cannot prevent their children from having problems**.

This means that, for both your own well-being and the sake of your teen, you need to work through your own feelings of powerlessness or inadequacy about having a child who is struggling. Move past the self-blame game. This, admittedly, can be difficult because many teens in their lowest moments will blame you for their pain. Know that what they say likely does not reflect what they feel. People often take out their stress on those they know will stand by them no matter what. You are defined by your unwavering presence—it matters most now, even if your teen pushes you away.

It is often said that parents are only as happy as their least happy child. This means that it takes work to display the outer strength and resolve on which your child can rely. You don't have to make it look easy. But at the end of the day, your teen should know you feel good about being a source of strength for them now, just as they will be a source of support for others, including you, in the future.

To move yourself to a calmer place, you may also have to work through the feelings of inadequacy some parents feel when they realize that they can't solve their teen's problems all on their own. When your child was 3 years old, nobody could make them feel better than you. Teens' problems are more complicated. Try to work past the disappointment that your child needs something more than you can give. Getting others involved is an act of caring, not of failure. Again, good and responsible parents find their children extra support and resources when needed; they are not responsible for their children's problems.

If you believe that seeking professional help is a positive action—an act of strength and self-awareness—your teen is more likely to see it that way. If, however, you have mixed feelings about seeking professional help, try your best to resolve these thoughts before talking to your teen. Adolescents may pick up on mixed emotions and it may make them resistant to seeking help. A first step to resolving your feelings is to follow the suggestions listed in the Guiding Your Teen to Understand the Benefits of Professional Support section of this chapter as if they were me speaking directly to you.

Taking this a step further, it is particularly meaningful now that you model help seeking. The more you talk out loud when you seek advice from others, the more it will become an accepted part of your family culture. This is not just about professional help; it includes turning to others to help solve problems. Doing so normalizes help seeking. Plus, you are demonstrating that you are consistently stronger and wiser as a result. In fact, precisely when your teen struggles, you deserve the extra support to gather your own internal resources to remain strong when you feel most vulnerable.

It is hard to be calm when your child is struggling. And our culture is filled with so much stigma about mental health and judgment about concerning behaviors that it is easier said than done to suggest you quickly overcome your own thoughts on these matters. It is a journey you need to take to be able to be fully supportive to your child, but you might need more time to get there than you have right now. Forgive yourself of your own humanity. Your unspoken ambivalence is what will confuse them. If you struggle, tell them you struggle. You might say, for example, "I am having a hard time with the difficulties that you are going through, and I don't believe I'm my best self right now. But I do know that I will stand by your side. And we will find the right professional to guide us through this. You deserve that."

Guiding Your Teen to Understand the Benefits of Professional Support

Your discussions about help seeking should highlight both your teen's strengths and how they will benefit from professional guidance. The points offered throughout this section come from decades of experience helping teens and families positively engage in support services. They answer many of the asked and unasked questions on teens' minds as they consider professional support. These points, at their core, are trying to make 3 things clear: (1) professional guidance can make a real difference, and there are people who know how to work well with teens; (2) emotional discomfort is treatable, and people who have difficult times during adolescence often possess great strengths that predict positive futures; and (3) they will not be on this journey alone; you will stand by their side but give them the privacy they desire.

Make It Clear That Treatment Can Work

Many teens may wonder: "How can it help? Why waste my time?" Hopelessness can be a temporary part of emotional distress. It may be hard for teens who battle with depression to see the light at the end of the tunnel or for those with severe anxiety to feel as if they will ever stop worrying. Perhaps the most important thing you can do to prepare your teen to seek help is to reinforce that treatment can work and is worth the investment. Help them understand professionals have years of training and that decades of research have developed strategies that work. If you know of people who have gained their strength and control back after support, share that with your child. You may choose to share with your adolescent that, while most people start a professional relationship to address a problem, many choose to extend their counseling relationship because they learn that professional guidance helps them to be happier and grow as a person.

Underscore That Time Invested Will Pay Off

Teens these days have plenty of obligations. They may feel as if "there's no time for this." If your teen is highly anxious, they may worry the time invested in counseling will make them fall behind in other areas of their lives. Their anxiety may make it difficult for them to hear your words. Your even-tempered calmness reinforces that their mental well-being must come first. Remind them the investment in learning how not to waste time and energy in worrying increases their efficiency and focus. And that, ultimately, it will lead to more time and higher levels of achievement. This will be true in the near term and the future.

Reinforce That Seeking Treatment Is an Act of Strength

When it comes to asking for help, some teens may think: "I can handle it. I don't need anybody else." It is critical that we do not undermine the help-seeking process by framing it as a sign of weakness. We start with the right language—it is not what they *need* but what they *deserve*. It is courageous to be able to clearly state, "I don't feel right, and I deserve to feel better." Knowing that you deserve guidance is an act of self-awareness, and people with insight often become the most successful and happy adults. We must make it clear that seeking help is an act of strength. And that strong people know that they can feel better, deserve to feel better, and will take the steps to feel better.

Even using this strength-based approach, some teens may still have difficulty overcoming the stigma that is (wrongly) associated with mental health. If this is the case with your teen, remind them that finding a mental health care professional is no different than going to a doctor to examine a swollen knee. A professional is a professional. We turn to professionals to benefit from their expertise.

Say This (about seeking help)	Not That
A strong person learns how to reach out to others.	A strong person handles tough times.
It'll take time. But your own strengths, and the support you'll get from those who care about you, will help you heal.	Just get past it. Let it go. Don't dwell or obsess on it.
Sometimes the strongest thing a person can do is seek professional help.	Strong people move on.
You deserve to feel better.	You need help!

Acknowledge That They Are Not Alone in Having Challenges

When we struggle, it is not uncommon to feel alone and to retreat into ourselves and believe help is impossible. It is important that your teen understands how common it is for people to go through periods of discomfort and that we all struggle sometimes. If your teen is feeling isolated, make it clear that they are not alone. This reinforces for them that professionals will know how to respond to their needs.

Let Them Know That They Will Not Be Alone in Overcoming Their Challenges

Some teens fear that, in receiving professional help, they will lose the supportive relationships they have relied on, such as family, friends, teachers, school counselors, clergy, or coaches. It is important, therefore, to state that seeking professional help doesn't mean giving up other critical support systems. Most critically, your teen must know you'll continue to stand by their side. In fact, guide your child to understand that, because they'll be able to focus on problems with the professionals and learn to relieve stress there, relationships with family and friends may be strengthened.

Highlight How Strong Feelings Now Lead to a Strong Adulthood Later

The very sensitivity and depth of caring that may trouble your teen now is what positions them to have a full, rich life in the future. You can acknowledge that it is difficult to feel so fully now but that people with intense feelings and deep sensitivity make the best friends, life partners, colleagues, and parents. To get there, though, they must learn to manage the complexity of their feelings, including uncomfortable ones like sadness or anxiety. Once they manage these emotions, their sensitivity will enable them to enjoy life more fully now and through adulthood. Professional guidance can help. Always frame your desire for your teen to seek support by emphasizing how you want them to be comfortable and to be their best self. Remind them that you don't expect them to be perfect, just poised to have a satisfying and meaningful life.

If they express their emotions clearly, underscore that this is a sign that they possess lifelong strengths. You might say, "You are wise enough to know that you are struggling. Too many people go through life pushing feelings away or making no real effort to understand themselves. I am proud that you are aware of how you feel and are strong enough to reach out." This helps your teen understand their power of self-awareness and personal advocacy.

Relationships With Professionals Are Special

If your teen says, "I don't need anybody feeling sorry for me," make it clear that empathy is not pity. Professionals do not pity the youth they serve. They serve because they want to and have gone through years of training to be able to do so.

Help your child understand that youth-serving professionals choose to work with adolescents because they care for and respect young people. Often, they went into the field because they knew somebody in their lives who needed support (or they themselves struggled as adolescents), so they are committed to making life better for young people.

Professionals Honor Privacy

Teens have a strong desire for privacy. They may say, "I don't want everybody to know my business." They might not be aware that professionals are legally and ethically obligated to honor their patients' privacy and serve without judgment. Make it clear that you also will honor the private nature of that relationship. Tell your teen that you will always be there to support them and that you hope to know as much about their life as they choose to share. You will look to them as the expert in their own life to share what you need to know. You always want to be there but are happy to know that they have another trusted adult to talk to.

Professionals Are Supportive

Your teen may wonder: "Why can't I just talk to you, Mom/Dad? Or why can't I just talk to my friends? They can relate to me better than any adult can."

The beauty of a relationship with a professional is that the teen never has to worry about the therapist's thoughts or feelings. They've likely heard it all, so they won't be shocked. They want to hear about your teen's feelings. They won't be disappointed, hurt, or angry. They are there to support your teen. Relationships with friends and family are different—your teen may worry about disappointing them or hurting the relationship and, therefore, withhold from sharing important experiences, thoughts, and feelings. Help your teens understand seeking help is an "and," not an "or." Professional guidance will never replace your love and support. Good friends can never be replaced. The professional is an additional person—with specialized training.

Counseling Is About Guidance, Not Being Repaired

Your teen may think: "I'll figure it out. I'll deal with my own problems. No one can ever know what I've been through anyway. How could they fix it?" Help your teen understand that professionals guide others to become stronger by using skills others already have and by teaching them new ones. Explain that counseling is a learning process that offers new information that can help them make good decisions, manage challenges, and work through uncomfortable feelings. Professionals are there for support, but your teen will do the real work. Professionals do not give answers or solve problems; rather, they find the strengths of each person and build upon them. Your teen will solve their own problems. But they will have the support to do so.

Professional Support Can Strengthen Other Relationships

When teens struggle, they may feel as though they have somehow failed, thinking, "I've messed everything up." It is common for people under stress to challenge the relationships most important to them. Why? Because it is only in the relationships that hold the greatest security that we can take the chance of revealing our most uncomfortable thoughts and feelings. It is not unusual, therefore, for teens to push friends and family away precisely when they need the greatest support. We must make it known that our love remains unwavering. That we understand how their behavior reflects the fact that they are going through something. And reinforce that a major benefit of counseling can be repairing and restoring relationships.

You Deserve Support Too

Parenting can be tough. Life presents challenges to all of us. And just as our children can experience emotional distress or mental health challenges, parents can also. You've just invested a lot of time and energy reading this book to learn how to be most supportive to your developing teen. If you want to maintain that energy, commit to caring for yourself. Your teen wants you to be well, and it adds to their security knowing that you are taking care of yourself. So for your sake, and for the sake of your adolescent, invest in your own health and well-being. Turn to friends and family. But recognize that everything we just discussed about the strength of seeking professional guidance may apply to you as well.

Finding the Right Professional

Let your teen know that you will support them to find the right fit for them. Consider asking your child's health care professional, school guidance counselor, or clergyperson for thoughts and recommendations. When they make suggestions on where to find the best support, your teen will more likely believe the recommended person is trustworthy. The following professional organizations can help you find the best treatment for your child: American Academy of Pediatrics (www.aap. org), American Counseling Association (www.counseling.org), American Psychological Association (www.apa.org), and Society for Adolescent Health and Medicine (www.adolescenthealth.org). Many professionals serve our families as units, recognizing that when families are strengthened, each individual benefits. The American Association for Marriage and Family Therapy (www.aamft.org) can help you find a therapist.

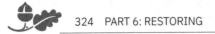

Understanding and Embracing the Parent Role

Professionals do not replace you. Your voice is the one that will reassure your teen that they will get through this. Your presence reminds them that you stand beside them now and long after this problem is a distant memory. Remember, help your teen know that this problem is temporary through the power of a single word. "I'll never feel OK again," becomes, "I haven't *yet* learned how to feel OK."

You have another role: to be the keeper of hope. It is awful to see your teen in pain. But did you want to raise a person who didn't feel? Who didn't care? The fact that your teen feels is what predicts that they will thrive in the future. They may wish they could shut down their sensitivity; your role is to remind them that their sensitivity is one of their greatest strengths. Guide them to understand that their challenge now is to learn to manage their rich capacity to feel, while assuring them that, when they do, they will be rewarded throughout life. Similarly, this is not the time to condemn their participation in unwise behaviors. That will push them away and prevent healing. Certainly, explain why you will not allow any dangerous behavior, but seek the root causes that are driving those behaviors. As you uncover the "why," you are likely to find a wonderful teen hiding behind these behaviors. Stay firmly committed in the knowledge that when they learn to manage their emotional self, their sensitivities and depth of their feelings predict a full, rich life.

Closing Thoughts

I magine if every parent of a tween was greeted by their friends and neighbors with the words, "Congratulations—you're having a teen!" In such a world, parents would look forward to the adolescent years as the opportunity to witness their children's astounding development. Parents would take the steps to prepare themselves for their irreplaceable role as guides to shape their children into caring, compassionate, confident, and resilient young adults. Adolescents would be surrounded by engaged, connected adults who would deepen their involvement when the teens strayed from being their better selves.

We can build that world together.

The subtitle of this book tells the story of what I hope you achieve during your child's adolescence. The goals are for you *to strengthen your family* and *raise a good person*. These lofty goals are best achieved with your full intention and active engagement. Teens deserve to be celebrated! They deserve nurturance and protection. They deserve our commitment to optimize their development. There will be some hard moments in the adolescent years, as there are in every stage of human development. There will be challenges between you and your teen, just as there are in all meaningful human relationships. But things that are hard are not without value. Challenges can be best met by building on existing strengths. Knowing all that is good and right about your teen is the key to helping your teen become their very best self. It is the critical first step to help you effectively engage in even the most challenging moments.

I hope that this is the beginning of your relationship with this book. Return frequently to these pages throughout the adolescent years to stay grounded in a strength-based philosophy, to understand each new stage of development, and to build your communication skill sets. I strongly suspect that, as you revisit these pages, you will find new strategies to apply each time, not because my words have changed but because *how* you apply these words will change to meet your teen's evolving needs.

Join the movement of concerned adults who commit to being teen advocates. We must build a nation in which every teen is developed to their potential. We must build communities in which every teen knows they can contribute to our collective well-being. We must build a bridge to a positive shared future by nurturing our teens today. Full stop.

I hope the journey we have taken together has helped you understand the truth about teens. Share these truths with all who will listen.

- **Truth No. 1**: Adults are the most important people in the lives of young people, and teens like adults.
- **Truth No. 2:** Adolescence is a time of astoundingly rapid brain development, and we can shape our children's future far into adulthood by nurturing that development.
- **Truth No. 3:** Adolescents are super learners, and they will learn more during this period of their life than at any other time that follows.
- **Truth No. 4:** Young people care deeply about safety and want to avoid danger but need guidance as they learn about risk.
- **Truth No. 5:** Teens can be as rational and thoughtful as adults when we talk to them calmly, acknowledge their intelligence, and recognize them as experts in their own lives.
- **Truth No. 6:** Adolescents are driven by idealism and committed to repairing the world.
- **Truth No. 7:** Parents matter!

Parents whose children are entering adolescence need to hear these truths. Don't let those who belittle adolescence with "survival guides" set the tone for them. Help these parents get started on the right foot by congratulating them as they enter these essential years.

Index

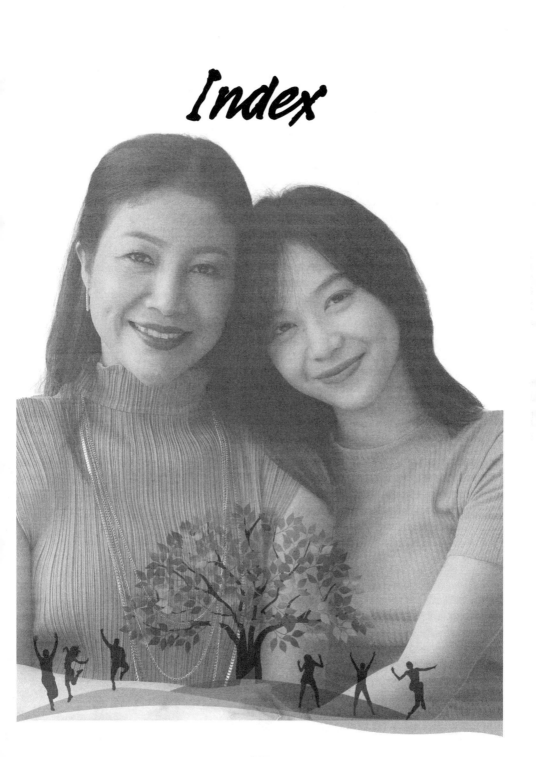

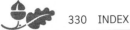

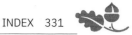

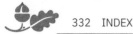

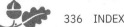